PUBLIC HEALTH IN THE 21ST CENTURY

SOCIAL DETERMINANTS AND MENTAL HEALTH

PUBLIC HEALTH IN THE 21ST CENTURY

Additional books in this series can be found on Nova's website
under the Series tab.

Additional E-books in this series can be found on Nova's website
under the E-books tab.

PUBLIC HEALTH IN THE 21ST CENTURY

SOCIAL DETERMINANTS AND MENTAL HEALTH

SABINE BÄHRER-KOHLER
EDITOR

Nova Science Publishers, Inc.
New York

Library of Congress Cataloging-in-Publication Data

Social determinants and mental health / editors, Sabine Bdhrer-Kohler.
p. cm.
Includes index.
ISBN 978-1-61324-353-4 (hardcover)
1. Social psychiatry. 2. Mental health--Social aspects. I. Bdhrer-Kohler, Sabine.
RC455.S5957 2011
362.2--dc22

2011012572

Published by Nova Science Publishers, Inc. † New York

CONTENTS

ABOUT THE AUTHORS

Dr. Sabine Bährer-Kohler: Holder of a Doctorate in Social Science (Dr. rer.soc)- University of Tübingen, a Diploma in Education - University of Education-Freiburg, and a Diploma in Social Work and Social Education– Protestant University of Applied Sciences- Berlin. Email: sabine.baehrer@datacomm.ch.

- Has her own company for counseling clients on how to deal with or prevent stress and burnout symptoms
- Lecturer at the University of Applied Science Bern Switzerland, on the subjects of dementia and life design, caregiver burden, social determinants and mental health
- Director of the International Psychogeriatric Association (USA)
- Representative to the WHO Advisory Group for the Revision of the ICD-10 Mental and Behavioral Disorders (Switzerland).

Dr. Simone Gonçalves de Assis: Latin American Center of Violence and Health Oswaldo Cruz Foundation-FIOCRUZ/ Health Ministry Rio de Janeiro, Brazil. Email: sgassis@globo.com.

Dr. Joviana Quintes Avanci: Latin American Center of Violence and Health. Oswaldo Cruz Foundation-FIOCRUZ/ Health Ministry, Rio de Janeiro, Brazil. Email: sgassis@globo.com.

Prof. Gary Bailey: International Federation of Social Workers, President. Bern, Switzerland, Simmons College School of Social Work Boston USA. Email: gary.bailey@simmons.edu.

Prof. (Assoc.) Dr. Sarah Melinda Dobie Buila: Southern Illinois University College of Education and Human Services, School of Social Work. Carbondale, USA. Email: sdbuila@siu.edu.

Prof. Dr. Francisco Javier Carod-Artal: Department of Neurology, Virgen de la Luz Hospital, Cueca, Spain. Email: fjcarod-artal@hotmail.com.

Prof. Dr. Jiska Cohen-Mansfield: Department of Health Promotion, School of Public Health , Herczeg Center on Aging, Tel-Aviv, Israel. Department of Health Care Sciences and of Prevention and Community Health, George Washington University Medical Center and School of Public Health, USA. Email: jiska@post.tau.ac.il.

Prof. Dr. David Conn: University of Toronto Department of Psychiatry and Baycrest Centre for Geriatric Care, Toronto-Ontario, Canada. Email: DConn@baycrest.org.

Prof. Dr. Luis Diaz-Serrano: University of Rovira i Virgili, Department of Economics, Reus, Spain. Email: luis.diaz@urv.cat.

Prof. Dr. Bernd Dollinger: University of Siegen, Faculty of Pedagogy and Psychology, Siegen, Germany. Email: dollinger@fb2.uni-siegen.de.

Prof. Dr. Eliane Jurkoswki: Southern Illinois University College of Education and Human Services, School of Social Work, Carbondale, USA. Email: etjurkow@siu.edu.

Prof. Dr. Urs Kalbermatten: University of Applied Science Bern, Institut of Gerontology, Bern, Switzerland. Email: urs.kalbermatten@bfh.ch.

Prof. Dr. Carlos Augusto de Mendonça Lima: Department of Psychiatry and Mental Health, Centro Hospitalar do Alto Ave, E.P.E., Guimarães, Portugal. Email: climasj@yahoo.com.

Raquel de Vasconcelos Carvalhaes de Oliveira: Laboratory of Clinical Epidemiology Research Institute Evandro Chagas/Oswaldo Cruz Foundation FIOCRUZ/Health Ministry, Rio de Janeiro, Brazil. Email: sgassis@globo.com.

Dr. Renata Pires Pesce: Oswaldo Cruz Foundation-FIOCRUZ/ Health Ministry, Rio de Janeiro, Brazil. Email: sgassis@globo.com.

Prof. Dr. Ignat Petrov: Bulgarian Association of Ageing, Sofia, Bulgaria. Email: ignatpetrov@yahoo.com.

Dr. Patryk Piotrowski: University Wroclaw, Wroclaw Medical University, Department of Psychiatry, Wroclaw, Poland. Email: patryk_p@psych.am.wroc.pl.

Dr. Anandamandiram Ramakrishnan: Faculty of Old Age Psychiatry, Royal College of Psychiatrists, Nottinghamshire Healthcare NHS Trust, Kirkby-in-Ashfield, United Kingdom. Email: rkrish33@gmail.com.

Silvia Schenker: Member of the Swiss Parlament, Basel, Switzerland. Email: kontakt@silviaschenker.ch.

Prof. Dr. Henning Schmidt-Semisch: University of Bremen, Department of Human and Health Science, Bremen, Germany. Email: schmidt-semisch@uni-bremen.de.

Terry L. Shirley: Southeast Missouri State University and Community Counseling Center Cape Girardeau USA.. Email: tlshirley1s@yahoo.com.

Dr. Alexandrina Petrova Stoyanova: University of Barcelona, Facultaty of Economics, Barcelona, Spain. Email: alexandrina.stoyanova@ub.edu.

Prof. Dr. Masatoshi Takeda: Osaka University Graduate School of Medicine, Faculty of Medicine, Department of Integrated Medicine, Osaka, Japan. President of International Psychogeriatric Association, USA. Email: mtakeda@psy.med.osaka-u.ac.jp.

Prof. Dr. I-Chen Tang: Department of Medical Sociology and Social Work, Chung-Shan Medical University, Taichung, Taiwan. Email: itang@csmu.edu.tw.

Prof. Dr. Richard Uwakwe: Faculty of Medicine College of Health Sciences, Nnmadi Azikiwe University Awka-Nnewi Campus, Awka, Nigeria. Email: ruwakwe2001@yahoo.com.

PD Dr. Henrike Wolf: University of Zurich, Department of Old Age Psychiatry and Psychiatry Research, Zurich, Switzerland. Email: hw@henrikewolf.de.

Prof. Dr. Hui-Ching Wu: National Taiwan University, Department of Social Work, Taipei, Taiwan. Email: hchingwu@ntu.edu.tw.

Prof. Dr. Joanna Wyka: Wroclaw University of Environmental and Life Science, Faculty of Food Sciences, Department of Agricultural Technology and Storage, Wroclaw, Poland. Email: wyka@wnoz.ar.wroc.pl.

PREFACE

The substance of this book is a in-depth discourse about health and, more particularly, mental health.

Mental health and mental illness are many-faceted and related to social, biological and psychological factors. [1] In this context, the aspect of the social determinants of health is perhaps the most complex and challenging of all. [2] The term 'social determinants of health' describes the conditions in which people are born, grow up, live, work and age. [3]

In this book, integrating the lifespan perspective, 28 credentialed authors and teams attempt to provide detailed evidence-based descriptions of social determinants and explain their context. At the end of the book, its perspective broadens. Authors from 14 countries worldwide present comprehensive scientific reports on the subject from diverse points of view and with diverse academic backgrounds integrating individual lifestyle factors, social and community networks and general socioeconomic, cultural and environmental conditions.

Next to the message of the book, there is a need to provide impulses for political implementation. This is why the editor has involved authors who deal explicitly with political implementation as well as international scholars to present findings and statements in the context of concepts, emerging evidence and practices to promote mental health and prevent mental disorders.

The editor concludes there is much that remains to be done in the field of mental health for all, especially in the context of social determinants.

[1] WHO (2010). Mental health: strengthening our response. http://www.who.int/mediacentre/factsheets/fs220/en/index.html.

[2] Tsouros, A.D. (2003). Foreword. In Marmot, M. Wilkinson, R. (Editors) (2003). Social Determinants of Health, The solid facts, second edition, p.5.

[3] WHO (2010). Social determinants of health. http://www.who.int/socialdeterminants/en.

In: Social Determinants and Mental Health
Editor: Sabine Bährer-Kohler
ISBN: 978-1-61324-353-4

Chapter 1

FOREWORD: INTRODUCTION TO THE BOOK

Sabine Bährer-Kohler
Behavioral Disorders, Switzerland
Bern University of Applied Science, Bern, Switzerland
Representative to the WHO Advisory Group for the Revision of the *ICD-10* Mental and
Director of the International Psychogeriatric Association, US

The substance of this book is a discourse about health and, more particularly, mental health.

In 1948 the World Health Organization (WHO) defined *health* as "a state of complete physical, mental, and social well-being and not merely the absence of disease or infirmity." [1][2] Beyond this, the WHO specified that *mental health* is defined as a state of well-being in which every individual realizes his or her own potential, can cope with the normal stresses of life, can work productively and fruitfully, and is able to make a contribution to her or his community. [3]

Mental health and mental illness are many-faceted and related to social, psychological and biological factors. [4]

In this context, the aspect of the social determinants of health is perhaps the most complex and challenging of all. [5]

The term 'social determinants of health' describes the conditions in which people are born, grow up, live, work and age, which includes the health system. [6]

This book is dedicated to these complex and continually varying determinants, keeping in mind that as early as 2005 the WHO instituted a commission to deal with the social determinants of health. [7]

There are several models for categorizing social determinants, including [8] [9] [10]. Dahlgren and Whitehead's model of health determinants [11] is helpful since it illustrates how various health influencing factors are embedded within broader aspects of society, [12] subdividing them into individual lifestyle factors, social and community networks and general socioeconomic, cultural and environmental conditions.

As the WHO documented in 2004, the clearest evidence is associated with indicators of poverty including low levels of education, and in some studies with poor housing and insufficient income. [13] Moreover increasing and persisting socio-economic disadvantages for individuals and communities are recognized risks factors impacting mental health. The *WHO MIND Project: Mental Improvement for Nations Development* document that common mental disorders are about twice as frequent among the poor as among the rich. [14]

In addition, there are other components such as these:

- The number of people in risk of falling into poverty has increased. [15]
- Unemployment will grow. [16]
- More people will be living in the world. [17]
- There will be more elderly people with their special needs [18] [19] such as protection from physical, sexual, financial, psychological abuse and neglect. Prevalence rates or estimates range from 4% to 6% [20].
- Mental diseases will spread and lifetime prevalences had increased [21] [22] [23], and mental and neurological disorders are responsible for around 13% of the global burden of disease. [24]
- An estimated 450 million people worldwide suffer from a mental disorder, 25% of individuals, develop one or more mental or behavioral disorders at some stage of life. [25] An estimated 76.3 million persons suffer worldwide from disorders related to alcohol abuse. [26]

In this book, whose content structure loosely follows that of the WHO publication entitled *Social Determinants of Health – the Solid Facts* [27], but nevertheless this book has its own individual content structure due in part to the integration of the lifespan perspective, 28 credentialed authors and teams attempt to provide detailed evidence-based descriptions of social determinants and explain their context. At the end of the book, its perspective broadens. Authors from 14 countries worldwide present comprehensive scientific reports on the subject from diverse points of view and with diverse academic backgrounds integrating individual lifestyle factors, social and community networks and general socioeconomic, cultural and environmental conditions.

- One of the articles, for example, will deal with childhood and mental health, as the foundations of mental health are laid in childhood.
- Another will sketch out aspects of the situation of adolescents and the impact of these aspects on mental health.
- Several articles in the book will discuss social determinants in old age. The world is rapidly ageing. While this is an important challenge for the developed world, 70% of all older people now live in low or middle-income countries. The elderly constitute a group in which environmental and social factors contribute greatly to active and healthy aging in societies. [28] At any rate, psychiatric morbidity in old age frequently coexists with physical illness and is likely to be further complicated by social problems. [29] One article will highlight the topic loneliness in older people, loneliness is of great importance to mental health not only in elderly people but also in other age groups. [30]

- One article will deal with aspects of access options to service facilities worldwide, others with chances of social participation and social capital. The article concerning social capital presents detailed data comes from the 2006 Spanish Health Survey.
- One article underlines the importance of social networks in the context of mental health. Social networks may have a protective effect on mental health by, for example, buffering individuals from the effects of stressful events. [31]
- Another will deal with social support. Social support is related to the ability to cope with stress and illness and has the potential to improve mental health. [32] [33]
- One article describe socioeconomic factors in the context of mental health from the individual, structural and political perspective.
- Yet other articles will highlight the importance of residential forms and nutrition for mental health. The WHO MIND Project: *Mental Improvement for Nations Development* document that people experiencing hunger are more likely to suffer from common mental disorders. [34]
- Another article, for example, will deal with prevention. Prevention is a subject that is referred to repeatedly because the prevention of mental disorders is obviously one of the most effective ways to reduce the burden. [35]

The chapters offer scientific descriptions and are readable at the same time, with a brief overview at the beginning of each chapter.

My wish as editor of this book is that the up-to-date, evidence-based accounts given in its articles may highlight social determinants that currently influence people with a mental disease, so that the quality of life of individuals and their relations may sustainably improve, well aware that there are many other social determinants that affect mental health.

Next to its scientific content, the book – in the editor's view – also needs to provide impulses for political implementation.

That is why I have involved authors who deal explicitly with political implementation as well as international scholars to present the book's findings and statements in the context of concepts, emerging evidence and practices to promote mental health [36], the WHO' concepts of prevention of 2004 [37] and the EU Framework for Action on Promotion of Mental Health and Well-Being of Children and Young People of 2009. [38]

But all stakeholders have important roles to play in the future- civil society, the governments, academic and research institutions, and bi- and multilateral agencies. [39]

A climate that respects and protects basic civil, political, socio-economic and cultural rights is fundamental to health and mental health promotion. Without the security and freedom provided by these rights, it is very difficult to maintain a high level of general health and mental health. [40]

Promoting mental health also depends largely on strategies. Specific ways to promote mental health include, analogous with the WHO's proposals- [41]

- "early childhood interventions (e.g. home visits for pregnant women, pre-school psycho-social activities, combined nutritional and psycho-social help for disadvantaged populations);
- support to children (e.g. skills building programmes, child and youth development programmes);

- socio-economic empowerment of women (e.g. improving access to education and microcredit schemes);
- social support for elderly populations (e.g. befriending initiatives, community and day centres for the aged);
- programmes targeted at vulnerable groups, including minorities, indigenous people, migrants and people affected by conflicts and disasters (e.g. psycho-social interventions after disasters);
- mental health promotional activities in schools (e.g. programmes supporting ecological changes in schools and child-friendly schools);
- mental health interventions at work (e.g. stress prevention programmes);
- housing policies (e.g. housing improvement);
- violence prevention programmes (e.g. community policing initiatives); and
- community development programmes (e.g. 'Communities That Care' initiatives, integrated rural development)."

The detailed proposals made by the WHO [41] [39] [37] [36] regarding intervention options as well as its entire promotion program should form part of training, professional development, courses, and national/international decisions in the health sector.

Moreover, each and every individual is important as well. One approach to promoting mental health is by self-management, because empowerment refers to the level of choice, a subject that will be presented in the book.

I know that professionals such as social scientists, social workers, sociologists, medical scientists, students, trainees, institutes, civil organizations, policy-makers and others interested in the subject, including myself, have been looking forward to such a book for a long time. I and my authors hope that this book will sustainably increase the general awareness of the subject of social determinants and mental health, especially as far as health inequities are concerned, for "social injustice is killing people on a grand scale." [42]

My heartfelt thanks to Julie, our daughter, and Jean-Luc, my husband, for assisting me in so many ways, to the authors for their contributions, and to the publishers for their excellent cooperation.

References

[1] Preamble to the Constitution of the World Health Organization as adopted by the International Health Conference, New York, 19-22 June, 1946; signed on 22 July 1947 by the representatives of 61 States (Official Records of the World Health Organization, no. 2, p. 100); and entered into force on 7 April 1948.

[2] Constitution of the World Health Organization (2006). Basic Documents, Forty-fifth edition, Supplement.

[3] WHO (2010). Mental health: strengthening our response. http:// www.who.int/mediacentre/factsheets/fs220/en/index.html, retrieved from WHO website 28 October 2010.

[4] WHO (2010). Mental health: strengthening our response. http://www.who.int/mediacentre/factsheets/fs220/en/index.html.

[5] Tsouros, A.D. (2003). Foreword. In Marmot, M. Wilkinson, R. (Editors) (2003). Social Determinants of Health, The solid facts, second edition, p.5.

[6] WHO (2010). Social determinants of health. http://www.who.int/socialdeterminants/en.

[7] WHO (2010). Social determinants of health. http://www.who.int/socialdeterminants/en.

[8] Hales, D., Lauzon, L. (2009). An Invitation to Health (2009-2010 Edition), Belmont: Wadsworth, Cengage.

[9] Lalonde, M. (1974). "A New Perspective on the Health of Canadians." Ottawa: Minister of Supply and Services.

[10] Centers of Disease Control and Prevention CDS (2011). Social Determinants and Health. Definition. Determinants of Health. http://www.cdc.gov/socialdeterminants/Definitions.html.

[11] Dahlgren, G., Whitehead, M. (1991). Policies and Strategies to Promote Social Equity in Health. Stockholm: Institute for Futures Studies.

[12] Mikkonen, J., Raphael, D. (2010). Social Determinants of Health. The Canadian Facts. http://www.thecanadianfacts.org.

[13] WHO (2004). Promoting Mental Health. http://www.who.int/mental_health/evidence/en/promoting_mhh.pdf.

[14] WHO (2007). Breaking the vicious cycle bewtween mental ill- health and poverty. www.who.int/mental_health/policy/development/1_Breakingviciouscycle_Infosheet.pdf./ Patel, V., Araya, R., de Lima, M., Ludermir, A., Todd, C. (1999). Woman, poverty and common mental disorders in four restructuring societies. *Social Science and Medicine*, 49:1461-1471.

[15] World Bank (2010). Poverty reduction & equity. http://www.web.worldbank.org, retrieved from Wordbank website 28 October 2010.

[16] OECD (2009). OECD Employment Outlook 2009: Tackling the Job Crisis. OECD Publishing.

[17] United Nations, Department of Economic and Social Affairs (2009). World Population Prospects. The 2008 Revision. Executive Summary. http://esa.un.org/unpd/wpp2008/pdf/WPP2008_Executive-Summary_Edited_6-Oct-2009.

[18] WHO (2004). What is the effectiveness of old-age mental health services? http://www.euro.who.int/__data/assets/pdf_file/0008/74690/E83685.pdf.

[19] Kinsella, K., Wan, H. (2008). U.S. Census Bureau, International Population Reports, P95/09-1, An Aging World. U.S. Government Printing Office,Washington, DC.

[20] WHO (2002). Abuse of the elderly. http://www.who.int/violence_injury_prevention/violence/world_report.

[21] World Health Organization (2004). Global Burden of Disease Study.

[22] World Health Organization (2000). International Consortium in Psychiatric Epidemiology. Cross-national comparisons of the prevalences and correlates of mental disorders. Bulletin of the World Health Organization. 78: 413-25.

[23] European Commission, Directorate-General for Health- Consumers (2008). Mental Health in the EU: Key facts, figures, and activities. A background paper.

[24] Global Forum for Health Research and World Health Organization (2007). Research capacity for mental health in low- and middle-income countries: Results of a mapping project, p. 3. http://www.who.int/mental_health/MHRC_FullText.pdf.
[25] WHO (2001). World Health Report. Mental Health: New Understanding, New Hope.
[26] WHO (2006). Alcohol consumption control- policy options in the south-east asia regio. http://www.searo.who.int/en/Section1430, retrieved from WHO website 6 April 2011.
[27] WHO (2003). Social Determinants of Health- the solid facts. Editors: Marmot, M., Wilkinson, R.G.
[28] WHO (2010). Our ageing world. http://www.who.int/ageing/en/.
[29] IPA (2010). http://www.ipa-online.org.
[30] Van Beljouw, I., Verhaak, P., Cuijpers, P., van Marwijk, H., Penninx, B. (2010). The course of untreated anxiety and depression, and determinants of poor one-year outcome: a one-year cohort study. *BMC Psychiatry*.10: 86.
[31] Kumar, S., Oakley Browne, M.A. (2008). Usefulness of the construct of social network to explain mental health service utilization by the maori population in new zealand. *Transcult Psychiatry*. Sep;45(3):439-54.
[32] Hewitt, B., Turrell, G., Giskes, K. (2010). Marital loss, mental health and the role of perceived social support: findings from six waves of an Australian population based panel study. *J Epidemiol Community Health*. Oct 21.
[33] Wills, T. A., Filer, M. (2001). Social networks and social support. In Baum, A., Revenson, T.A., Singer, J.E. (Eds.), Handbook of health psychology (p. 209-234). Mahwah, NJ: Erlbaum.
[34] WHO (2007). Breaking the vicious cycle bewtween mental ill- health and poverty. www.who.int/mental_health/policy/development/1_Breakingviciouscycle_Infosheet.pdf/ Patel, V., Araya, R., de Lima, M., Ludermir, A., Todd, C. (1999). Woman, poverty and common mental disorders in four restructuring societies. *Social Science and Medicine*, 49:1461-1471.
[35] WHO (2004). Prevention of mental disorders, effective interventions and policy options. http://www.who.int/mental_health/evidence/en/prevention_of_mental_disorders_sr.pdf.
[36] WHO (2004). Promoting mental health: concepts, emerging evidence, practice : summary report / a report from the World Health Organization, Department of Mental Health and Substance Abuse in collaboration with the Victorian Health Promotion. Foundation (VicHealth) and the University of Melbourne. http://www.who.int/mental_health/evidence/en/promoting_mhh.pdf.
[37] WHO (2004). Prevention of mental disorders, effective interventions and politics options. http://www.who.int/mental_health/evidence/en/prevention_of_mental_disorders_sr.pdf
[38] EC Europa (2009). Framework for Action on Promotion of Mental Health and Well-Being of Children and Young People. http://www.ec.europa.eu/health/ph_determinants/life_style/mental/docs/framework_young.pdf.
[39] WHO (2010). Mental Health and Development: Targeting people with mental health conditions as a vulnerable group. http://www.who.int/mental_health.
[40] WHO (2010). Mental health: strengthening our response. http://www.who.int/mediacentre/factsheets/fs220/en/.

[41] WHO (2010). Mental health: strengthening our response. http://www.who.int/mediacentre/factsheets/fs220/en/.
[42] WHO (2008). Closing the gap in a generation. Commission on Social Determinants of Health. Final Report.

In: Social Determinants and Mental Health
Editor: Sabine Bährer-Kohler
ISBN: 978-1-61324-353-4

Chapter 2

THE SOCIAL DETERMINANTS OF MENTAL HEALTH: AN INTERNATIONAL PERSPECTIVE

Gary Bailey
International Federation of Social Workers, Bern, Switzerland
Simmons College School of Social Work Boston, US

Mental health is an integral part of health; indeed, there is no health without mental health. Mental health is more than the absence of mental disorders.[1]

"If there is no struggle, there is no progress."

The son of a slave woman and an unknown white man, "Frederick Augustus Washington Bailey" was born in February of 1818 on Maryland's eastern shore in the United States. He spent his early years with his grandparents and with an aunt, seeing his mother only four or five times before her death when he was seven. (All Douglass knew of his father was that he was white.) During this time he was exposed to the degradations of slavery, witnessing firsthand brutal whippings and spending much time cold and hungry. When he was eight he was sent to Baltimore, Maryland, USA to live with a ship carpenter named Hugh Auld. There he learned to read and first heard the words abolition and abolitionists. "Going to live at Baltimore," Douglass would later say, "laid the foundation, and opened the gateway, to all my subsequent prosperity." Douglass spent seven relatively comfortable years in Baltimore before being sent back to the country, where he was hired out to a farm run by a notoriously brutal "slave breaker" named Edward Covey. And the treatment he received was indeed brutal. Whipped daily and barely fed, Douglass was "broken in body, soul, and spirit."

On January 1, 1836, Douglass made a resolution that he would be free by the end of that year; and he planned his escape; but early in April he was jailed after his plan was discovered. Two years later, while living in Baltimore and working at a shipyard, Douglass would finally realize his dream: he fled the city on September 3, 1838. Travelling by train, then steamboat, then train, he arrived in New York City the following day. Several weeks later he had settled in New Bedford, Massachusetts, USA living with his newlywed bride (whom he met in Baltimore and married in New York) under his new name, Frederick Douglass. Douglass would continue his active involvement to better the lives of African Americans. He conferred with President Abraham Lincoln during the U.S. Civil War and recruited northern blacks for the Union Army. After the War he fought for the rights of women and African Americans alike.[2]

On August 3, 1857, Frederick Douglass delivered a "West India Emancipation" speech at Canandaigua, New York, USA on the twenty-third anniversary of the event. Most of the address was a history of British efforts toward emancipation as well as a reminder of the crucial role of West Indian slaves in their own freedom struggle. However shortly after he began Douglass sounded a foretelling of the coming Civil War in the United States of America when he uttered two paragraphs that became the most quoted sentences of all of his public orations. It began with the words, "If there is no struggle, there is no progress."

"Let me give you a word of the philosophy of reform. The whole history of the progress of human liberty shows that all concessions yet made to her august claims have been born of earnest struggle. The conflict has been exciting, agitating, all-absorbing, and for the time being, putting all other tumults to silence. It must do this or it does nothing. If there is no struggle there is no progress. Those who profess to favor freedom and yet deprecate agitation are men who want crops without plowing up the ground; they want rain without thunder and lightning. They want the ocean without the awful roar of its many waters. This struggle may be a moral one, or it may be a physical one, and it may be both moral and physical, but it must be a struggle. Power concedes nothing without a demand. It never did and it never will. Find out just what any people will quietly submit to and you have found out the exact measure of injustice and wrong which will be imposed upon them, and these will continue till they are resisted with either words or blows, or with both. The limits of tyrants are prescribed by the endurance of those whom they oppress." [3]

In a speech delivered on 28th September 1948, in Paris, France, Eleanor Roosevelt said : "The development of the ideal of freedom and its translation into the everyday life of the people in great areas of the earth is the product of the efforts of many peoples. It is the fruit of a long tradition of vigorous thinking and courageous action. No one race and no one people can claim to have done all the work to achieve greater dignity for human beings and great freedom to develop human personality. In each generation and in each country there must be a continuation of the struggle and new steps forward must be taken since this is preeminently a field in which to stand still is to retreat. [4]

Ten years later in remarks she made at the presentation of a booklet on human rights, *In Your Hands*, to the United Nations Commission on Human Rights, at the United Nations, in New York City, Mrs. Roosevelt famously said: "Where, after all, do universal human rights begin? In small places, close to home - so close and so small that they cannot be seen on any maps of the world. Yet they are the world of the individual person; the neighborhood he lives in; the school or college he attends; the factory, farm, or office where he works. Such are the places where every man, woman, and child seeks equal justice, equal opportunity, equal dignity without discrimination. Unless these rights have meaning there, they have little meaning anywhere. Without concerted citizen action to uphold them close to home, we shall look in vain for progress in the larger world". [5]

Important are the basic instruments concerning Human Rights:

1. Charter of the United Nations (1945);
2. The Universal Declaration of Human Rights (1948);

3. The Covenants on Human Rights (1966) a) International Covenant on Civil and Political Rights b) International Covenant on Economic, Social and Cultural Rights;
4. The International Convention on the Elimination of All Forms of Racial Discrimination (1965);
5. The Convention on the Elimination of All Forms of Discrimination against Women (1979);
6. The Convention against Torture and other Cruel, Inhuman and Degrading Treatment or Punishment (1984);
7. The Convention on the Rights of the Child (1989) and; 8. The International Convention on the Protection of the Rights of all Migrant Workers and Members of their Families (1990). [6]

THE SOCIAL DETERMINANTS OF HEALTH

The social determinants of health are viewed by many as the conditions into which people are born, grow, live, work and age, including the health system. In large part these circumstances are shaped by the distribution of money, power and resources at global, national and local levels, which are themselves influenced by policy choices. The social determinants of health are mostly responsible for health inequities - the unfair and avoidable differences in health status seen within and between countries.

In his classic book, *The Sane Society*, published in 1955, the psychologist Erich Fromm proposed that: "health in a comprehensive sense, and the free and full development of human potential seem unattainable in the existing social context…when people are forced to adjust to an insane reality which frustrates their material, social, and psychological needs, they tend to develop various forms of ill health and to defend themselves by escaping or by acting aggressively… the insanity of the current social context is insane".

Responding to increasing concern about these persisting and widening inequities, the World Health Organization (WHO) established the Commission on Social Determinants of Health (CSDH) in 2005 to provide advice on how to reduce them. The Commission's final report was launched in August 2008, and contained three overarching recommendations:

1. Improve daily living conditions;
2. Tackle the inequitable distribution of power, money, and resources;
3. Measure and understand the problem and assess the impact of action. [7]

Much of what we understand in the area of health comes from research in the field of epidemiology: the scientific study of patterns of health and illness within a population; a wide range of mental health disorders, but also on reactions to national crises and traumatic events.

The research on psychiatric epidemiology shows that mental disorders are common throughout the world, affecting tens of millions of people each year; and that only a fraction of those affected receive treatment. While many mental disorders are common globally, their burden of illness is particularly concentrated amongst those who experience disability due to serious mental illness (SMI). The data presented from the United States National Survey on Drug Use and Health (NSDUH), defines SMI as:

- -Mental, behavioral, or emotional disorder (excluding developmental and substance use disorders)
- -Diagnosable currently or within the past year
- -Of sufficient duration to meet diagnostic criteria specified within the 4th edition of the Diagnostic and Statistical Manual of Mental Disorders (DSM-IV)
- -Resulting in serious functional impairment, which substantially interferes with or limits one or more major life activities.

Mental illness includes issues such as:

- Anxiety Disorders
- Attention Deficit Hyperactivity Disorder (ADHD, ADD)
- Autism Spectrum Disorders (Pervasive Developmental Disorders)
- Bipolar Disorder (Manic-Depressive Illness)
- Borderline Personality Disorder
- Depression
- Eating Disorders
- Generalized Anxiety Disorder
- Obsessive-Compulsive Disorder (OCD)
- Panic Disorder
- Prevention
- Post-Traumatic Stress Disorder (PTSD)
- Schizophrenia
- Social Phobia (Social Anxiety Disorder) and Suicide Prevention. [8]

These are disorders which occur in children and adolescents, older adults, women and men. The most common forms of interventions have included psychotherapy, medication and social empowerment/action. [9]

In its International *Policy on Health*, the International Federation of Social Workers (IFSW) asserts that "health is an issue of fundamental human rights and social justice and binds social work to apply these principles in policy, education, research and practice. All people have an equal right to enjoy the basic conditions which underpin human health. These conditions include a minimum standard of living to support health and a sustainable and health promoting environment. All people have an equal right to access resources and services that promote health and address illness, injury and impairment, including social services. IFSW demands and works towards the realization of these universal rights through the development, articulation and pursuit of socially just health and social policies. [10]

IFSW has also long known that poverty and its ramifications contribute to the disproportionate evidence of mental health issues amongst some populations and communities when compared to those of greater affluence. The IFSW Policy on Poverty Eradication and the Role of Social Workers states in part that:

2.1 The effects of poverty are often reflected in a multitude of the vulnerable groups such as; youths, children, women, elderly, disabled, refugees, migrants, homeless and all those at risk. Children suffer amongst other deprivations, from hunger and malnutrition. Half the deaths of pre-school children are attributed to the intersection between malnutrition and infectious diseases. Even in wealthiest countries, 40 to 50 million children are growing up in relative poverty. Women comprise the majority of those affected by poverty. They are afforded fewer educational opportunities, have maternal responsibilities and are subjected to forced labor, trafficking and other forms of violence. The elderly comprise the fastest growing segment of the world's population, and this group will quadruple by year 2050 from 600 million to 2 billion. The elderly are subject to poverty because of lack of work opportunities and in many societies there are no political or social arrangements for their security and survival.

2.2 The disabled in some circumstances are removed from society entirely to live in an institutionalized, marginalized and abused existence. Refugees, migrants, immigrants, homeless and ethnic minorities are groups experiencing similar exclusion from the opportunities of the major society and consequently suffer from poverty and other attendants indignities. Indigenous people are particularly at risk for poverty, are often stateless and lack a voice within the countries where they reside. Often invisible in large urban areas or segregated in distant reservations, indigenous people often suffer from high unemployment which contributes to their extreme poverty in developing countries or relative poverty in more developed countries. Urban and rural dwellers experience different, but equally oppressive, forces leading to poverty, urban dwellers from lack of competitive skills and rural people from lack of available work. Those who live in areas most vulnerable to natural disasters are usually poor. And as survivors they are left with no access to resources. The poor who survive armed conflict are generally displaced. Armed conflicts have been increasing within states, and most victims are civilians, poor and consequently made poorer. Widespread evidence confirms that pandemics and poverty are mutually interwoven and have disastrous consequences. [11].

According to the WHO, mental health is an integral and essential component of health. The WHO constitution states: "Health is a state of complete physical, mental and social well-being and not merely the absence of disease or infirmity." An important consequence of this definition is that mental health is described as more than the absence of mental disorders or disabilities.

Multiple social, psychological, and biological factors determine the level of mental health of a person at any point of time. Persistent socio-economic pressures are recognized risks to mental health for individuals and communities. The clearest evidence is associated with indicators of poverty, including low levels of education. Poor mental health is also associated with rapid social change, stressful work conditions, gender discrimination, social exclusion, unhealthy lifestyle, risks of violence and physical ill-health and human rights violations.

There are also specific psychological and personality factors that make people vulnerable to mental disorders. Lastly, there are some biological causes of mental disorders including genetic factors and imbalances in chemicals in the brain. [12].

Strategies and Interventions

Mental health promotion involves actions to create living conditions and environments that support mental health and allow people to adopt and maintain healthy lifestyles. These include a range of actions to increase the chances of more people experiencing better mental health.

As Dr. Bährer-Kohler has written in her foreword to this book , "a climate that respects and protects basic civil, political, socio-economic and cultural rights is fundamental to mental health promotion. Without the security and freedom provided by these rights, it is very difficult to maintain a high level of mental health. Promoting mental health depends largely on intersectional strategies." [13].

To paraphrase Douglass yet again: *"If there is no struggle, there is no progress.* This struggle may be a moral one, or it may be a physical one, and it may be both moral and physical, but it will be a struggle. Power concedes nothing without a demand. It never did and it never will".

REFERENCES

[1] WHO. *http://www.who.int/mediacentre/factsheets/fs220/en/index.html* retrieved from WHO website 31 March 2011

[2] Public Broadcasting Service (PBS). *http://www.pbs.org/wgbh/aia/part4/4p1539.html* retrieved from PBS website 31 March 2011

[3] Frederick Douglass.(1857). *Two Speeches by Frederick Douglass* (Rochester).

[4] Eleanor Roosevelt.(1948). *The Struggle for Human Rights.*

[5] Eleanor Roosevelt (1958). *In your hands : A Guide for Community Action for the Tenth Anniversary of the Universal Declaration of Human Rights.*

[6] IFSW. *http://www.ifsw.org/p38000212.html* retrieved from IFSW website 31 March 2011

[7] WHO. *http://www.who.int/social_determinants/en/* retrieved from WHO website 31 march 2011

[8] The National Institute of Mental Health (*NIMH*). *http://www.nimh.nih.gov/health/topics/social-phobia-social-anxiety-disorder/index.shtml* retrieved from NIMH website 31st March 2011

[9] The National Institute of Mental Health (*NIMH*) *.http://www.nimh.nih.gov/health/topics/child-and-adolescent-mental-health/index.shtml* retrieved from NIMH 31 March 2011

[10] IFSW. *http://www.ifsw.org/p38000081.html* retrieved from IFSW website 31 March 2011

[11] IFSW. *http://www.ifsw.org/p38002089.html* retrieved from IFSW website 31 March 2011

[12] WHO. *http://www.who.int/mediacentre/factsheets/fs220/en/index.html* retrieved from WHO website 31 March 2011

[13] WHO. *http://www.who.int/mediacentre/factsheets/fs220/en/index.html* retrieved from WHO website 31 March 2011.

In: Social Determinants and Mental Health
Editor: Sabine Bährer-Kohler
ISBN: 978-1-61324-353-4

Chapter 3

The Present and Future Importance of Social Determinants, Aspects of Political Implementation for Switzerland

Silvia Schenker
Member of the Swiss Parlament, Basel, Switzerland

Mental illness is a widespread phenomenon. Various studies suggest that almost one in two persons suffers from some mental illness or other in the course of his or her life. The danger is particularly great in transitional phases, such as starting school, puberty, starting employment and retirement as well as in critical situations, such as getting divorced, losing your job and experiencing violence.

In addition, people's mental health is influenced by their level of education and their economic situation. You will have a better chance of retaining your mental health if you are well educated, if your material situation is secure, if you are embedded in your own social network, and if your family has been living in the same cultural environment for generations.

This insight is slowly making headway on the international plane and also in Switzerland. Even politics can no longer turn a blind eye. The issue of mental health has been on the political agenda of the European countries and the WHO since 1995. Held in Helsinki, Finland, from January 12 to 15, 2005, the European ministerial WHO conference on mental health developed a plan of action for its promotion. Recommended by the WHO to its member countries for implementation, the entire range of measures contained in the action plan is intended to contribute toward promoting people's mental health. (1)

In Switzerland, too, mental health is being taken seriously. In 2004, the Swiss National Health Policy Institute developed a national strategy for mental health. Quite a number of the recommendations contained in it are addressed to politics and the authorities in charge. Among other things, the strategy suggests reducing institutional discrimination and creating a legal foundation for providing self-help organizations with the funds they need. (2)

Now, more than 5 years after the strategy was developed, the track record is disillusioning. It is true that various activities have been launched, but they have not been harmonised and, consequently, never been embedded in a national strategy: yet another proof that the federalist system is not without its problems in Switzerland.

Nevertheless, efforts are being made at the national level. When it was found that the number of people that have been pensioned off because of some mental illness had increased markedly, measures designed to ensure that affected persons are identified and supported as early as possible were reviewed and introduced in the course of a revision of the disability insurance system. Early diagnosis, early intervention, and integration measures are financed by the disability insurance and implemented flexibly and adaptively in conformance with the will of the legislative power. Moreover, attempts are made to sensitize employers and assist them on request. Another measure under review is to re-integrate people who are already receiving a pension into the labor market. There are supporting measures designed to ensure the highest possible level of security for those concerned.

Together with the institutions involved, the disability insurance endeavors to re-integrate people with mental problems into the labor market. The main reason for this is that the insurance has been making a loss for several years and has racked up a considerable debt. If its endeavors should actually bear fruit, and if it should really succeed in keeping more mentally ill people in employment, the persons concerned would stand to benefit as well.

Next to support and assistance designed to benefit those concerned at the individual level, more and more steps are being taken to de-stigmatize mental illness. Besides removing its stigma, the early diagnosis of mental illness is to be promoted as well. Alliance Against Depression, an action program originally developed in Germany, was first introduced in Switzerland in the canton of Zug in 2003, where particular attention was paid to senile depression which is under a powerful taboo. After all, depression is frequently diagnosed too late or not at all. What is more, elderly people with depression have a double stigma to contend with, old age and depression. Meanwhile, the Alliance Against Depression has spread to six Swiss cantons. It supports sensitization as well as prevention, health promotion, and self-help. 'Depression has many faces' – this is one of the key messages of the public campaigns waged by the various alliances against depression. Another message of equal importance is that depression is treatable. The intention is to motivate the people concerned to seek the assistance of doctors and therapists.

The fourth public health report for the canton of Bern shows how unequally health chances are distributed. The report clearly states that this holds particularly true for mental health. For this reason, its authors envisioned various field of action and measures aimed at improving the health chances of the socially disadvantaged. Objectives include not only cutting poverty in half and integrating migrants but also strengthening and empowering the family. (3)

Parents and Schools Strengthen Children (ESSKI), a program developed by the Social Work University (FHNW), promotes psychosocial health at primary schools by reinforcing the competences and resources of teachers, pupils and parents. The program was first put to the test at schools in Basle. It was found that although the approach is appropriate, it did not appeal sufficiently to families with a migration background. Work on this will begin in the next phase. (4)

A comprehensive study of a large number of files on persons who were awarded a pension by the Swiss disability insurance for mental reasons revealed important insights. The study says that the mental problems of a large proportion of the insured originated in childhood or adolescence. (5) To sustainably improve and change the support of mental health, therefore, intervention must begin much earlier and in a much denser network.

As public health is greatly influenced by social determinants, public health cannot be maintained and promoted by health policy alone. Educational policy, social policy, and other political fields must make their own contribution. This, however, still remains to be acknowledged by political actors. The tendency to consider each political field separately is still far too dominant. Moreover, coordination is rendered difficult by the fact that in Switzerland, the federal as well as the cantonal governments are responsible for social policy.

Switzerland lacks national health targets and related strategies. This gap will be closed by the Federal Act on Prevention and Health Promotion that has already been adopted by the Federal Council and is now being debated in parliament. Since promoting mental health is among the objectives of the Prevention Act, it would also serve to support the endeavors of various players who advocate improving the mental health of the Swiss population. The Act might improve the chances of highly praiseworthy initiatives undertaken by cantonal governments, institutions, and organizations and help to disseminate important information.

Thus, Switzerland might take another step toward the goal of promoting mental well-being for all.

REFERENCES

[1] *Europäischer Aktionsplan für psychische Gesundheit.* (2005). Helsinki, Finland.

[2] *Nationale Gesundheitspolitik Schweiz*, Nationale Strategie zum Schutz, zur Förderung, Erhaltung und Wiederherstellung der psychischen Gesundheit der Bevölkerung in der Schweiz, 2004.

[3] Vierter Gesundheitsbericht des Kantons Bern, 2010, *www.gef.be.ch.*

[4] Sandmeier, A., Schönenberger, M., & Schmid, H. (2009). Schlussbericht zur Evaluation von ESSKI-Z - Eltern und Schule stärken Kinder im Kanton Zug. *Olten: Hochschule für Soziale Arbeit FHNW.*

[5] Baer, N., Frick, U., Fasel, T. (2009). *Dossieranalyse der Invalidisierung aus psychischen Gründen. Liestal.*

In: Social Determinants and Mental Health
Editor: Sabine Bährer-Kohler
ISBN: 978-1-61324-353-4

Chapter 4

PSYCHO-SOCIAL DETERMINANTS OF MENTAL HEALTH

Elaine T. Jurkowski
Southern Illinois University College of Education and Human Services
School of Social Work, Carbondale, US

The former United States Surgeon General, Dr. David Satcher, identified one's mental health as one's psychological state on a continuum, fluctuating based upon a variety of factors, both internal and external to the person (USDHSS, 2000). In addition, various theoretical perspectives help understand the complexity of one's mental health functioning. Understanding these factors and accompanying theories that underlay the basis of an integrated and healthy mental or psychological state is crucial in building prevention and intervention programs to help strengthen one's mental health at micro (individual), meso (group), and macro (community) levels. This chapter will address the social determinants of health and how these interplay within one's mental health, and will also discuss psychological theories and how these theories impact the psycho-social determinants of one's mental health.

SOCIAL DETERMINANTS

In some spheres, the traditional notion of health and mental health of an individual has been attributed to the germ theory (McKeown, 1973). Dr. Thomas McKeown, in efforts to reshape the British health care system, challenged this traditional notion and argued that the behavior and lifestyle of the individual played a role in one's physical and mental health, as well as factors such as environment and genetics. Although McKeown's perspective and divisions are not the only way to conceptualize factors that impact one's health and mental health, Marc Lalonde, The Minister of Health in Canada (1981) built upon McKeown's theory to articulate five main criteria which undergird the health of individuals. These determinants articulated in his health plan for Canadians (Lalonde, 1981) have been embraced by the World Health Organization in a variety of seminal documents, but most recently have been used to help identify social determinants of health (2005, 2008). These social determinants include economics, behavior/lifestyle, genetics, environment, and social networks. While there is significant documentation within the literature to suggest that these factors have a significant impact on one's health, the literature summarized in various reports exploring mental health conditions, etiology, and epidemiology (WHO, 2008; USDHHS, 2000) also suggests that these factors individually or in combination also contribute to one's mental health.

Economics

The literature has well documented the relationship between poverty and mental disorders in low and middle income countries (Lund et al, 2010). Lund and colleagues (2010) conducted a meta-analysis of 115 epidemiologic studies to examine the interplay between common mental disorders and poverty, and continue to substantiate the role that economics plays in promoting mental health. They found within their analysis of variables in their meta-analysis, that 77% of these studies found a consistent relationship between inadequate income and mental disorders. It has long been established in developed countries that there is a relationship between poor mental health outcomes and poverty (Saraceno & Barbui, 1997; Saraceno, Levav & Kohn, 2005, McPherson & McGibbon, 2010). In addition to poverty, other factors related to one's economic status such as unemployment (Weich & Lewis, 1998), low income, social class, and socio-economic status (SES) (Lorant et al., 2003) have demonstrated an association with poor mental health outcomes, or the presence of common mental health disorders (depression, anxiety, and somotaform disorders). Although a systematic review and series of meta-analysis studies conducted on the relationship between poverty and mental health outcomes concluded poverty is associated with poor mental health outcomes in lower and middle income countries as well (Araya, Lewis, Rojas & Fritsch, 2003; Jayakady & Stauffer, 2002; Patel, Araya, de Lima, Ludermir and Todd, 1999, Patel & Kleinman, 2003), more recently there is some debate about which factors actually contribute the most to one's mental health. Factors such as food insecurity, financial stress, and housing may play a larger role than income, social class, and socio-economic status, especially within lower and middle class countries due to a perspective that a deprivation of one's basic needs occurs. (Havenaar et al, 2008; Patel, Kirkwood, et al, 2008; Patel, Fisher & Cohen, 2006; Sabin et. al., 2003; and Seino, et. al, 2008). These factors (food insecurity, financial stress, and housing) may contribute to a more global sense of deprivation, which then contributes to poorer mental health outcomes for common mental health disorders such as depression, anxiety, and somotaform disorders (Barnes, Wright, Noble and Dawes, 2007). In one case, poverty may be a lack of access, as seen in higher income countries, but deprivation may result in unmet needs for not only people suffering from mental distress, but those living within entire communities (Toye & Infanti, 2004), thus impacting the conditions within one must seek interventions. These studies cut across several continents and countries, to include South Africa (Havenaar, Geerlings, Vivian, Collinson & Robinson, 2008; Barnes, Wright, Noble & Dawes, 2007; Brazil, Chile, Indonesia, Lesotho, Pakistan, Zimbabwe (Patel & Kleinman, 2003); Latin America and Britain (Araya, Lewis, Rojas & Fritsch, 2003), Mexico, South America (Sabin, 2003) and Afghanistan (Seino et. al., 2008).

Dsashiff, DiMicco, Myers, and Sheppard (2009) argue that professionals need to remain active in advocacy efforts to address the impact that poverty plays in one's mental health across the lifespan, but especially adolescents. This group appear to be most vulnerable to mental health issues, since all too often they are expected to take on adult roles or responsibilities while still working on their own development, with often limited resources financially. Poverty, along with these stressors can also lead to adolescent risk behaviors (USDHHS, 2000) and increased crime (McLeod & Shanahan, 1996).

Economics also plays a pivotal role in access to mental health services. In countries where consumers pay a fee for service or where mental health services are a commodity, the issues of health disparities and access to services becomes an issue (USDHHS, 2000). Economics further plays a role in the provision of mental health services, due to six separate economic barriers that impact how services can be obtained (Knapp et. al., 2006). Economically oppressed communities, or governments, place a lower priority on mental health services than countries or communities which are economically well off, and economic barriers will have a greater impact in six distinct areas when seeking to obtain mental health services. These barriers include problems obtaining information, insufficient resources, problems of resource distribution, inappropriate resources, inflexible resources, and poor timing of the intervention of resources for mental health concerns (Knapp et. al., 2006).To further illuminate this point, in a study which examined data from the World Health Organization, fewer than one third of countries identified that a budget for mental health services or infrastructure existed (Milne & Robertson, 1998). These authors also found that of the remaining countries that identified the availability of mental health resources, more than one third of these countries spent one percent or less of their public health budget on services for mental health issues (Milne & Robertson, 1998).

Behavior/Lifestyle

A number of factors related to one's lifestyle and health behavior/practices will impact one's mental health outcomes. While we often think about the relationship between individual behavior and health outcomes, models designed to help understand health behavior can also be used to understand community behaviors toward prevention and health promotion. While health behavior may affect lifestyle, specific lifestyle behaviors related to nutrition, substance abuse, and self-management also play a role in mental health outcomes *(*Harbottle and Schonfelder, *2008).*

Health behavior theorists have examined the roles of behavior/lifestyles on one's mental health status and have concluded that there is a relationship between one's behavior and lifestyle and positive mental health outcomes. The *Health Belief Model* (Rosenstock, 1974, Becker, 1974) helps explain the role of lifestyle based upon human motivation. Perceived seriousness and perceived susceptibility play a role into how people handle and attend to factors which promote or detract from optimal mental health conditions. In like manner, Ajzen's work to identify a "*Theory of Reasoned Action*" has been utilized in numerous studies to help identify some of the antecedents that lead to help-seeking and health promotion behaviors related to mental health conditions. Their theory suggests that individuals will integrate preventative or help-seeking behaviors into their lifestyle which will impact their mental health status, when the cultural context within which they live supports their behaviors. Thus, if there is a stigma or taboo associated with mental health, one's will not view any intervention in a positive light (Ajzen, 1991).

Prochaska & Diclemente (1983) identified six stages of change which impact one's readiness to participate in change regarding smoking behavior. While their original work examined one's behaviors in relation to addiction behavior, the stages of pre-contemplation, contemplation, preparation, action, evaluation, and termination are relevant in how people participate in their own self care and within treatment for mental health disorders (Prochaska, DiClemente & Norcross, 1992; Prochaska & Velicer, 1997; Rochlen, Rude & Baron, 2005; Derisley & Reynolds, 2000).

Social learning theory or social cognitive theory (Rosenstock, Strecher & Becker, 1988) theorized that learning and behavior result from events or a series of reinforcements and expectations. Individual behaviors are guided by individual expectations, but ultimately may be controlled by external expectations, or expectations from others. Internal and external locus of control will have an impact on one's behavior; however the expectations of others will greatly influence the outcome (Rosenstock, Strecjer & Becker, 1988). Bandura (2005) built upon the components of social cognitive theory to evolve a model of self-regulatory behavior. Self-regulation is a complex psychosocial process and refers generally to efforts of a person to alter or maintain his or her responses through such coping processes as self-monitoring, evaluation, control, goal setting, self-reward, and expression of emotion, especially in challenging circumstances (Bandura, 1997; Baumeister & Vohs, 2004; Taylor & Stanton, 2007).

The health promotion literature has well documented the success or failure of health interventions targeting mental health based upon these theories (Glanz, Rimmer and Viswanath, 2008). Zhou et al. (2010) worked with 2,441 people over the age of 60 in China to assess the impact of dietary and lifestyle changes on one's mental health. The researchers developed an individualized intervention, based upon the Transtheoretical model and particular stage of change identified. After a nine-month intervention, the intervention group improved significantly on measures of mental health and emotional status, pointing to the importance of understanding compliance behavior through the lens of a theoretical framework for behavior. Similarly, Rochlen, Rude, and Baron (2005) evaluated participants within a short-term counseling setting at a post-secondary institution in Texas, USA. They found that clients in the pre-contemplation stage were not as likely to succeed as those in later stages of readiness for behavioral change. The self-regulatory model was used for teaching children skills to strengthen their ability to control emotional skills, within an elementary school setting in Rochester, NY, USA. In a sample of 226 kindegarten – 3rd grade students, children were taught a set of skills to maintain their emotional control using a variety of skill development and modeling exercises, based upon self-regulation. Children receiving the intervention had a 46% mean decrease in disciplinary referrals and a 43% decrease in suspensions during the 4-month intervention period (Wyman, Cross, Brown, Yu, & Eberly, 2010).

Unfortunately, some cultures or settings utilize the notion that one is personally responsible for their own health and mental health (Jurkowski, 2008) and shift the burden of responsibility for mental health on the individual, rather than the state, or government or social/structural factors. Thus, any deficits or maladaptive behavior is a result of the individual and their lifestyle, which results in a societal perspective of "blaming the victim" (Ryan, 1971, 1976). Although this term was coined to help understand ghetto formation and intergenerational poverty in Ryan's work, "Blaming the Victim" (1971, 1976), the work provides a theory to help us understand how our institutions divert social responsibility for caring or addressing social issues, and shift this responsibility to the individual. Unfortunately, the individual may have limited control over the social and cultural situation/response to their issues (Janoff-Bulman, Timko, & Carli, 1984). Rappaport, Davidson, Wilson, and Mitchell (1975) further suggested that professionals and interventions all too quickly also "blame the environment" as well, and suggested that both attitudes impede an understanding of how to harness human behavior to change one's maladaptive behavior.

Biology/ Genetics

Early scientific studies to understand schizophrenia through twin studies helped lead rise to the interplay between genetics and psychopathology. These early studies have continued to be substantiated and continue to help reinforce the linkage between genetics and mental health disorders such as depression, schizophrenia, or bi-polar disorder (Cooper, Field, Goswami, Jenkins & Sahakian, 2010; de Lara et al, 2010; Meyer-Lindenberg, 2010; Nijmeijer, 2010; Sprangers, M. et al, 2010; Toulopoulou et al, 2010). Developed countries have embraced the outcomes of these studies; however, most recently scientists have begun to suggest that there is an interplay between understanding the relationship between genetics and cultural and societal nuances (Edwards, 2010).

A meta-analysis of evidence was reviewed to identify if there was a link between schizophrenia and bi-polar disorder (Van Shellenberg & de Candia, 2009) and to decide if these genes co-exist within families. Within the 2,326 studies identified, findings suggested that there was evidence that families were more likely to have a continuing of genetic coding linking schizophrenia and bi-polar disorder. Rather than one discrete gene responsible for a specific diagnostic category of mental illness, these genes operate along a continuum.

Hyman (2000a) advanced our understanding of the relationship genetics played in relationship to causation for mental illness. He suggested that a simple cause-effect relationship contributed by a single gene was no longer realistic, due to the complexity of our understanding of the interplay between genetics and its interaction with non-genetic factors in explaining behavioral developments. Hyman (2000b) also argued that we cannot understand brain functioning without understanding the intricate relationship between the brain and behavior and genetic forces, as well as the interaction with the environment.

International clinicians, educators, and theorists need to understand the cultural contexts in efforts to support the role that genetics can play in one's mental health before this may be largely accepted, especially within developing contexts.

Environment

The context of one's environment has also long been linked to one's overall health and subsequently, one's mental health (NIMH, 1998). The arguments supporting the nurture component of the "nature or nurture" environments and its relationship to one's health and mental health status point to the importance of environment and its linkage with one's mental health. In the United States, a number of studies were conducted post Hurricane Katrina to identify how one's environment and neighborhood impacted one's mental health. Kloos and colleagues (2009) evaluated 109 people who had relocated to South Carolina as following Katrina, to determine if a neighborhood relocation intervention would have any impact on their stress levels. Results revealed that perceived neighborhood factors and satisfaction with host relationships were related to positive mental health outcomes (Kloos et al., 2009). Neighborhood social climate partially mediated several mental health outcomes. Other studies conducted in Finland and Canada have pointed to the correlations between one's physical environment and health or mental health, and one's neighborhood environment and its relationship to mental health outcomes, as well (Andrersson, Bjorngaard, Kasperson, Wang, Skre & Dahl, 2010; Jackson, Langille, Lyons, Hughes & Martin, 2009, Truong & Ma, 2006).

The "natural" or "green" environment also has an effect on one's self esteem. Pretty, Peacock, Sellens, and Griffen (2005) examined how exposure to nature had positive effects on physical and mental health. In their control trial, five groups of 20 subjects were exposed to a sequence of 30 scenes projected on a wall during an exercises session on a treadmill. Four categories of scenes were tested: rural pleasant, rural unpleasant, urban pleasant, and urban unpleasant, while a control group was running without exposure to images. Both rural and urban pleasant scenes produced a significantly greater positive effect on self-esteem than the exercise-only control. This shows the synergistic effect of green exercise in both rural and urban environments. By contrast, both rural and urban unpleasant scenes reduced the positive effects of exercise on self-esteem. The rural unpleasant scenes had the most dramatic effect, depressing the beneficial effects of exercise on three different measures of mood. It appears that threats to the countryside depicted in rural unpleasant scenes had a greater negative effect on mood than already urban unpleasant scenes.

Studies also suggest that the environmental toxins and pollutants can have an adverse effect on one's mental health. Guo and colleagues (2007) examined the impact of arsenic in drinking water, using subjects from 13 counties within Mongolia, China. They found that there was a direct correlation between the pollutants and poorer mental health outcomes.

The work context represents another environment, which deserves mention as having an impact on one's mental health and well-being. Simmons and Swanborg (2008) examined the work environment, and relationship between psychosocial job characteristics and depressive symptoms for US workers using a 2002 national database. For working non-poor employees, high psychological demands and low supervisor and coworker support were associated with depressive symptoms.

Social Networks

Lastly, social networks and supports play a pivotal role as a social determinant to one's mental health. Peer support and group intervention strategies have been well documented within the literature as strategies to help facilitate stronger mental health outcomes during intervention trials (NIMH, 1998; USDHHS, 2000). Studies have also documented the negative effects of loneliness and isolation on mental health outcomes. Although the literature makes the case for the relationship between social support and positive mental health outcomes, Nemeroff, Medlarsky, and Meyer (2010) question to what extent personality plays a role in utilizing social networks to moderate stress and distress. They hypothesized that personality impacted to what extent social networks were utilized, and concluded that one's perception of power and ability to be empowered play a key role in successfully navigating resources when in a stress mode.

Rapp (1998) argued that labels, deficits, and pathology, environmental deficits, and blaming the victim lead to a cycle of oppression for people living with mental illness. He provided empirical evidence to support the use of a "strengths based" approach that builds on the individual's social networks, builds a positive supportive environment, and creates a personal care plan based upon individual needs and goals.

The value of a strength's based approach and mutual support/participation was further explored by Pistrang, Barker, and Humphreys (2008). These researchers reviewed empirical studies on whether participating in mutual help groups for people with mental health problems leads to improved psychological and social functioning. To be included, studies had to satisfy four sets of criteria, covering: (1) characteristics of the group, (2) target problems, (3) outcome measures, and (4) research design. The 12 studies meeting these criteria provided evidence that mutual help groups benefit people with three types of problems: chronic mental illness, depression/anxiety, and bereavement. Positive outcomes were reported by nine studies, and none of the studies found negative effects as a result of participation in mutual aid groups. More high-quality outcome research is needed to evaluate the effectiveness of mutual help groups across the spectrum of mental health problems.

Thus far we have examined how specific determinants of mental health impact mental health outcomes for individuals. These determinants included economics, behavior/lifestyle, genetics, environment, and social lifestyle. In addition, our understanding of psycho-social determinants of mental health can be broadened through our understanding of psychological theories which underlie human behavior. From this point of view, thus, it may be helpful to understand the role that psychological theories play in contributing to determinants of mental health.

Psychological Theories Which Contribute to Determinants of Mental Health

Over the past century, a number of advances have been identified and articulated into theory within the field of psychology and science, to help explain human behavior. These theories have been exceedingly useful in helping to understand human behavior and one's mental health, and in helping experts build intervention strategies in efforts to support one's mental health. An understanding of these theories can assist greatly in the development of community based intervention strategies for people with mental health concerns. These theories include behaviorism psychoanalytic perspectives, genetics, information processing perspectives, psycho-social stages of development, selective optimization, and a life-span developmental approach (USDHHS, 2000; Belsky, 1993). This section will briefly discuss these theories, and will identify how they help us build our understanding of how these theories contribute to the psycho-social determinants of one's mental health.

A. Behavioral Perspectives

The concept of behaviorism involves many aspects, specifically that "behaviorists do not believe there is any such thing as a defined, age-related change" (Belsky, 1999). Traditional behaviorism focuses on the impact of nurture, or the environment, and decidedly ignores the effects of nature, or genetics. Traditional behaviorism states that behaviors are learned through two different forms—classical and operant, or instrumental, conditioning, coined by B.F.Skinner (Kimble, 1993). Classical conditioning is associated with primitive forms of learning; this is most often associated with Pavlov's famous dogs. Classical conditioning involves an involuntary response (salivation) caused by an unconditioned stimulus (food)—this response can be also be provoked through a conditioned stimulus that occurs at the same time as the unconditioned stimulus (bell sound with food). Operant conditioning occurs as conscious responses to rewarded, or reinforced, stimuli. This type of conditioning can involve several varying "schedules of reinforcement," including rewards after every response, rewards at expected times, and irregularity in rewards, each of which causes a different pattern of behavior and teaches "persistence". Traditional behaviorists utilize these two types of conditioning, as well as reinforcement and extinction (the loss of a behavior over time), to explain changing and persisting behaviors through the lifespan, acquired through a trial and error process. Traditional behavioral concepts are used to explain behaviors such as behavioral outbursts in young children, suicide rates, domestic violence, and mental and physical decline in nursing homes, etc. as behaviors formed through various reinforcements (Belski, 1993). Mental disorders were conceived as learned and reinforced with some form of incentive for maladaptive behavior. These behaviors had the potential to be unlearned through behavior modification (Kazdin, 1996, 1997).

The cognitive/social learning approach is a theory created approximately 30 years ago by psychologist Albert Bandura, who realized that classical and operant conditioning could not fully explain behaviors (Bandura, 1977). Bandura's idea was that learning transpires often without rewards in a form of observation, or modeling, in which the imitator chooses which behaviors to model and continue. Cognitive behaviorism generally follows many of the principles of traditional behaviorism, specifically the belief that nurture effects behavior far more than nature. In opposition, cognitive behaviorists view people as active, not reactive, and study cognitions and perceptions. Another feature of cognitive behaviorism is the idea of self-efficacy, or the belief in one's own capabilities, particularly in performing adequately at specific tasks. Bandura affirms that efficacy is what drives behavior; high self-efficacy results in high action and vice a versa (1997). Cognitive behaviorists use these theories to explain perspectives on non-reinforcing or reinforcing events, such as viewing setbacks or failures as temporary or lasting. Cognitive behavior concepts are used to describe behaviors such as children imitating behavior, a speedy recovery, mid life careers, and retreating from communication because of poor memory linked to aging as resulting from changing self-efficacy. There appear to be three main benefits of behavioral theory: it is optimistic in identifying and easily reversing problem behaviors; it has global applicability; it is action-oriented and involves frameworks for improving quality of life (Bandura, 1997).

B. Psychoanalytic Perspective

Sigmund Freud's psychoanalytic perspective on aging believes that the basic personality is formed in early childhood and involves three different facets; the instinctive id, the logical ego, and the moral superego (Freud, 1924). Freud also stated that parents are responsible for learning and life-long mental health, and thus effect ego development (Belsky, 1993). These theories explain unconscious motivations which describe behaviors throughout the aging process. Freud's psychoanalytic perspective is age-hostile because Freud says that nothing changes very much after childhood (Freud, 1924).

C. Behavioral/Genetic Perspective

The behavioral genetic perspective came about because neither behaviorism nor psychoanalysis explain why there is so much variation of behaviors person to person (Ploman & McLearn, 1993). Behavioral genetics are just that; these theorists look at the influence that genetics have on behavior. In order to accomplish this, behavioral geneticists perform multiple studies, including twin studies. Twin studies involve the comparison of identical twins, who share 100% of their genes, to fraternal twins, who share only 50% of their genes with the obvious idea that if a trait is influenced by genetics, then identical twins should be more alike in their behaviors than fraternal twins (Ploman & McLearn, 1993). These studies are scored and subsequently correlated according to a correlation coefficient. This number is then subtracted for the two groups of twins, and then doubled to define heritability, or the degree to which variations in that trait can be attributed to genetic influences. Heritability is not applied individually; rather, it is applied across populations.

An issue with twin studies is that it is difficult to separate environmental influences from genetics since twins are generally raised together, and often treated more alike by parents/family since they are more alike (38). In the 1980s, the Swedish adoption/twin study of aging identified 99 identical twins and 229 fraternal Swedish twins separated and adopted into different families before the age of 10 and then reunited over the age of 50. These sets of twins were vigorously tested, and their responses compared and tested against twins raised together. Results from these tests found that heritabilities vary from quality to quality and trait to trait, and that the highest heritability appeared to be in cognition. A realization of these studies is that, "as we approach the outer limits of behavior, who we are as people is less determined by our life experiences and more heavily influenced by our genes". Twin studies have found, too, that the heritability of illness is lower in groups of older people than in groups of younger people, meaning that illness in younger years is more likely due to heritability while illness in later life is more likely caused by the aging process and environmental factors. It is important to understand that both nature and nurture play a role in determining behavior (Bouchard, 1994; Ploman & McLearn, 1986). Overall, we may see patterns of a pre-disposition for a mental health diagnosis between family members, which is accounted for through this theoretical approach.

D. Information-Processing Perspective

The information-processing perspective through the lifespan is dedicated to understanding thought processes and conceptualizes the mind as a kind of computer, explaining behavior at every stage of life through research. This perspective has been most useful in explaining cognitive-decline related to the aging process (Belsky, 1993). Conversely, it also explains the rapid speed at which children pick up information, learn and mimic the world around them. The mind encodes messages through a series of neurotransmitters. This process is most efficient in young children, and through "wear and tear" slows down as one ages USDHHS, 2000).

E. Erik Erikson's Psychosocial Crises

Erikson's theories address psychosocial concerns and issues relating to identity and relationships based upon a series of life stages (Erikson, 1963). Erikson opposed Freud's belief that human nature is ruled by the unconscious and that growth stops at the age of five, and established a theory that defines eight life tasks (psychosocial crises) that are applied to an approximate age-range, and which are experienced by every person, and build upon each other. Using this developmental approach, a person cannot master a given stage until the previous stages have been successfully passed through. Each stage incorporates a physical, emotional, and psychological stage of development, and incorporates specific developmental task at each stage. Infants are confronted with trust/mistrust; toddlers process through autonomy while pre-schoolers begin to take initiative. In contrast, school-aged children develop a sense of self worth through activity and "industry"; adolescents attempt to identify their own unique identity, while young adults seek out intimacy. Two principles utilized within Erikson's theory during adulthood include generativity and ego-integrity. Generativity is a crucial aspect of mid-life, where the commitment to guiding the development of other people becomes a priority. Ego-integrity occurs in later life and involves the acceptance of the current situation and past experiences in order to be at peace with impending death. Interventions based on psychosocial crises are found in clinical work with people, based upon their life stages. For example, interventions with people who are older adults focus particularly on reminiscence or life review in nursing homes and assisted living (Erikson, 1963).

F. Carl Jung's Passage toward Maturity

Jung divides life into two parts: puberty to mid-thirties (youth) and forty and beyond (adult), but majorly emphasizes the second part of life, which focuses on introspection and contemplation because the passions of youth have been calmed. This shift to maturity in mid-life, says Jung, provides psychological wholeness where the personality is finally fully accepted and integrated (Mattoon, 1987). This often leads to less differentiation between male and female behavior, but despite this, Jung's theories had no major impact on researchers of the aging process (Belsky, 1999).

G. Selective Optimization with Compensation

Paul Baltes' theory involves three major components; contemporary, or the focus of energy on most important life activities; optimization, where hard work to perform well in these areas is evident; and compensation, in which we rely on external resources to help us with things we cannot do ourselves (Marsiske, Lang, Baltes & Baltes, 1995).Baltes (1993) suggests that as people grow older, they prioritize which activities that they will focus upon,let those activities of lesser importance go, and compensate through the use of resources outside of their personal self. In this approach, one must have insight and power to be able to identify which activities are of utmost importance, and discern how to focus their energy on areas which they have the most ability, and will have the most impact. Individuals at earlier stages in their lives may not utilize this approach due to the fact that they need to develop insight into their behaviors, prior to being able to selectively differentiate what activities to prioritize.

H. Life-Span Developmental Approach

Behaviors are best described and understood through the lens of the contextualizing, life-span developmental approach, which embraces all of these points of view, and decides that diversity is the best strategy to follow in understanding age change (Baltes & Willis, 1977; Dixon, 1992). The life-span approach recognizes that change throughout the llifespan, from infancy into old age, is both multidirectional and multidimensional and that patterns of behaviors follow diverse forms which focus on the total context (life situation of the person). The purpose of the life-span approach is to describe, explain, and optimize behavior across developmental stages throughout one's life. If one does not master these tasks developmentally at earlier years, or mediate negative life events, they affect one adversely at a later point in one's life. This adverse effect can severely impact one's mental health and well being, until resolved. It also may occur at various points in time across one's life span (Baltes & Willis, 1977).

In conclusion, various theories help explain human behaviors, and contribute to the development of adaptive or maladaptive behavior. Different approaches call for different types of interventions. For example, a behaviorist approach as described in section A and B, would utilize a behavior modification approach, targeting the individual level. Psychotherapy may be more appropriate if using a Jungian view in diagnosing behaviors. Cognitive-behavioral approaches may be more appropriate when addressing unmet stages of development such as Erickson's stages (USDHHS, 2000). These theories are also helpful to use as a lens to identify different therapeutic approaches to diagnosis and intervention across disciplines. Moreover, the theories help us to create a canvas to understand some of the psycho-social determinants of mental health.

Summary

In this chapter we have examined the role and interplay between specific social determinants and their impact on mental health. Factors such as economics, behavior/lifestyle, genetics, environment, and social networks, all contribute to one's mental health. Economics will play an essential role at the macro or community level, since service availability or access impacts the ability to mediate psycopathology, and impact mental health outcomes. As Knapp (2006) points out, problems obtaining information, insufficient resources, problems of resource distribution, inappropriate resources, inflexible resources, and poor timing of the intervention of resources for mental health will have an impact on the prevalence of mental health disorders within the community, and the ability to optimize one's treatment. The will to finance programs and services are also pivotal in building interventions.

Behavior/lifestyle plays an integral role in one's self management of psychopathology and mental illness. While some responsibility may lay with the individual (Ryan, 1971, Rappaport, 1975), systems of mental health services also benefit from integrating health behavior and health promotion frameworks into the development of individual, programmatic, and policy interventions. As Glanz, Rimer, and Viswnah (2008) point out, many successful community based initiatives have been developed using one of the health behavior frameworks as a conceptual and theoretical framework.

Environment, genetics, and social support also factor into the equation as factors to consider as social determinants of mental health. A Strengths Based approach which facilitates the individual empowerment and self-management can move the individual to independence much more quickly than medical model approaches, because the approach is assets based, does not stress upon one's limitations, and does not label or stigmatize the individual (Rapp, 1998). Conceptually, in the majority of cases, as pointed out by Rapp (1998) a strengths-based approach builds social networks, empowers and promotes self-esteem for the individual, improves case management outcomes and helps create conditions for effectiveness.

In addition, we can understand mental health through the lens of a range of behavioral theories. These lay out a theoretical foundation not only for behavior and mental health outcomes, but also to serve as a guide for how interventions can be developed. Investments should be made at the policy levels within state and national health entities to support initiatives which target building an infrastructure to support the mental health needs of constituents within communities, based upon these principles. Similarly, public health entities should embrace the fact that just as there are social determinants of public health, there are social determinants of mental health, which can be of extreme use within the development of policy programs and services to promote positive mental health outcomes.

References

Ajzen, I., (1985) "From Intentions to Actions: A Theory of Planned Behavior." In J.Kuhl and J. Beckman (eds.) *Action Control: From cognition to behavior.* Heidelberg: Springer-Verlag.

Andersson, H.W., Bjorngaard, J.H., Kasperson, S.L., Skre, I., Dahl, T. (2010). The effects of individual factors and school environment on mental health and prejudiced attitude among Norwegian adolescents. *Social Psychiatry and Psychiatric Epidemiology. 45*(5). 569-577.

Araya, R., Lewis, G., Rojas, G., & Fritsch, R. (2003). Education and income: Which is more important for mental health? *Journal of Epidemiology and Community Health, 57*, 501-505.

Baltes, P. B. (1993). The aging mind: Potential and limits. *The Gerontologist, 33.* 580-594.

Baltes, P.B., & Willis, S.L. (1977). Toward psychological theories of aging and development. In J. Birren & K. W. Schaie (Eds.), *The handbook of the psychology of aging* (pp. 128-154). New York: Van Nostrand-Reinhold.

Bandura, A. (2005). The primacy of self-regulation in health promotion. *Applied psychology: An international review. 54*(2). 245-254.

Bandura, A. (1977). Self-efficacy: Toward a unifying theory of behavioral change. *Psychological Review,* 84, 191-215.

Bandura, A. (1997). *Self-efficacy: The exercise of control.* New York: Feeman.

Barnes, H., Wright, G., Noble, M., & Dawes, A. (2007). *The South African index of multiple depreviation for children.* CapeTown: HSRC Press. Baumeister & VohsBecker, M.H. (1974). The health belief model and personal health behavior. *Health Education Monographs,* (2), 4.

Belsky, J. (1999).*The psychology of aging: Theory, research, and interventions.* 3rd Edition. Belmont: Brooks Cole Publishing, Co.

Bouchard, T.J. (1994), Genes, environment, and personality. *Science, 264,* 1700-1701.

Dashiff, C., DiMicco, W., Myers, B., Sheppard, K. (2009). Poverty and adolescent mental health. *Journal of Child and Adolescent Psychiatric Nursing, 22*(1), 23-32.

DeLara, C. L., Cruceanu, , Mamdani, F., Lebel, V., Yerko, V., Becki, A., Young, L.T., Rouleau, G., Grof, P., Alda, M., Turecki, G., (2010). Implication of synapse-related genes in bipolar disorder by linkage and gene expression analyses. *International Journal of Neuropsychopharmacology, 13*(10), 1397-1410.

Derisley, J. & Reynolds, S. (2000). The transtheoretical stages of change as a predictor of premature termination, attendance and alliance in psychotherapy. *The British Journal of Clinical Psychology, 39*(4), 371-382.

Dixon, R.A. (1992). Contextual approaches to adult intellectual development. In R.J. Sternberg & C.A.Berg (Eds*). Intellectual development*, (350-380). London: Cambridge University Press.

Edwards, J.G. (2010). A transnational approach: A commentary on "lost in translation: Limitations of a universal approach in genetic counseling". *Health and Mental Health Counseling, 19* (1) 7-8.

Erikson, E.H. (1963). *Childhood and society.* New York: Norton Publishers.

Freud, S. (1924). On psychotherapy. *Collected papers. (Vol.1)* London: Hogarth Publishers.

Glanz, K., Rimer, B.K., & Viswanath, K. (2008*). Health behavior and health education: Theories, research and practice.* CA: John Wiley and Sons, Inc.

Guo, J. X., Hu, L., Yand, P. Z., Tanabe, K., Miyatalre, M., Chen, Y., (2007). Chronic arsenic poisoning in drinking water in Inner Mongolia and its associated health effects. *Journal of Environmental Science and Health, 42*(12), 1853-1858.

Harbottle, L., & Schonfelder, D. (2008). Nutrition and depression: A review of the evidence. *Journal of Mental Health, 17*(6). 576 – 587

Jurkowski, E.T. (2008). *Policy and Program Planning for Older Adults*. NY, NY: Springer Publishing Company.

Havenaar, J., Geerlings, M.I., Vivian, L. Collinson, M., & Robertson, B. (2008). Common mental health problems in historically disadvantaged urban and rural communities in South Africa: prevalence and risk factors. *Social Psychiatry and Psychiatric Epidemiology, 43,* 209-215.

Hyman S.E., (2000a). The genetics of mental illness: implications for practice. *The Bulletin of the WorldHealth Organization, 78*(4), 455-463.

Hyman, S.E. (2000b). National Institute of Mental Health goals for behavioral science. *Experimental and clinical psychopharmacology, 8*(3), 271-272.

Jackson, L., Langille, L, Lyons, R., Highes, J. Martin, D., & Winstanley, V. (2009). Does moving from a high poverty to lower-poverty neighborhood improve mental health? *Health and Place, 15*(4), 961-970.

Janoff-Bulman, R., Timko, C., & Carli, L. (1984). Cognitive biases in blaming the victim. (1985). *Journal of Experimental Social Psychology, 21*(2), 161-177.

Jayakody, R., Stauffer, D., (2002). Mental health problems among single mothers: Implications for work and welfare reform. *Journal of Social Issues, 56*(4), 617-634.

Kimble, G.A. (1993). Evolution of the nature-nurture issue in the history of psychology. In R. Plomain & G.E. McLearn (Eds.) *Nature, nurture, and psychology*. Washington, DC: American Psychological Association.

Kloos, B., Flory, K., Hankin, B., Cheely, B., Segal, M., (2009). Investigating the roles of neighborhood environments and housing-based social support in the relocation of persons made homeless by Hurricane Katrina. *Journal of Prevention & Intervention in the Community, 37*(2), 143-154.

Knapp, M., Funk, M., Curran, C., Prince, M., Grigg, M., & McDaid, D. (2006). Economic barriers to better mental health, practice and policy. *Health Policy and Planning, 21*(3), 157-170.

LaLonde, M. (1981). *A New Perspective on the Health of Canadians: A working document*. Ottawa: Government of Canada.

Lorant, V., Deliege, D., Eaton, W., Robert, A., Philippot, P., & Ansseau, M. (2003). Socio-economic inequalities in depression: a meta-analysis. *American Journal of Epidemiology, 157,* 98-112.

Lund, C., Breen, A, Fisher, A.J., Kakuma, R., Corrigall, J., Joska, J., Swartz, L., & Patel, V. (2010). Poverty and common mental disorders in low and middle income countries: A systematic review. *Social Science and Medicine*, 71, 517-528.

Marsiske, M., Lang, F.B., Baltes, P.B., & Baltes, M.M., (1995). Selective optimization with compensation: Life-span perspectives on successful human development. In R.A.Dixon & L. Backman (Eds.), Compensating for psychological deficits and declines: Managing losses and promoting gains, (35-79). Mahwah: NJ:Erlbaum.

Mattoon, M.A. (1981). *Jungian psychology in perspective.* NY: Free Press Publishing.

McLeod, J.D. & Shanahan, M.J. (1996). Trajectories of poverty and children's mental health. *Journal of Health and Social Behavior, 37*(3), 207-220.

McKeowan, T. (1971). A historical appraisal of the medical task, from "*Medical History and Medical Care*", Oxford University Press.

McPherson, C.M. & McGibbon, E.A. (2010). Addressing the determinants of child mental health: Intersectionality as a guide to primary health care renewal. *Canadian Journal of Nursing Research, 42*(3) 50-64.

Meyer-Lindenberg, A. (2010). Neurogenetic risk mechanisms of schizophrenia: An imaging genetics approach. *Advances in Schizophrenia research,* in Gattaz, Wagner, F. & Busatto, G. (Eds.) New York, NY: Springer Science and Business Media.

Milne, M., & Robertson, B. (1998). Child mental health services in New South Africa. *Child Psychology and Psychiatry Review, 3,* 128-134.

National Institute of Mental Health (1998). *Genetics and mental disorders; Report of the National Institute of Mental Health's Genetics Workgroup.* Rockville, MD.

Nemeroff, R., Medlarsky, E., & Meyer, J.F. (2010). Relationships amoung social support, perceived control, and psychological distress in later life. *International Journal of Aging and Human Development, 71*(1), 69-82.

Nijmeijer, J.S, Arias,-Vadsqiez, A., Rommeise, N., Altink, M.E., Anney, R. J.L., Asherson, P., Banaschewski, T., Buschgens, C., Fliers, E.A., Gill, M., Minderaa, R., Poustka, L., Sergeant, J., Buitelaar, J., Franke, B., Ebstein, R.P., Miranda, A., Mulas, F., Oades, R.D., Roeyers, H.,Rothernberger, A., Sonuga-Barke, E.J.S., Bteinhausen, H.C., Faraone, S.V., Hartman, C.A. (2010) Identifying loci for the overlap between attention – deficit/hyperactivity disorder and autism spectrum disorder using a genome-wide QTL linkage approach.. *Journal of the American Academy of Child and Adolescent Psychiatry, 49*(7), 675-685.

Patel, V., Araya, R., deLima, M., Ludermir, A. & Todd, C. (1999) Women, poverty and common mental disorders in four restructuring societies. *Social Science and Medicine, 49,* 1461.

Patel, V., Fisher, A., & Cohen, A. (2006). Social and cultural determinants of mental health. In R. Murray, K.Kendler, P. McGuffin, S. Wessely & D. Caslte (Eds.), *Essentials of Psychiatry* (2nd ed.). Cambridge: Cambridge University Press.

Patel, V., Kirkwood, B.R., Pednekar, S., Weiss, H., & Mabey, D., (2006). Risk factors for common mental disorders in women. Population based longitudinal study. *British Journal of Psychiatry, 189,* 547-555.

Patel, V., & Kleinman, A. (2003). Poverty and common mental disorders in developing countries. *Bulletin of the World Health Organization, 81,* 609-615.

Pistrang, N., Barker, C., & Humphreys. (2008). Mutual help groups for mental health problems: A review of effectiveness studies. *Journal of Community Psychology. 42* (1/2), 110-121.

Plomin, R., & Mcclearn, G.E. (1993). *Nature, nurture and psychology.* Washington, DC: American Psychological Association.

Pretty, J., Peacock, J., Sellens, M., & Griffin M. (2005). The mental and physical health outcomes of green exercice. *International Journal of Environmental Health Research, 15*(5), 319-337.

Prochaska, J. O., DiClemente, C. C., & Norcross, J. C. (1992). In search of how people change. *American Psychologist, 47,* 1102-1114.

Prochaska, J. O., & DiClemente, C. C. (1983). Stages and processes of self-change of Smoking: Towardan integrative model of change. *Journal of Consulting and Clinical Psychology, 51,* 390-395.

Prochaska, J. O., & Velicer, W.F. (1997). The transtheoretical model of health behavior change.*American Journal of Health Promotion, 12,* 38-48.

Rapp, C.A. (1998). *The Strengths Model: Case management with people suffering from severe and persistent mental illness.* New York: Oxford University Press.

Rappaport, J. Davidson, W.S., Wilson, M.N., & Mitchell, A. (1975). Alternatives to blaming the victim on the environment: Our places to stand have not moved the earth. *American Psychologist, 30*(4), 525-528.

Rochlen, A.B., Rude, S.S., & Baron, A. (2005). The relationship of client stages of change to working alliance and outcome in short-term counseling. *Journal of College Counseling, 8*(1), 52-64.

Rosenstock, I.M., Strecher, V.J., Becker, M.H. (1988). Social learning theory and the Health Beliefmodel. *Health Education Quarterly, 15*(2), 175-183.

Rosenstock, I. (1974). Historical Origins of the Health Belief Model. *Health Education Monographs*, *2*(4).

Ryan, (1971, 1976).*Blaming the Victim.* NY: Vintage Books.

Sabin, M., Lopes, C.B., Nackerud, L., Kaiser, R., & Varese, L. (2003). Factors associated with poor mental health among Guatemalan refugees living in Mexico 20 years after civil conflict. *JAMA, 290*, 625-642.

Saraceno, B., & Burbui, C. (1997). Poverty and mental illness. *Canadian Journal of Psychiatry, 42,* 285 290.

Saraceno, B., Levav, I., & Kohn, R. (2005). The public mental health significance of research on socio economic factors in schizophrenia and major depression. *World Psychiatry, 4,* 181-185.

Seino, K., Takano, T., Marshal, T., Hemat, S., & Nakamura, K., (2008). Prevelence of and factors influencing posttraumatic stress disorder among mothers of children under five in Kabul, Afghanistan, after decades of armed conflicts. *Health and Quality of Life Outcomes, 6,* 29.

Sprangers, M.A.G., Bartels, M., Veenhoven, R., Baas, F., Martin, N.G., Mosing, M., Movas, B., Ropka, M.E., Shinozaki, G., & Swaab, D. (2010). Which patient will feel down, which will be happy? The need to study the genetic disposition of emotional states. *Quality of Life Research: An international Journal of Life Aspects of Treatment, Care and Rehabilitation, 19*, (10). M1429-1437.

Taylor, S.E. & Stanton, A.L.(2007). Coping resources, coping processes, and mental health. *Annual Review of Clinical Psychology, 3,* 377-401.

Toulopoulou, T., Goldberg, T., Rebollo, M., Picchioni, M., Rijsdijk, F., Stahl, D., Cherney, S., Sham, P., Faraone, S.V., Tsuang, M., Weinberger, D., Seidman, L.J. Murray, R.M. Impaired intellect and memory: A missing link between genetic risk and schizophrenia. *Archives of General Psychiatry, 67*(9), 905-913.

Toye, M., & Infanti, J. (2004). *Social inclusion and social economic development: Literature Review.* Victoria, BC: The Canadian CED Network.

Truong, K.D., & Ma, S. (2006). A systematic review of relations between neighborhoods and mental health. *Journal of Mental Health Policy and Economics, 9*, 137-154.

United States Department of Health and Human Services(USDHHS). (2000). *The Surgeon General's Report on Mental Health.* MD; US Government Printing Office.

Van Snellenberg, J.X., de Candia, T.(2009). Meta-analytic evidence for familial co aggregation of schizophrenia and bipolar disorder. *Archives of Gen Psychiatry, 66*(7). 748-755.

Weich, S., & Lewis. G. (1998). Poverty, unemployment and common mental disorders: population based cohort study. *British Medical Journal, 317*, 115-119.

World Health Organization. (2008). *Closing the gap in a generation: Health equity through action on the social determinants of health*. Geneva: WHO Printing Office.

World Health Organization Commission on Social Determinants of Health. (2005). *Action on the social determinants of health: Learning from previous experiences.* Geneva: WHO Printing Office.

Wyman, P.A., Cross, W., Brown, C.H., Yu, Q., & Eberly, S. (2010). *Journal of Abnormal Child Psychology, 38,* 707-720.

Zhou, B., Chen, K., Yu, Y., Wang, H., Zhang, S., & Zheng, W. (2010). Individualized health intervention: Behavioral change and quality of life in an older rural Chinese population. *Educational Gerontology, 36*(10/11), 919-939.

In: Social Determinants and Mental Health
Editor: Sabine Bährer-Kohler
ISBN: 978-1-61324-353-4

Chapter 5

Discrimination and Mental Health

Urs Kalbermatten
University of Applied Science Bern
Institut of Gerontology, Bern, Switzerland

Abstract

Our professional literature tells us as an indisputable fact that stigmatization and discrimination may impair mental health. So far, discrimination has mostly been examined from the perspective of the victim. Interpreting discrimination as an interactive process, the author points out that there is particular need for action on the discriminators' side, for they need to become more sensitive to the interpersonal perception of their behavior, and to become aware of the effects of their actions.

The interaction between discrimination and mental health is discussed in greater detail in the context of age discrimination. Based on relevant studies, the author shows how this interaction has been investigated in daily life and, more specifically, in the context of nursing. The article concentrates on analyzing the discriminating players, a necessarily sophisticated research project in which the author presents the research designs used, including video-taped observations and case vignettes. Results indicate that caregivers do not recognize age discrimination for what it is; instead, they believe that any discriminatory action is traceable to personal reasons and the working conditions prevailing in institutions. Programs to promote mental health should accord particular weight in research and implementation to the social factor as it is explained in this chapter on discrimination.

Introduction

In the very first lines of its report entitled 'Promoting mental health' (2004, 3), the WHO assigns a pivotal role to the importance of social relations for mental health: '… to foster activities in the field of mental health, especially those affecting the harmony of human relations.' Therefore, if we wish to promote mental health we need to pursue a holistic approach, and interventions should relate to people in their everyday interpersonal relations.

The WHO (2004) believes that in this context we should be interested not only in manifestations of illness but also, and more than before, in healthy people, asking ourselves how we might mitigate interpersonal and social factors that foster mental illness. Science should concentrate more on this field, formulating theoretical concepts and conducting specific studies so that preventive steps can be taken.

Any definition of health needs to include not only personal elements but also those components of the environment to which man is exposed. 'Mental health promotion involves actions that support people to adopt and maintain healthy lifestyles and create supportive living conditions or environments for health.' (WHO, 2004, 5) This contribution highlights this concern in the context of older people, a particularly vulnerable population group which in recent years has moved into the focus of discrimination (e.g. as a burden on society or a cost factor) and whose negative experiences, even in their immediate social relations, may threaten their mental health. Discrimination may cause older people to develop mental disturbances or depressive symptoms, withdraw from public life, or fall mute. Discrimination forms a critical event in life if, for example, certain population groups are unable to pursue their objectives, are marginalized, or are treated worse than others. Ongoing discrimination and the experience of powerlessness may threaten mental health. While the age groups affected are increasingly criticizing discrimination, it is not an issue for the discriminating interaction partners. Although the scientific debate on age discrimination has been expanding in recent years, there is still a general dearth of studies that focus on discriminatory interactive action. The subject is normally discussed from the victims' perspective. If, however, the victims of discrimination are very old people who are no longer able to defend themselves effectively and depend on the assistance of others, the perpetrators will have to be induced at long last to change their behavior by moving them into the focus of the discussion. There is a wide range of social systems that are capable of contributing materially to mental health. To foster mental health, we need shared social values and attitudes, and we need to respect people's fundamental rights. Something must be done in this field because most of those who discriminate against others are not aware of the consequences of their actions and the threat they represent to the mental health of their fellow human beings.

Discrimination Defined as Interactive Action

Discrimination against a particular group of people evolves as a process that builds up over decades and is joined by individuals who are often unaware of having done so. There is nearly universal agreement that discrimination is not exclusively a cognitive or emotional phenomenon, and that it expresses itself in concrete actions vis-à-vis individuals or groups.

Discrimination is interpreted as treating someone inequitably not because of his or her actions but because of some group characteristic (Kalbermatten-Schmid, 2003).

Discrimination is necessarily founded on some interpersonal perception based on a simple act such as, for example,

- the distinction of colors (black, red, gray) or
- gender differentiation.

To groups of persons distinguished in this manner, labels and stereotypes are affixed that are frequently derogatory. Discriminatory action is controlled by thoughts, feelings, value concepts, stigmatization, and prejudice (e.g. a negative image of old age). Once these have been projected by science and the media for a long time, they turn into social representations that are supported and/or suffered uncritically and tacitly. Apparently, this background makes it easier to provide a different grade of medical care for a specific group of persons, ration their benefits, or refuse them the right to privacy or self-determination. Frequently, discrimination is related to a certain acceptance in society. In most cases, there is neither any empathy with the feelings of the targets of discrimination nor any readiness to adopt their perspective. Discriminatory actions in everyday life furnish another incentive because they remain without consequences. Among other things, discrimination may disturb the balance of the mind, impair people's joy of life, or lead to social disintegration.

To identify discrimination, it is crucial whether we adopt the perspective of the victim or that of the detached observer. Most contributions and studies focus on the victim. The perpetrator's actor-centered view has been playing a marginal role in research so far. It has been emphasized that most players are unaware of the effects of a discriminatory act, and that they themselves would not designate such an act as discriminatory. Brauer & Clemens (2010, 33) suggest the following: 'To prove or disprove a case of ageism, it is ultimately irrelevant from a structural point of view whether or not actors are aware of the discriminatory and stereotyping content of their actions.' What is experienced as discrimination crucially depends on the perspective adopted, that of the victim or the observer. As we are looking at an interactive process, we need to know more about how actors deal with the matter, how far they are able to perceive the social category of discrimination, and how they interpret their own actions that are perceived as discriminatory by others. This, too, is part of the information we need if we wish to take steps against discriminatory action.

Discrimination we define as an interactive action involving an actor who executes and/or initiates an act of discrimination and an affected individual or target group which interprets this act as discriminatory. For a more profound understanding, we may consult the social representations of reference systems. Perspectives may either converge or diverge. Disclosing the various perspectives may initiate a process of mutual understanding. Beelmann & Jonas (2009, 23) also refer to these interpersonal processes: 'Conversely, the concept of discrimination is defined from the perspective of the victim. It needs to be negotiated between victims, perpetrators, and unaffected groups as the perspectives of the various positions may occasionally diverge widely.'

Discrimination means unjust treatment of groups and individuals that are disadvantaged and marginalized without any reason founded in fact. As a general rule, the ability to implement discrimination is predicated on social, economic, political, or journalistic power. In most cases, discrimination conveys at least short-lived benefits on the actor by, for example, saving costs, gaining time, assisting in decision-making, or obtaining public attention. It may also take the form of contact avoidance, obstruction of access to goods and positions, boycotts, or personal defamation. Discrimination may equally well be an act of commission or omission.

Discrimination of Older People

Currently, interest in age discrimination is growing in the German-speaking regions (see Rothermund & Mayer, 2009; Beelmann & Jonas, 2009), although the focus is mostly on discrimination in the labor markets (Brauer & Clemens, 2010). Relatively little systematic research is done on everyday discrimination as practiced by insurances, government authorities, banks, healthcare professionals, or caregivers. Age discrimination concerns everybody; sooner or later, we all switch from the out-group to the in-group. Whereas fighting handicap-, race- or gender-related discrimination is an obvious and well-known issue, we are not as well informed about and ready to take action against age discrimination. The matter is exacerbated by concepts of age used in the everyday and, more specifically, the scientific language, such as 'disengagement theory' and 'retirement', which place older people away from the mainstream of society. We should seriously ask ourselves whether these terms, which have remained almost unchallenged so far, do not reflect a discriminatory attitude. We should reposition old age in society and introduce into our societal discourse more adequate metaphors to describe this phase of life, metaphors that express the value of age and emphasize integration and participation by older people. Together with images of deficiency, retirement as a metaphor might form a cognitive seedbed for age discrimination. Gerontology is now faced with the challenge of generating new theories about old age and another language to describe it. After all, the *Survey of everyday people* (Kalbermatten-Schmid, 2003) shows that older people do also feel discriminated by the language used by scientists and experts who talk about the burden of the old, societal senescence, false demographic facts, and the cost of old age. Collier (2005) similarly points out that social representations of old age are negative and disrespectful. Old people are attributed with physical, cognitive and sexual dysfunctions. 'Old' is often used as a generic term describing negative human traits, such as pig-headedness, conservatism, lethargy, forgetfulness, grumpiness etc., while 'young' is the stereotype for positive attributes.

It is a specific of age discrimination that, because it is not so evident in the societal discourse, it became a legal issue in Europe later than other kinds of discrimination, and legal prosecution is rare. There are EU countries that actually practice rationing of medical services for older people. Forming a particularly vulnerable population group, older people are highly dependent on the support of institutions and their families, and their only reaction to discrimination often is helplessness and withdrawal.

Macnicol (2006) discusses important issues relating to age discrimination. It operates both directly and indirectly, institutionally as well as statistically. According to Macnicol (2006), age discrimination represents a complex multi-faceted phenomenon whose prevalence is difficult to assess. He calls for developing an awareness of age discrimination and inquiring more closely into the reasons for it. Older people are marginalized and their economic status is curtailed. Employment and health care are the key subjects of age discrimination. In health care, discrimination may lead to rationing and jeopardize access to certain medical services.

Age discrimination is difficult to prosecute legally because the onus of proof is normally on the victim. Perpetrators are rarely prepared to admit to discriminatory behavior. In research, it is easy to obtain innumerable examples of age discrimination from our surveys. But we know hardly anything about the perpetrators.

DISCRIMINATION AND MENTAL HEALTH

The WHO (2004, 12) has defined mental health as follows: 'A state of well-being in which the individual realizes his or her own abilities, can cope with the normal stress of life, can work productively and fruitfully, and is able to make a contribution to his or her community.' Regular confrontation with actions perceived as discriminatory impairs and threatens mental health. However, discrimination has been rarely discussed in this context so far, and there are few studies that analyze the effect of discrimination on health. When older people complain about discrimination, they suffer from it. We need to take them seriously, identify the sources of discrimination, and intervene. We must not belittle discrimination because thwarted ambitions as well as the loss of behavioral control and mastery of the environment are regarded as factors that influence mental health and are particularly badly affected by discrimination. This is why it is important to analyze discriminatory and harmful actions and inform potential perpetrators about the consequences of their doings.
Discrimination must be graded as a risk factor for mental health.

The WHO (2004, 24) names the following 'Key determinants of mental health: social inclusion, freedom of *discrimination* and violence, and economic participation.' The key element in the promotion of mental health is social inclusion.

In the field of mental health, older people experience specific impairments. P. Macdonald, a psychotherapist, writes (2010, 14): 'Discrimination is the most common form of prejudice experienced by those aged over 55, and this has a negative impact on confidence and self-esteem, with many older people facing barriers to participation in public and private life. (…) Older people are also vulnerable to rejection by health professionals.' He also draws attention to the fact that in relative terms, older people are more widely affected by depression than other age groups because their experiences of situations capable of triggering depression are more numerous. 'Social isolation is a major risk factor for poor mental health. (…) The realization that some goals are no longer achievable can cause distress and lead to depression or feeling of deprivation.' (Macdonald, 2010, 15). He also points out that symptoms of depression, such as anxiety or agitation, may be misinterpreted as Parkinson's disease, dementia, etc. Discrimination may also keep older people from achieving their goals or cause them to develop some mental illness, fall mute, or withdraw into social isolation.

In the context of discrimination, older people need sound emotional and social support. Martindale (2007) describes how older people try to get the attention of caregivers and tell them about their needs. Carers should encourage older people to talk about their feelings, their fears and any negative thoughts. This may serve to mitigate depression, relieve isolation, and avoid discrimination. In the daily practice of nursing, it is important to support older people, listen to them, take their fears seriously and adopt the perspective from which they view their situation in life in order to maintain the mental health of those who are in need of support.

In her article 'Latent discrimination in mental health care' Collier (2005, 42) points out that older people are denied proper care because of institutionalized ageism: 'Contemporary mental health policy and practice seem to have a blind spot when it comes to people over 65.'As Burns et al. (2002) and Collier (2005) emphasize, clinical depression is the most prevalent mental disturbance among older people. The needs of older people suffering from various mental illnesses are largely ignored.

According to Burns et al. (2002), statistics covering people over 65 who suffer from psychoses are difficult to find. Surveys ignore them once they are 74 or older. Having analyzed 2874 articles published in 6 journals on mental health and nursing, Collier (2005) found that only 18 articles (0.6%) addressed functional mental disorder-related subjects in the 65+ age group. According to Collier, the problem with age discrimination is that mentally impaired old people are ignored. Thus, a clientele that is particularly vulnerable but invisible is socially excluded.

Nursing old people is often called the most unpopular form of care. Is that something to do with society's attitude about the value of older people, the inevitable erosion, or the stereotypes that say that older people are incompetent, disengaged or inflexible? Collier (2005, 45) concludes that 'there is a gaping hole in the nursing literature in relation to the care of people with functional mental disorders aged over 65. (...) In addition, the expectancies of older people should be investigated to find out what we are really working with.'

Hirsch (2005) argues that there is nothing new in the debate about whether society can afford to give the same intensive and qualified health care to old people. Even now, there are some countries whose health system features age-based rationing. Many old people complain that they feel disadvantaged by medical professionals because of their age. 'Thus, for example, there are doctors who deny necessary diagnostic or therapeutic measures to patients because of their age. Moreover, it is still difficult for an 80-year-old to find a psychotherapist.' (Hirsch, 2005, 55) He too points out that older people are often diagnosed wrongly, especially where mental disturbances are involved. 'Fixing your perspective and, consequently, your mindset on "old" leads to omissions in diagnosis as well as in treatment, rehabilitation, and care that are harmful to the patient and, more importantly, increase the cost total. What is needed is not determined by the elderly but by younger people for whom it is difficult to adopt the perspective of the old. Older people who are mentally ill suffer the additional still-negative stigma of being "mental". (...) Those who are old, mentally ill, and in need of care are all too often cast out by our society.' (Hirsch, 2005, 57/58)

Among other issues, Hirsch (2005) discusses rationing in medical care, distinguishing between the explicit denial of services to certain groups of persons as in Great Britain, where the over-70s are not entitled to dialytic treatment, and implicit rationing, meaning restricted medical care. 'The introduction of an age limit may appear superficially acceptable, yet it is discriminatory and without any foundation in fact. Calendar age, according to gerontologists, is not a meaningful indicator for therapeutic indicators.' (Hirsch, 2005, 63) Independently of age, the criterion for treatment should be a patient's mental and physical condition. According to Hirsch (2005), rationing is an age-specific phenomenon, for clinical care expenses decline with increasing age.

Hirsch (2005) points out that because of their age, old people encounter various discriminatory prejudices that are commonly countenanced in public as well as in institutions and organizations. He names the following reasons for the development of prejudices against old age and older people:

- Difficulties with adopting their view
- Historically evolved aversions and aggressions against older people
- Unrealistic perceptions of the life-world of older people
- Derogatory language used in describing old age and old people

In their study 'Social human rights of older people in nursing', Aichele and Schneider (2006) found that institutions do fail to provide for elementary needs such as nutrition, intake of liquids, incontinence provision and decubitus prophylaxis. Based on the data available to them, the authors estimate that basic care in human dignity is not assured for older people in Germany.

According to the WHO (2002, 3), the correlation between mental disorders in old people and discrimination merits particular attention: 'Both WHO and WPA have recognized that the stigma and discrimination attached to mental disorders are strongly associated with suffering, disability and economic losses.' Among other things, the WHO (2002, 20) recommends that professionals

- 'Ensure that their own practice is free from stigma and discrimination.
- Ensure that all educational and continuing professional development curricula contain training to develop awareness of stigma and discrimination.
- Ensure that local workplace policies are in place to identify and reduce stigma and discrimination.'

Studies on Discrimination in the Health Service

Several studies dealing with age discrimination have been conducted within our working group. Kalbermatten-Schmid (2003) systematically analyzed 281 cases of age discrimination from the point of view of the persons affected, using a category system. Eight cases concerned symbolic discrimination (e.g. in media coverage), 121 were graded as structural discrimination (institutions, laws, unsuitable buildings etc.), and there were 143 cases in which personal discrimination was ascribed by the respondents to one or more persons. The cases of personal discrimination involved direct interaction with, for example, caregivers (23 cases) or doctors (16 cases). What the older people especially criticized was that these professional groups tended to be guided mainly by technical and economic considerations. As 120 cases relate to the public health system, we will now discuss two studies from that sector that contain in-depth analyses in which the views of potential discriminators were investigated.

Opinion polls about autonomy and self-determination in institutions paint a relatively positive picture from the perspective of caregivers as well as patients if we consult long-term memory data gathered through questionnaires or interviews. However, as these often do not jibe with everyday observations, Ament-Kistler (2007) carried out a study at two nursing centers where caregiving situations were recorded on videotape. These recordings were analyzed and certain scenes (mobilization, eating, washing, and technical tasks) were shown to the staff for interpretation. Ament-Kistler (2007) intended to demonstrate the effect of the caregivers' communication behavior on the scope of self- and co-determination of older people. Results show that patients were basically involved in all activities. In 58 cases, they were instructed how to do certain things, and there were only 9 cases in which they were not involved at all. However, instances of genuine self-determination on the part of the patients were observed only rarely. Caregivers are trusted profoundly, and patients feel safe and well. However, it was observed that while information was often (17 times) given in advance, there is a markedly greater number of cases (51) in which it was only given during the activity itself – which is actually too late. As many activities were routine, there was no need to ask for permission or consent in every instance. However, there were situations in which the patients really should have been informed in advance to give them a chance to decide about their preferences for themselves. In 82 cases, patients were asked about their opinion and given time to answer. There were only 7 instances in which caregivers did not wait for an answer. However, there were 4 cases in which we observed that caregivers disregarded what patients had to say, although no complaints were made by them. In 81 cases, baby talk – characterized by the shortening and simplifying of words – was recorded.

Following Ament-Kistler (2007), we may say that the general run of the interactions investigated is characterized by impoverished language. It was found that communication itself is not as critical as the frequent lack of necessary information. In other cases, caregivers asked autonomy-related questions without waiting for an answer. Caregivers appear to know what is good for a patient and inform them inadequately or not at all about what they are doing. The reason they give is that they do not have enough time to wait for a decision or discuss it with a patient. Information is given either selectively or not at all whenever caregivers fear that the patient might reject it. Things are rarely done in spite of a patient's refusal, and then only if caregivers believe that the action contemplated is prophylactic. The caregivers investigated agree that co-determination is important, adding that they question, reinforce, encourage and inform their patients to achieve it. The data of this explorative study show that co-determination is not really that big a problem. But it also reveals cases where asking patients for their consent would have made sense, and others where that question was asked only after the beginning of an activity.

Brohan et al. (2010) similarly highlight the importance of the interactive component of stigmatization and discrimination. To understand discrimination, it is important that the experiences and actions of both victims and perpetrators should be taken into consideration. Ament-Kistler (2007) reports that the caregivers' self-image differs from that which emerges from the CCTV documentation. The caregivers are in control in most cases, and cases are relatively rare in which patients are involved in decisions to an extent that permits them to take a hand. Nevertheless, the atmosphere that prevails in the sequences observed may reasonably be called friendly, relaxed and agreeable. The majority of the patients are contented, as confirmed by the interviews. Patients are dealt with politely and respectfully, although the language used shows a certain degree of impoverishment. Information extracted from Ament-Kistler's (2007) study could be used to develop interventions or training for nursing staff in order to avoid such actions and support the caregivers.

An in-depth analysis of the perspective of caregivers regarding their understanding of discrimination in nursing was completed by Schär-Büttikofer (2009). Its purpose was to acquire information about how caregivers perceive the phenomenon of age discrimination, which was then to be used to develop action recommendations for dealing with older patients in everyday nursing. She investigated the mechanisms and reasons that lead to older people being treated inequitably. In agreement with the results of our literature search presented previously, she found that there is virtually no data about the perspective of discriminating persons or groups. For ethical reasons, the study involved no video confrontations, and the persons included were not directly involved. From that group, 50 representatives were selected and given 5 written descriptions of discriminatory situations. They were then asked the following questions: Can we identify any awareness of discrimination in caregivers? Are various forms of discrimination recognized as such? Is there a discernible influence of professional seniority? What reasons are given? What features characterize such situations?

Answers were evaluated systematically with the aid of a category system specially developed for the investigation. The system contains three levels of reasons: professional, personal, and institutional. Each level contained various dimensions to which various categories were assigned. The professional level, for example, contained three dimensions: theoretical knowledge, professional behavior, and professional responsibility. Another detailed category system was developed for analyzing the responses.

Some selected results should be presented at this point. The answers to a question about the potential reasons for dissatisfaction on the part of patients and their relations showed that the respondents were able to understand their view. To a large extent, the reasons given relate to the personal sphere, which means that the understanding for this behavior is not based on professional references or institutional targets. One exception is a situation which involves rationing to save material, where the reason is seen to be partly rooted in faulty professional behavior. In their daily work, caregivers perceive themselves as beset by various claims: those of the patients, their own needs, the structures and demands of their institutions, and those of other professions. This is the framework within which they are supposed to ensure that everything runs as smoothly, efficiently, and cost-effectively as possible. In the caregivers' opinion, the most prevalent reasons for patient dissatisfaction are these: not being taken seriously, inadequate communication, and the system of values. A question about the reasons for the caregiver's behavior yielded highly diverse answers.

- There are two situations in which the professional level comes to the fore: lack of professional competence and lack of reflection about one's own actions.
- In situations involving rationing, the reason is mostly attributed to the institutional level; ethical aspects are occasionally mentioned as well.
- In two situations, personal reasons dominate, such as stereotype perception, exercise of control and mental stress.
- At the institutional level, some situations clearly show the extent to which the time and cost factor is used in explanation.
- While lack of time is not regarded as a major reason, it is thought to be important for the emergence of such situations.

An additional question asked at the end inquired about features which the various situations had in common. Such features emerged in the following categories:

- Not taking people seriously, a negative mindset, and stereotyping old age. This might be taken as evidence that age discrimination is recognized indirectly, although no more than 4 caregivers out of 50 explicitly designated it as such or related it to the patients' age. Schär-Büttikofer (2009) interprets this as meaning that although inequitable treatment is noticed, it is not regarded as a grave matter.
- Effects on nursing quality are not recognized either. The fact that scarcity of time and staff was mentioned so often may be regarded as indicating that the staff situation at institutions encourages discriminatory actions.

This turns the personal level into a major common denominator between the situations. Therefore,

- Professional development and
- Regular reflection in teams might prove highly rewarding in our effort to reduce discrimination.
- However, these results also reflect a societal phenomenon that cannot be tackled exclusively at the individual level: society needs to develop the way in which we deal with old age, and it needs to grow more sensitive to discriminatory behavior towards old people.

CONCLUSION

According to the WHO (2004), social determinants are closely associated with mental health. To maintain and improve mental health, therefore, there is a great need for intervention in the social environment. Using age discrimination as an example, it has been shown that it is necessary to intensify our research into the perpetrators' perspective. Studies from the nursing sector have been quoted in support.

- Programs of prevention and intervention should focus not only on the individual awareness of the people concerned but also on dyadic and wider social contexts (groups, fields of activity, institutions).
- We should create a sensitized and supportive environment and promote health policies that operate along those lines.
- The detailed proposals made by the WHO (2004) regarding intervention options as well as its entire promotion program should form part of the discourse and training in general and the gerontological discourse and training in particular.
- In most cases, perpetrators do not recognize discrimination explicitly or designate it as such. Consequently, we need to sharpen their awareness of discrimination, make them take the experience of age discrimination seriously, and pay more heed to its harmful effects on mental health.

If we do want to promote mental health, discrimination must not be accepted in any walk of life.

REFERENCES

Aichele, V. & Schneider, J. (2006). Soziale Menschenrechte älterer Personen in der Pflege. Berlin: *Deutsches Institut für Menschenrechte.*

Ament-Kistler, K. (2007). *Das Kommunikationsverhalten Pflegender und die Auswirkung dieses Verhaltens auf die Möglichkeit der Mitbestimmung älterer Menschen.* Masterarbeit. Bern: Berner Fachhochschule.

Beelmann, A. & Jonas, K. J. (2009). (Hrsg.) *Diskriminierung und Toleranz*. Wiesbaden: Verlag für Sozialwissenschaften.

Brauer, K. & Clemens, W. (Hg.) (2010). *Zu alt? "Ageism" und Altersdiskriminierung auf dem Arbeitsmarkt*. Wiesbaden: Verlag für Sozialwissenschaften.

Brohan, E. Slade, M., Clement, S. and Thorncroft, G. (2010). Experiences of mental illness stigma, prejudice and discrimination: a review of measures. *Health Services Researches*. 10-80.

Burns, A. et al. (2002). *Mental Health in Older People, in Practice*. London: Royal Society of Medicine Press.

Collier, E. (2005). Latent age discrimination in mental health care. *Mental health practice*, vol 8 no 6 42 – 45.

Hirsch, D. R. (2005). Diskriminierung im Alltag älterer Menschen: Gesundheitswesen. In *Kuratorium Deutscher Altershilfe*. (Hrsg.) Altersdiskriminierung – Alterspotenziale. (55 - 70) Köln: Kuratorium Deutscher Altershilfe.

Kalbermatten-Schmid, E. (2003). *Altersdiskriminierung in der Schweiz. Diplomarbeit*. Bern: Berner Fachhochschule.

Macdonald, P. (2010). Caring for older person. *Practice Nurse*, Feb 12, 39, 14 – 16.

Macnicol, J. (2006). *Age Discrimination. An Historical and Contemporary Analysis*. Cambridge: Cambridge University Press.

Martindale, B. (2007) Resilience and vulnerability in later life. *Br J Psychother*, 23 (2), 205 - 216.

Rothermund, K. & Mayer, A.-K. (2009). Altersdiskriminierung. *Erscheinungsformen, Erklärungen und Interventionsansätze*. Stuttgart: Kohlhammer.

Schär-Büttikofer, U. (2009). Altersdiskriminierung in der Akutpflege. Auf den Spuren eines Phänomens. *Master of Advanced Studies in Gerontology*. Berner Fachhochschule.

WHO – WPA (2002). *Reducing stigma and discrimination against older people with mental disorders*. Geneva: World Health Organization and World Psychiatric Assoziation.

WHO (2004). *Promoting Mental Health. Concepts – Emerging Evidence – Practice*. Geneva: World Health Organization.

In: Social Determinants and Mental Health
Editor: Sabine Bährer-Kohler

ISBN: 978-1-61324-353-4
©2012 Nova Science Publishers, Inc.

Chapter 6

Social Capital and Mental Health Exploring the Impact of Individual and Community Social Capital on Mental Health Status in Spain

***Alexandrina P. Stoyanova*[1] *and Luis Diaz-Serrano*[2]**
[1]University of Barcelona, Facultaty of Economics Barcelona, Spain
[2]University of Rovira i Virgili, Department of Economics, Reus, Spain

Introduction

Research on the social determinants of health and well-being has been on the agenda of scientists, health professionals and policy makers for some time. Social capital is one of the more recent perspectives through which health outcomes and disparities have been analysed.

Social interactions are hypothesised to have major implications for mental health outcomes, and better understanding of the true relationship between the two is required in order to design policies and programmes, across society as a whole, to improve health and reduce health inequalities by influencing community social resources (McKenzie and Harpham, 2006).

Mental Health

Mental health disorders are among the major (chronic) health problems. Poor mental health may negatively impact general well-being, and may also increase the risk of social and economic problems. Many individuals who suffer from mental illness also present physical diseases. Moreover, mental disorders are associated with poor quality of life (Alonso et al, 2004; Katschnig et al, 2006; Evans et al, 2007), may lead to functional limitations or reduce healthy self-care conducts. The social disadvantages of mental problems include the increased probability of poor mental health among individuals within the vulnerable population strata, such as unemployed, homeless and immigrants. The total annual cost of living with a long-term mental health condition has been estimated at over Euro 2,000 for each European household (McDaid, 2009). The indirect costs are twice the direct ones (those incurred by the health system). The major financial burden of mental disorders comes from productivity losses due to work absenteeism, premature retirement and withdrawal from the labour force, as well as from opportunity costs paid by caregivers (family members – partners, parents or children – who may have to give up work or education because of care commitments).

The lifetime prevalence of mental disorders in the Spanish adult population is estimated at around 20%, while 12-month prevalence is 8.4% (Haro et al, 2006). These figures are similar to those in many developed countries (Somers et al, 2006; Wittchen and Jacobi, 2005). For example, an international study reports that the 12-month prevalence of mental disorders in Europe is 9.6%, while lifetime prevalence is almost 25% (Alonso et al, 2004). The figures from the United States are quite different. Kessler et al (2005a) showed that nearly half of the Americans (46.4%) presented mental health disorders at some point in their life. More than one-forth of the Americans have been affected by at least one psychological disorder in the past 12 months (Kessler et al, 2005b; WHO, 2009). Depressive episodes and anxiety conditions are among the most frequent types of mental health problems affecting approximately one in every ten Spaniards at some time in their lifetime. Recent data from the WHO (WHO, 2009) revealed that Spain and Italy are among the countries with lower prevalence of depressive and anxiety disorders (12-month prevalence of below 7%), while France, New Zealand or the United States tended to have higher estimates (12-month prevalence ranging from just below 14% to above 19%).

Women face a greater risk of poor mental health than men for a variety of reasons, some biological – e.g. differences in coping mechanisms – and some related to social aspects, such as having to play several roles, which may cause psychological stress. (Alonso et al, 2004; Somers et al, 2006).

What is Social Capital?

In spite of the conceptual controversies surrounding the term 'social capital' (Arrow, 2000; Navarro, 2002; Sobel, 2002; Szreter and Woolcock, 2004) – the norms, values and institutions that shape interactions within and between social networks – it is becoming increasingly relevant as an explanatory factor in many socio-economic phenomena, including health and healthcare (Masinko and Starfield, 2001; Islam et al., 2006; Scheffler and Brown, 2008).

Some authors still disagree over whether social capital is an individual characteristic or a community attribute, and whether it should be considered a public good (Glaeser et al, 2000; Kawachi et al, 2004; Yang, 2007). Individual social capital can be viewed as a person's social characteristics (Durlauf, 2002), and measured by the level of trust, membership in social networks, or participation in different community groups or activities. Meanwhile, community social capital is defined as the extent and density of trust, cooperation, and associational links and activity within a given population. However, some recent studies (Anderson et al, 2004), provide evidence supporting the conceptualization of social capital as both an individual and a collective attribute.

Irrespective of its nature (individual or collective, or both), social capital can be disaggregated into two main components: structural (objective and measurable) and cognitive (subjective and intangible) (Harpham et al, 2002; Grootaert and Van Bastelaer, 2002). While the structural dimension refers to membership of formal voluntary organizations and participation in informal networks, the cognitive aspects of social capital refer to individual perceptions of support, trust, reciprocity and cooperation. The two components are likely to interact. Cognitive components of social capital help shape its structural framework, while the structural social capital can form or transform the cognitive framework. In other words, cognitive social capital acts as the underlying base and foundation for the components of structural social capital, while the presence of structural components may reinforce the cognitive aspects (Cullen and Whiteford, 2001).

Exploring the Health-Social Capital Binomial

Social capital is theoretically hypothesised to exert a positive effect on health. At least three mechanisms by which social interactions translate into health benefits have been identified in the literature (Scheffler and Brown, 2008).

- First, social capital channels health-related information to community members, encouraging better health habits, such as a healthy diet (Poortinga, 2006) and regular exercise (Lindström et al, 2001 and 2003; Stahl, 2001, Addy et al, 2004, Haughton McNeill et al, 2006; Mummery et al, 2008), and limiting the influence of risk-related conducts (tobacco use (Lindström et al, 2003; Brown et al, 2006, etc.); alcohol consumption (Poortingga, 2006; Weitzman and Chen, 2005); illicit drug taking (Lundborg, 2005).
- Second, social capital may promote easier access to higher quality health (and social) care (Mohseni and Lindstrom, 2007).
- Lastly, social capital is linked to health through its influence on psychosocial processes. It is considered to provide emotional support, ensure social acceptance and help develop self-confidence and boost self-esteem, all of which mitigate stress and improve mental health (Scheffler et al., 2007).

Increasing empirical evidence supports the theoretical considerations and reveals that higher stock of social capital is, in general, associated with better physical and mental health, lower mortality and reduced suicide rates (e.g., Kawachi *et al.*, 1997 and 1999; McKenzie *et al.*, 2002; Cullen and Whiteford, 2001; Patel, 2010). Nevertheless, some studies also highlight the adverse consequences (negative externalities) some social networks may exert on the community as a whole, but especially on the health of vulnerable subgroups in the population, such as single mothers, immigrants, adolescents, ethnic and religious minorities, etc. (Maycock and Howat, 2007; Rose, 2000; Storr et al, 2004; Takashi and Magalong, 2008).

In terms of mental health, there is relatively less research specifically focusing on how it may interact independently with social capital. De Silva *et al.* (2005) offer a systematic review on the association between mental health and social capital. The majority of the studies analyse mental disorders common in adults, although some employ alternative indicators of mental health, such as indices of depression or psychosis. The findings vary depending on the social capital indicators employed in the analyses. The ambiguity of the results may be explained by the fact that the true relationship between mental health and social capital is highly complex and varies between settings (Kawachi and Berkman, 2001; McKenzie et al., 2002; De Silva, 2006). Stoyanova and Diaz-Serrano (2009a, 2009b) provide the only empirical evidence on the beneficial impact of social capital on mental health in the Spanish population.

This chapter aims to examine the impact of different forms of social capital on the physiological health of Spanish adults. The complexity of social capital is captured by the use of multidimensional indicators. Separate analyses by gender are performed to ensure the comprehensiveness of the investigation.

Data and Variables

The data comes from the 2006 Spanish Health Survey, which is based on a representative nationwide sample of 28,954 individuals aged 16 and over. The survey includes self-reported information on health status, morbidity, disability, accidents, use of health services, drug consumption, lifestyles and health-related behaviours, social relations and various socio-economic characteristics (referring both to the individual and to the head of the household). The participants were randomly selected by means of a multiple-stage random sampling strategy.

Outcome Variables: Mental Health Status Indicators

We use two alternative outcome variables for psychological health status[1]. The first indicator is based on the 12-item version of the General Health Questionnaire (GHQ-12), which is a commonly used measure for assessing self-assessed mental health that identifies the possible existence of psychological health conditions such as worries, anxiety and depression (Goldberg and Williams, 1988). The GHQ-12 ranges from 0 to 12, where 0 indicates no risk of poor mental health and 12 shows a high risk. The total score is calculated as the sum of the positive answers to the twelve questions regarding problems of mental concentration, sleep disorders caused by worries, feelings of uselessness, ability to take decisions, feelings of tension/oppression, inability to cope with difficulties, enjoyment of daily activities, ability to face problems adequately, lack of happiness and loss of self-confidence. A mean GHQ-12 score of 1.62 was obtained in the full sample (with 45% of the individuals indicating at least one of 12 items). Women were found to be at greater risk of psychological distress than men, with GQH-12 scores of 1.91 and 1.17, respectively. If we consider the binary version of the GHQ-12 indicator[2], 50.3% of women gave a positive

[1] We initially defined three indicators. The mental health risk based on the GHQ-12, (self-perceived) poor mental health and diagnosed poor mental health. The correlation between self-assessed and diagnosed poor mental health measures was quite high. In fact, only 3% of the individuals who reported a poor psychological status were not certified as being in poor mental health by a health professional. It is therefore not surprising that the econometric analyses produced similar results. In the final version of this chapter, we have only included the findings based on the more objective mental health indicator.

[2] The GHQ-12 index is transformed into a binary variable in order to obtain directly comparable results between the two alternative mental health measures used in the econometric specification.

answer to at least one of the twelve questions, while this proportion fell to 36.8% among men. Gender differences highlighting the higher prevalence of mental-health problems among women compared to men have been previously found in numerous studies using Spanish data (e.g., Cortés et al., 2004; Haro et al., 2006), as well as in a wide number of international studies (e.g. Piccinelli and Wilkinson, 2000; Rosenfield, 1982; Simon, 2002).

The second outcome variable, *Poor mental heath*, is a binary indicator taking the value 1 if the individual has been diagnosed by a doctor as suffering from any depression, anxiety or any other mental disorder episode during the last twelve months. Around 17% of Spanish adults are or have been in poor psychological health, with significant gender differences being apparent. The share of women presenting mental health problems (21.9%) is more than double that of men (9.2%).

Table 1. Mental health status

Variable	Women	Men	Total
Mental health indicator (GHQ-12)	1.91	1.17	1.62
Mental health risk (based on GHQ-12)	50.3%	36.8%	44.9%
Poor mental health	21.9%	9.2%	16.9%

Explanatory Variables

The vector of covariates includes two groups of variables, i.e. individual characteristics and community-based social capital indicators. The set of individual variables can be split into three groups, i.e. socio-demographic characteristics (household income, age, education, employment status and social class based on occupation), health-related behaviours (body mass index, alcohol consumption, smoking habits and physical activity) and individual social capital.

Most variables show important divergences by gender. The men in the total sample are on average younger than the women (49.2 versus 51.6 years of age). To check the hypothesis that mental well-being decreases with age[3] we included two covariates in the estimations, namely, age and age squared.

The beneficial impact of marriage and co-habiting on health, supported by existing evidence (Gardner and Oswald, 2004), is controlled for by five dummy variables describing the respondent's marital status: married (63.8% of the men and 62.2 % of the women), single (27.3% versus 16.1% in favour of men), widowed (5.1% and 16.8% in each sub-sample) and divorced/separated (3.8% among men and 4.9% among women).

Numerous studies have shown the relevance of educational qualifications as a health-enhancing and health-protecting factor. No significant gender differences are observed. However, there are slightly more university graduates among the men than among the women (16.0% versus 14.6%). However, the percentage of women with no education is significantly higher than the percentage among men (15.6% versus 10.9%, respectively).

[3] Previous research shows that the elderly are at greater risk of suffering from depression, anxiety or of becoming addicted to drugs or alcohol.

Five variables are included in the group of health-related factors capturing the effect of lifestyle on health: i) smoking habits, ii) the body mass index (BMI) of the respondent, iii) the amount of physical exercise in everyday life and iv) physical exercise in the respondent's leisure time. Some of the health-related behaviours present substantial gender differences. One third of the men smoke on a regular or occasional basis, while 22.1% of the women do so. However, about 65% of women have never smoked, whereas the percentage among men is below 35%. The BMI reveals that overweight and obesity are more serious problems among men (35.2% can be considered overweight and 15.6% have a BMI of above 30 kg/m^2) than among women (21.7% weight above the average, and 13.9% are obese). Finally, men do more physical activity in both their everyday life and their leisure time (64.1%) than women (58.4%).

Table 2. Health-related behaviours

Variable	Women	Men	Total
Smoker	22.1	33.7	26.7
Ex-smoker	13.6	31.6	20.7
Non-smoker	64.4	34.7	52.6
BMI<19.5	2.5	0.6	1.7
19.5<BMI<25.8	47.8	42.5	45.6
25.8<BMI<30	21.7	35.2	27.1
BMI>30	13.9	15.6	14.6
Sit all day	31.7	37.3	33.9
Stand all day	57.6	41.5	51.2
Heavy physical activity (+walk and carrying weight)	10.7	21.3	14.9
Regular or occasional physical activity in leisure time	58.4	64.1	60.6

Table 3. Individual social capital

Construct	Survey question	Women	Men	Total
Talk	Do you have the opportunity to talk to someone about problems at work or home	4.60	4.57	4.59
	Do you have the opportunity to talk to someone about personal and family problems	4.60	4.56	4.59
	Do you have the opportunity talk to someone about financial problems	4.59	4.54	4.57
Care	Can you count on people who worry about you?	4.64	4.60	4.62
	Do you receive love and affection?	4.66	4.63	4.65
	Do you receive help when you are sick in bed	4.65	4.71	4.67
Interact	Do friends and relatives visit you?	4.15	4.08	4.12
	Do you receive invitations to enjoy othe people's company?	4.31	4.31	4.31
	Do you receive useful advice when something happens?	4.47	4.40	4.44
Help	Do you receive help around the house?	3.90	3.99	3.93
	Do you receive praise and recognition in the workplace?	3.88	3.88	3.88

Note: Elicited responses are based on a five-point scale: 1. Much less than I wish; 2. Less than I wish; 3. Fair; 4. Almost as much as I wish; 5. As much as I wish. This table contains the mean values of the responses.

Individual social capital encompasses self-perceived emotional and instrumental support[4] as revealed by eleven survey questions. These are grouped into four factors using principal component analysis[5]. The first construct (*talking*), based on three variables, reflects the opportunity to share personal, economic and work-related concerns. The second construct (*care*) covers three questions regarding access to care, trust and reliance, and perception of love and affection. The third factor (*interaction*) is associated with three variables covering the degree of the individual's social interaction. Finally, the fourth factor (*help*) is related to two questions on receiving recognition in the workplace and help with domestic issues. Table 3 contains the survey questions included in each construct, as well as the mean values of the responses by gender and for the sample as a whole. Previous evidence reveals the positive effect of social interactions, and especially emotional contacts with family, relatives and close friends, on the overall (physical and mental) health of the individual (e.g. Kawachi and Berkman, 2001, Boreham et al., 2003; Petrou and Kupek, 2008).

Community social capital measures are aggregated at a regional level (17 Spanish Autonomous Regions). They are constructed based on Putnam (1993). To do so, we use the Spanish files of the World Values Survey for 1995, 2000 and 2005. Putnam (1993, p. 167) defines social capital as features of social organization, such as trust, norms, and networks, which can improve the efficiency of society by facilitating coordinated actions. Based on this definition, we use three sets of variables covering the three dimensions of social capital

[4] Emotional support refers to the opportunity to receive care and be involved in emotional interactions, while the instrumental component reflects access to information, advice, and material help.

[5] There is quite a strong correlation between the individual social capital variables. We use principal component analysis in order to collapse them into four orthogonal factors. This procedure allows us to avoid overlapped effects and multicolinearity in the econometric estimates..

mentioned in Putnam (1993). As usual, social trust is proxied using the responses to the question; "*Generally speaking, would you say that most people can be trusted or that you need to be very careful in dealing with people?*" Social norms are considered using four questions where individuals are asked to report whether they find the following actions acceptable: i) Claiming government benefits to which you are not entitled, (ii) Avoiding a fare on public transport, (iii) Cheating on taxes if you have a chance, and (iv) Someone accepting a bribe in the course of their duties. Finally, we use the individuals' associational activities within church/religious organizations, art/ music or educational organizations, labour unions, political parties, environmental organizations, professional organizations and humanitarian or charitable organizations.

Our community social capital indicators are constructed by averaging the variables mentioned above by region, and applying a principal component analysis to the aggregated variables for social norms and associational activities. Some studies have already used factor analyses to capture the multidimensional aspect of social capital (Onyx and Bullen, 2000; Bjornskov and Svedsen, 2003, Bjornskov, 2006). This procedure reveals the latent dimensions of a set of variables by grouping correlated attributes (attributes that may reflect a shared underlying trait). Some authors have expressed doubts about the validity of the instruments obtained using the factor analyses (Hair at al, 1998), because of the uncertainty in identifying the underlying factors and in determining the total number of factors. However, the development of a generally accepted method for constructing a valid and reliable social capital index is still in its early stages (Islam et al, 2008). Despite this criticism, we believe that factor analysis is a suitable technique since it prevents overlapping effects and other technical shortcomings derived from using a large number of generally correlated variables. The principal component analysis allows us to identify three different factors. The first factor (CSCF1) is related to associational activity within church/religious organizations, political parties, environmental organizations and professional organizations. The second factor (CSCF2) is associated to all the variables regarding social norms. Finally, the third factor (CSCF3) includes associational activity in educational, humanitarian and charitable organizations. We assign the same value to each of these indicators for all individuals residing in the same region.

EMPIRICAL MODEL

A random-effect probit specification (Greene, 2000) is used to model the probability of being at risk of suffering from mental health disorders or of being in poor mental health. To determine the effect of social capital beyond those of the usual health determinants, the mental health outcomes were first regressed on the individual's socio-demographic characteristics and health lifestyles, and then on individual and community social capital indicators[6]. In total, we developed four non-linear models, one separate equation for men and

6 It should be noted that the community social capital measures only vary at a regional level. In order to disentangle their impact on the mental health from that of other regional variables, it is therefore necessary to consider specific-regional effects. These effects can be accounted for by two alternative estimation models - a multilevel regression (Goldstein 1987 and 1991) and a random-effects probit specification (Green, 2000). The two estimation techniques provided similar results. Given that the multilevel technique does not allow

women (to assess whether the social capital effects differ with gender) and one for each mental health outcome (to guarantee the comprehensiveness of the analysis).

RESULTS

Table 4 shows the association between mental health, individual factors and social capital indicators. The estimated results[7] for the two measures of mental health and for men and women are reported.

Table 4. Estimates of the determinants of the propensity to mental health risk and the probability of poor mental health

		Mental Health Risk		Diagnosed Poor Mental Health	
		Women	*Men*	*Women*	*Men*
Socio-demographic	Logarithm of monthly income	-0.0578*	-0.0371*	-0.0421*	-0.0036
	Age	-0.0034**	-0.0035***	0.0190*	0.0074*
	Age squared	0.0000**	0.0000	-0.0002*	-0.0001*
(Base: higher education)	Without studies	0.0741*	0.0479***	0.0797*	-0.0005
	Primary education	0.0010	0.0076	0.0328**	0.0054
	Secondary education	0.0064	0.0128	0.0268**	0.0115
(Base: Working)	Working (on sick leave >3 months)	0.2505*	0.3737*	0.1652*	0.1444*
	Unemployed	0.0596*	0.1343*	0.0485*	0.0475*
	Retired	0.0632*	0.0822*	0.0831*	0.0912*
	Student	0.0345	-0.0497***	0.0670**	-0.0274***
	Homework	0.0208	-0.0779	0.0382*	-0.0087
	Other	0.1381*	0.1241**	0.1084**	0.1218**
Life-style	Body Mass Index	0.0030*	-0.0020	0.0043*	0.0003
(Base: all the day sited)	Stand up all day (no major effort)	-0.0483*	-0.0809*	-0.0443*	-0.0259*
	Walking, moving, carrying heavy items	0.0159	-0.0517*	-0.0173	-0.0332*
	Major physical effort	0.0913*	-0.0392***	0.0110	-0.0210**
(Base: physical act. leisure)	No physical activity in leisure time	0.0307*	0.0175***	0.0057	0.0127*
Individual social capital	*Talk* (opportunity to talk about problems)	-0.0437*	-0.0433*	-0.0178*	-0.0061*
	Care (receive care, love, affection)	-0.0421*	-0.0304*	-0.0176*	-0.0097*
	Interact (social life and leisure)	-0.0729*	-0.0720*	-0.0225*	-0.0118*
	Help (recognition and help)	-0.0776*	-0.0570*	-0.0172*	-0.0081*
Community social capital	*Trust*	0.0494	0.0609	0.0168	0.0177
	Associational	-0.0175*	-0.0140*	-0.0069	-0.0029
	Social norms	-0.0232*	-0.0196*	0.0025	-0.0021
	Charity	-0.0372*	-0.0417*	-0.0238*	-0.0153*
	Log-likelihood	-8,867	-6,000	-6,614	-2,691
	N	13,812	9,816	14,008	9,954

Notes: (*) Significant at 1% level; (**) Significant at 5% level; (***) Significant at 10% level
Reported values are estimated marginal effects, and therefore indicate the increase in the probability with an additional unit in a given covariate. For dummy variables, the increase in the probability is caused by the change from 0 to 1.

marginal effects to be computed, here we only present and discuss the findings of the random-effects specification.

7 Table 4 displays the estimated marginal effects instead of the estimated parameters.

Mental Health Risk Propensity

- Age is found to exert the most surprising effect on the estimates of propensity to mental health risk. It is determined to be U-shaped for women and negative for men.
- Income is an important protective factor against exposure to mental health risks. The effect is significantly stronger for women.
- Education seems to play a minor role, since only those without studies present higher propensities of physiological health risks compared to individuals with at least primary studies.
- Retirement and unemployment are conditions clearly associated with a higher probability of mental health risk for the two sub-samples.

The impact of health-related behaviours differs between genders. Body mass index (BMI) exerts a statistically significant positive effect only on women, i.e. overweight and obese women are more exposed to mental health risks than women with normal weight. On the other hand, smoking habits increase the probability of suffering mental health disorders in men, but do not significantly affect women. Physical activity has a positive influence on maintaining mental health among both men and women. Moreover, active women are more likely to maintain good mental health than men.

Social capital indicators provide interesting results. The individual measures of social capital report a negative and statistically significant effect on the probability of being at risk of mental illness among both population groups. The perception of a lack of social interactions or help when in need exerts the greatest detrimental effect on psychological health. Except for the variable *Trust*, all remaining community social capital indicators turned out to significantly reduce the probability of mental health risks for men and women. The lack of significance of the *Trust* indicator can be explained by its high correlation with the factor associated to social norms. When only the *Trust* measure is included in the model, its estimated effect becomes negative, but it does not become statistically significant in determining the mental health risk propensity.

Probability of Poor Mental Health

The results regarding the probability of suffering a poor mental health episode are somehow different from those obtained for the mental health risk propensity. Elderly men and women are more prone to mental health disorders than the younger age groups. The effect of age on physiological health is an inverted U-shape, i.e. positive but decreasing. There are notable differences between men and women. Among women, the probability of having poor mental health starts to decrease at the age of 49, while among men this happens at the age of 38. This result indicates the higher exposure (that last longer) to poor mental health conditions of women compared to that of men. Income significantly reduces the probability of being diagnosed with an adverse mental health condition, but only among women. The result does not necessarily mean that material well-being does not exert a beneficial impact on men's mental health, but may indicate that men seek psychological care less often and as a consequence have fewer diagnosed episodes. Education exerts a protective effect on women's mental health status, but does not significantly influence men's psychological conditions. People belonging to vulnerable groups of the population, such as the unemployed or the retired, are again found to be more likely to suffer from poor mental health conditions.

Lifestyle behaviours exert differential impact on men's and women's mental health status. Excess weight (measured by the BMI) and smoking habits are only significantly deteriorating women's mental health, but does not affect men's one. On the contrary, greater physical activity in daily life and leisure time reduces the probability of suffering bad mental episodes only for men

A significant association is found between mental health status and individual social capital for women and men.

- Social support and satisfactory interactions with family, relatives and friends help improve the physiological health of individuals. The effect of individual social capital variables is stronger among women than among men.
- The greater effect among women is observed for the factor *Interact* (visits, invitations for leisure and useful advices), while for men the most significant is the influence of the factor *Talk*.
- Finally, the variables regarding community social capital presented a much more modest effect on reducing the probability of poor mental health. Only one of the factors regarding community associational activities (participation in charitable or educational associations) turned out to be statistically significant for both genders, though again it was stronger for women than for men.

CONCLUSION

The main objective of this chapter was to elicit the relevance of various dimensions of social capital for adults' mental health status and thus shedding more light on the complex (and ambivalent) relationship between them (McKenzie and Harpham, 2006). Additionally, separate analyses by gender were carried out based on the well-known fact that the determinants of health, and of psychological well-being in particular, for men and women differ not only in their significance, but also in their magnitude. Our results stress the role of all individual social capital indicators on the propensity to mental health risk and on the probability of being in poor mental health. The influence is stronger among women, which confirms existing evidence suggesting that women invest more than men in social relations and in establishing and preserving emotional support (Cheng and Chan, 2006).

Unlike the individual aspects of social capital, the behaviour of the community dimensions differed widely depending on the mental health outcome analysed. Neither generalised trust nor associational activities related to church, political parties, environmental or professional organizations thus seem to significantly influence an individual's probability of experiencing an adverse psychological episode. This result is consistent with some recent empirical individual-level studies showing that activity in voluntary organisations is only very weakly associated with generalised trust (Claibourn and Martin, 2000; Stolle, 1998; Uslaner, 2002). Contrary to Putnam's explanation, associational activity only creates benefits for members, but this does not extend to outsiders, i.e. it does not generate positive externalities.

However, our findings also at least partially support Putnam's claim, since individuals are less prone to suffering any mental health disorder in regions with a higher percentage of residents participating in educational or charity associations. This result is true for men and women, but the impact is significantly stronger for the latter. A noteworthy result is the significant impact of community social capital on propensity to the risk of mental health. Spaniards residing in regions characterised by higher levels of associational activism, widely accepted and respected social norms and engaged in charitable behaviour are less subject to mental health risks.

Bearing in mind the common controversies related to social capital measures used in empirical research, some of which are also valid here (Arrow, 2000; Navarro, 2002; Sobel, 2002; Szreter and Woolcock, 2004), the analyses presented in this chapter allow us to conclude that: (i) women are more subject than men to mental health problems; (ii) individual social capital plays a crucial role in protecting an individual's psychological well-being; and, (iii) community social capital, due to its multidimensional nature, is revealed as a more effective tool in preventing mental health disorders than as an instrument for "treating" those in poor mental health. The first result calls for gender-oriented mental health policy initiatives. Focusing on policies that enhance individual social capital could be beneficial not only at an individual level, but could also exert a positive effect on community health, or on the distribution of health among the various members or groups in the society. The main implication of the latter conclusion is that although community social capital should not be considered a cure- all pill, encouraging associational activities and participation in educational and civic initiatives (policy measures that are relatively less resource-consuming compared to others) could potentially reduce the prevalence of psychological conditions, and contribute to improving the general health of the population.

Acknowledgments

Financial support from Spanish Ministry of Education (grant number SEJ2007-66318) is gratefully acknowledged.

References

Addy, C.L., Wilson, D.K., Kirtland, K.A., Ainsworth, B.E., Sharpe, P., & Kimsey, D. (2004). Associations of perceived social and physical environmental support with physical activity and walking behaviour. *American Journal of Public Health*, *94*(3), 440–443.

Alonso, J., Angermeyer, M.C., Bernert, S., et al. (2004). Prevalence of mental disorders in Europe: results from the European Study of the Epidemiology of Mental Disorders (ESEMeD) project. *Acta Psychiatrica Scandinavica, Suppl. 109*(420): 17-29.

Arrow, K. (2000). Observations on social capital. In P. Dasgupta, & I. Serageldin (Eds.), *Social Capital: A Multifaceted Perspective*, (pp. 3-5). Washington, DC: The World Bank.

Becker, G.S., & Murphy, K.M. (2000). *Social economics. Market behaviour in a social environment*. Cambridge, MA: The Belknap Press of Harvard University Press.

Bjornskov, C., & Svendsen, G.T. (2003). *Measuring social capital: Is there a single underlying explanation?* Working Paper 03-5. Department of Economics, Aarhus School of Business, Denmark.

Boreham, R.M., Stafford, M., & Taylor, R. (2003). *Health Survey for England 2000: Social Capital and Health*. London: The Stationery Office.

Borjas, G.J. (2003). Welfare Reform, Labor Supply, and Health Insurance in the Immigrant Population. *Journal of Health Economics*, *22*(6), 933-958.

Brown, T., Scheffler, R., Sukyong, S., & Reed, M. (2006). The empirical relationship between community social capital and the demand for cigarettes. *Health Economics*, *15*, 1159-1172.

Burström, B., & Fredlund, P. (2001). Self-rated health: is it a good predictor of subsequent mortality among adults in lower as well as in higher social classes? *Journal of Epidemiology and Community Health*, *55*(11), 836-840.

Cheng, S., & Chan, A. (2006). Socialsupport and self-reted health revised: is there a gender difference in later life? *Social Science and Medicine*, *63*, 118-122.

Claibourn, M., & Martin, P.S. (2000). Trusting and joining? An empirical test of the reciprocal nature of social capital. *Political Behavior*, *22*, 267– 291.

Cullen, M., & Whiteford, H. (2001). *The interrelations of social capital with health and mental health*. Canberra: Commonwealth of Australia.

De Silva, M.J., McKinzei, K., Harpham, T., & Hutty, S.R. (2005). Social capital and mental illness: a systematic review. *Journal of Epidemiology and Community Health*, *59*(8), 619-627.

Devillanova, C. (2008). Social Networks, Information and Health Care Utilization: Evidence from Undocumented Immigrants in Milan. *Journal of Health Economics*, *27*(2), 265-286.

Dowd, J.B., & Zajacova, A. (2007). Does the predictive power of self-rated health for subsequent mortality risk vary by socioeconomic status in the US? *International Journal of Epidemiology*, *36*, 1214-1221.

Durlauf, S.N. (2002). On the empirics of social capital. *The Economic Journal*, *112*(483), 459-479.

Evans, S., Banerjee, S., Leese, M., & Huxley, P. (2007). The impact of mental illness on quality of life: A comparison of severe mental illness, common mental disorder and healthy population samples. *Quality of Life Research*, *16*(1), 17-29.

Folland, S. (2008). An economic model of social capital and health. *Health Economics, Policy and Law*, *3*, 333-348.

Gardner, J., & Oswald, A. (2004). How is Mortality Affected by Money, Marriage and Stress? *Journal of Health Economics*, *23*, 1181-1207.

Glaeser, E.L., Laibson, D., & Sacerdote, B. (2000). An economic approach to social capital. *The Economic Journal*, *112*(483), 437-458.

Greene, W.H. (2000). *Econometric Analysis* (4th edition). Upper Saddle River, NJ: Prentice-Hall.

Goldstein, H. (1987). Multilevel covariance component models. *Biometrika*, *74*, 430-431.

Goldstein, H. (1991). Nonlinear multilevel models with an application to discrete response data. *Biometrika*, *78*, 45-51.

Grootaert, C., & Van Bastelaer, T. (2002). Understanding and Measuring Social Capital: A Synthesis of Findings and Recommendations from the Social Capital Initiative [E-working paper].

http://www.usaid.gov/our_work/economic_growth_and_trade/eg/forum_series/social-capital.pdf.

Haro, J.M., Palacín, C., Vilagut, G., et al. (2006). Prevalencia de los trastornos mentales y factores asociados: resultados del estudio ESEMeD-España. *Medicina Clínica* (Barcelona), *126*(12), 445-451.

Harpham, T., Grant, E., & Thomas, E. (2002). Measuring social capital within health surveys: key issues. *Health Policy and Planning*, *17*(1), 106-111.

Haughton McNeill, L., Kreuter, M.W., & Submanian, S.V. (2006). Social environment and physical activity: A review of concepts and evidence. *Social Science and Medicine*, *63*(4), 1011-1022.

Huisman, M., Van Lenthe, F., & Mackenbach, J. (2007). The predictive ability of self-assessed health for mortality in different educational groups. *International Journal of Epidemiolo*gy, *36*, 1207-1213.

Idler, E.L., & Beyamini, Y. (1997). Self-rated health and mortality: a review of twenty-seven community studies. *Journal of Health and Social Behaviour*, *38*, 21-37.

Idler, E.L., & Kasl, S. (1995). Self-ratings of health: Do they also predict change in functional disability? *Journal of Gerontology and Social Science*, *50*B, S344-S353.

Islam, K., Merlo, J., Kawachi, I., Lindström, M., & Gertham, U.-G. (2006). Social capital and health: Does egalitarianism matter? A literature review. *International Journal for Equity and Health*, *5*(3), 1-28.

Islam, M.K., Gertham, U.-G., Gullberg, B., Lindström, M., & Merlo, J. (2008). Social capital externalities and mortality in Sweden. *Economic and Human Biology*, *6*, 19-42.

Katschnig, H., Freeman, H., & Sartorius, N. (Eds.) (2006). *Quality of Life in Mental Disorders* (2th edition). Chichester, UK: John Wiley & Sons.

Kawachi, I., & Berkman, L.F. (2001). Social ties and mental health. *Journal of Urban Health*, *78*(3), 458-467.

Kawachi, I., Kim, D., Coutts, A., & Subramanian, S. (2004). Commentary: Reconciling the three accounts of social capital. *International Journal of Epidemiology*, *33*(4), 682-690.

Kessler, R,C,, Berglund, P.A., Demler, O., Jin, R., & Walters, E.E. (2005a). Lifetime prevalence and age-of-onset distributions of DSM-IV disorders in the National Comorbidity Survey Replication (NCS-R). *Archives of General Psychiatry*. *62*(6), 593-602.

Kessler, R.C., Chiu, W.T., Demler, O., & Walters, E.E. (2005b). Prevalence, severity, and comorbidity of twelve-month DSM-IV disorders in the National Comorbidity Survey Replication (NCS-R). *Archives of General Psychiatry*, *62*(6), 617-627.

Lindström, M., Hanson, B.S., & Östergren, P.O. (2001). Socioeconomic differences in leisure time physical activity: the role of shaping participation and social capital in shaping health related behaviour. *Social Science and Medicine*, *52*(3), 441-451.

Lindström, M., Moghaddassi M., & Merlo, J. (2003). Social capital and leisure time physical activity: a population-based multilevel analysis in Malmö, Sweden. *Journal of Epidemiology and Community Health*, *57*(1), 23–28.

Lindström, M., Moghaddassi, M., Bolin, K., Lindgren, B., & Merlo, J. (2003). Social capital and daily tobacco smoking: a population-based multilevel analysis in Malmö, Sweden. *Scandinavian Journal of Public Health*, *31*(6), 444-450.

Lochner, L, & Moretti, E. (2004). The effect of education on crime: evidence from prison inmates, arrests, and self-reports. *American Economic Review*, *94*, 155-189.

Lundborg, P. (2005). Social capital and substance use among Swedish adolescents – an explorative study. *Social Science and Medicine*, *61*(6), 1151-1158.

Macinko J., & Starfield B. (2001). The Utility of Social Capital in Research on Health Determinants. *The Milbank Quarterly*, September, *79*(3), 387-427.

Maycock, B.R., & Howat, P. (2007). Social capital: implications from an investigation of illegal anabolic steroid networks. *Health Education Research December*, *22*(6), 854-863.

McDaid, D. (Ed.) (2009). Bridging the gap between physical and mental health. Brussels: Mental Health Platform.

McKenzie, K., Whitley, R., & Weich, S. (2002). Social Capital and mental health. *The British Journal of Psychiatry*, *181*, 280-283.

McKenzie, K., & Harpham, T. (2006). *Social Capital and Mental Health*. London: Jessica Kinglsey Publishers.

Milligan, K., Moretti, E., & Oreopoulos, P. (2004). Does education improve citizenship? Evidence from the U.S. and the U.K. *Journal of Public Economics*, *88*, 1667-1695.

Morreti, E. (2004). Estimating the social returns to higher education: evidence from longitudinal and repeated cross-sectional data. *Journal of Econometrics*, *121*, 175-212.

Mummery, W.K., Lauder, W., Schofield, G., & Caperchione, C. (2008). Associations between physical inactivity and a measure of social capital in a sample of Queensland adults. *Journal of Science and Medicine in Sport*, *11*(3), 308-315.

Navarro, V. (2002). A critique of social capital. *International Journal of Health Services*, *32*, 423-432.

Onyx, J., & Bullen, P. (2000). Measuring social capital in five communities. *Journal of Applied Behavioural Science*, *36*, 23-42.

Patel, V. (2010). Building social capital and improving mental health care to prevent suicide. *International Journal of Epidemiology*, *24*, 1-2.

Petrou, S., & Kupek, E. (2008). Social capital and its relationship with measures of health status: evidence from the Health Survey for England 2003. *Health Economics*, *17*(1), 127-143.

Piccinelli, M., & Wilkinson, G. (2000). Gender differences in depression. *British Journal of Psychiatry*, *177*, 486-492.

Poortinga, W. (2006). Do health behaviours mediate the association between social capital and health? *Preventive Medicine*, *43*, 488-493.

Putnam R. (2000). *Bowling Alone. The Collapse and Revival of American Community*. New York: Simon and Schuster.

Rose, R. (2000). How much does social capital add to individual health: A survey of Russians. *Social Science and Medicine*, *51*(9), 1421-1435.

Rosenfield, S. (1982). Sex Roles and Societal Reactions to Mental Illness: The Labeling of 'Deviant' Deviance. *Journal of Health and Social Behavior*, *23*, 18-24.

Simon, R.W. (2002). Revisiting the relationship among gender, marital status, and mental health. *The American Journal of Sociology*, *107*(4), 1065-1096.

Sobel, J. (2002). Can we trust social capital. *Journal of Economic Literature*, *40*, 139-154.

Somers, J.M., Goldner, E.M., Waraich, P., & Hsu, L. (2006). Prevalence and incidence studies of anxiety disorders: a systematic review of the literature. *Canadian Journa lof Psychiatry*, *51*(2), 100-113.

Stahl, T., Rutten, A., Nutbeam, D., Bauman, A., Kannas, L., Abel, T., Luschen, G., Rodriquez, D.J., Vinck, J., & Van der Zee, J. (2001). The importance of the social environment for physically active lifestyle-results from an international study. *Social Science and Medicine*, *52*(1), 1–10.

Stolle, D., (1998). Bowling together, bowling alone: the development of generalized trust in voluntary associations. *Political Psychology*, *19*, 497– 525.

Storr, C.L., Chen, Y., & Anthony, J. (2004). "Unequal opportunity": neighbourhood disadvantage and the chance to buy illegal drugs. *Journal of Epidemiology and Community Health*, *58*(3), 231-237.

Stoyanova, A., & Díaz-Serrano, L. (2009a). El Impacto Diferencial del Capital Social sobre la Salud Mental de la Población Autóctona y los Inmigrantes residentes en Cataluña. *Gaceta Sanitaria*, *23*, 93-99.

Stoyanova, A., & Díaz-Serrano, L. (2009b) Dissentangling the link between health and social capital: a comparison of immigrant andnative-born populations in Spain, mimeo.

Szreter S., & Woolcock, M. (2004). Health by association? Social capital, social theory, and the political economy of public health. *International Journal of Epidemiology*, *33*(4), 650-667.

Takashi, L.M., & Magalong, M.G. (2008). Disruptive social capital: (Un)Healthy socio-spatial interactions among Filipino men living with HIV/AIDS. *Health & Place*, *14*, 182-197.

Uslaner, E.M. (2002). *The Moral Foundations of Trust*. Cambridge, UK: Cambridge University Press.

Weitzman, E.R, & Chen, Y. (2005). Social capital's risk modifying effects on measures of heavy alcohol consumption, alcohol abuse, harms, and second-hand effects; national survey findings. *Journal of Epidemiology and Community Health*, *59*(4): 303-309.

Wittchen, H.U., & Jacobi, F. (2005). Size and burden of mental disorders in Europe-a critical review and appraisal of 27 studies. *European Neuropsychopharmacology*, *15*(4), 357-376.

World Health Organisation (2009). The WHO Mental Health Survey Initiative. *Presentation at the 2009 IFPE Congress,* Vienna (Austria).

http://www.hcp.med.harvard.edu/wmh/IFPE_WMH.pdf

Woolcock, M. (1998). Social capital and economic development: Towards a theoretical synthesis and policy framework. *Theory and Society*, *27*, 151-208.

Yang, K. (2007). Individual social capital and its measurement in social surveys. *Survey Research Methods*, *1*(1), 19-27.

In: Social Determinants and Mental Health
Editor: Sabine Bährer-Kohler

ISBN: 978-1-61324-353-4

Chapter 7

SOCIAL PARTICIPATION AND MENTAL HEALTH

Francisco Javier Carod-Artal
Department of Neurology, Virgen de la Luz Hospital, Cuenca, Spain

INTRODUCTION

According to the World Health Organization's *International Classification of Functioning, Disability, and Health*, Participation has been defined as a person's involvement in a life situation. Participation is conceived as the result of a complex interaction among factors including a person's disease, the individual's body structure and function, and their activity performance [1].

Community participation has been increasingly recognized as a social determinant of mental health. Several epidemiological studies have documented a link between social participation, subjective wellbeing and mental health [2,3]. Participating in social and civic life has been found to be a protective factor against physical and mental diseases [4] and mortality, including from suicide [5].

Getting involved with others may protect against anxiety and depression, reduce stress and improve self esteem. Active and continuous community participation has been associated with a lower frequency of psychosocial distress and mental disturbances in young [6] and elderly people [7]. Leisure and religious activity participation has been associated with lower frequency of depression and an increased satisfaction with life among older adults [8]. Physical activity and sports participation has been linked with improved mental and social well-being, including reduced risk of depression and suicidality [9]. By contrast, psychological distress may be related to low levels of participation. Lack of contact with friends, and the loneliness associated with friendlessness, may be a precursor to depression [10].

In addition, participation in some types of social activities may reduce mortality and cognitive function impairment in the elderly [11]. The level of social engagement may be protective against a decline in mental health among women living alone [7].

Lack of Participation and Social Exclusion

The concepts of social and community participation may overlap with social exclusion and social capital, respectively. In fact, lack of participation is usually assessed in most of dimensions of social exclusion (such as consumption, production, political engagement and social interactions). Some indicators of social exclusion (housing, education, income, employment, social support and neighbourhood deprivation) overlap with restrictions in community participation and are associated to lower mental health [12].

Several studies worldwide have reported a low level of participation among people with mental illness [13,14]. For example, community-based schizophrenia patients may suffer poverty and experience more social isolation, discrimination and exploitation in the workplace [15].

Participation snd Structural Social Capital

Social capital is a way of describing social relationships within societies, and consists of five main characteristics: community networks; civic engagement and participation; local civic identity (sense of belonging, solidarity); reciprocity and sense of obligation to help others; and trust in the community.

According to Putnam, social capital can be divided into a cognitive/perceptual component (trust) and a behavioural one (participation); they are referred to as cognitive and structural social capital respectively [16]. Participation is known as the structural component of social capital ("what people do"), whereas cohesion is deemed as the cognitive component ("what people feel").

Individual capital social is usually measured by asking individuals about their participation in social relationships and their perceptions of the quality of those relationships. By contrast, ecological social capital may be assessed by aggregating the responses of individuals in population surveys to the community level.

Evidence of significant inverse association between levels of cognitive and structural social capital and mental health has been reported [17,18]. In addition, gender and socio-economic differences have been found to be important determinants [3,4,19].

Causal association between lower socio-economic position in early life and poorer health across the life span has been reported [20]. Social origins seem to play a major role for inequality in educational attainment and in other cultural areas such as cultural participation in adolescence and adulthood. In fact, a good part of intergenerational transmission in earnings, education and occupational outcomes may be mediated via parent's impact on children's cognitive development [21].

People with intellectual disabilities have poorer physical and mental health and are more likely to be exposed to poverty during childhood [22,23]. A socially significant proportion of the increased risk of poorer health among children and adolescents with intellectual disabilities has been attributed to their increased risk of socio-economic disadvantage [23]. Several risk factors for ill health among people with intellectual disabilities have been reported and include poor nutrition and diet, medication, obesity and physical inactivity [24]. In addition, overweight/obesity, gastroesophageal reflux, urinary tract infections and dysphagia are more frequent in individuals with cerebral palsy. Functional impairment severity has been associated with health status among older persons with intellectual disability and cerebral palsy [25].

A higher overall level of social participation has been reported in women, whereas middle life circumstances (busy working parents) may be associated to less time to extensive community participation [3]. Self-rated health may be affected by social capital and income inequality cross-nationally [26].

MEASUREMENT OF PARTICIPATION

A) Categories

Community participation comprises several categories including informal social connectedness, civic engagement, and political participation. Each one may contain multiple types of participation that can be measured directly and quantified in terms of frequency and duration [27].

Activities associated to an active social life with family, friends, neighbours, and workmates are included under the concept informal social connectedness. Social life resulting from participation in organised aspects of community life such as work, church or community is included under the concept civil engagement. Organising community activities, attending meetings, and doing voluntary work are some examples [28]. Other cores of analysis include social participation as space of citizenship and policy formulation; oriented to attention of collective needs; and decision taking [29].

Table 1. Types of community participation

Contact with immediate household
Contact with extended family
Contact with friends
Contact with neighbours
Social contact with workmates
Adult learning
Religious participation
Organised community activities
Voluntary sector activity
Giving money to charity
Active interest in current affairs
Expressing opinions publicly
Community activism
Political protest

B) Questionnaires to Assess Participation

Components of participation can be mapped over time. Subjective aspects of participation, such as perceived quality of social relationships arising from involvement in leisure activities can also be assessed. Questionnaires specifically developed to assess participation are scarce. The Australian Community Participation Questionnaire has been developed to measure 14 types of participation (table 1) and may be an adequate instrument of assessment [27].

Social relationships and autonomy can be assessed in health-related quality-of-life scales such as QOLIBRI, a disease-specific quality-of-life measure in traumatic brain injury. The scale was sensitive to areas of life amenable to intervention, such as accommodation, work participation, mental health and functional outcome [30].

Participation and Disability. Stroke as a Paradigm

Chronic disabling neurological diseases usually provoke a deep impact on health. Lower levels of participation may be result of an interaction between factors of patient's social and physical environment [1].

People with chronic neurological diseases are limited in many types of participation, such as contacts with family, friends and neighbours; socialization with workmates; church activities; adult learning activities; civic engagement; and community activism.

In addition, cognitive and emotional factors associated to disabling progressive diseases may limit participation and activism in the community. Neurological degenerative diseases, such as Alzheimer's and Parkinson's disease, can present with apathy and/or depressive symptoms and restrict community participation at early stages.

Rehabilitation strategies may re-enforce social and participation level. Patients with major neurological impairment who receive rehabilitation care may achieve modest improvements in their levels of community participation [31].

Communication, mobility, self-care, domestic life, personal relationships and community and social participation are deeply affected in stroke survivors. In the last decade, several epidemiological studies, focused on the biopsychosocial model of stroke, have observed a link between social support, social participation and mental health in stroke survivors and their caregivers [32]. Approximately between 30 and 50% of stroke survivors have post-stroke depression [33]. One third of spouses (caregivers) of stroke patients suffer from anxiety. Burden, subjective well being and mental health of stroke caregivers are correlated with social support and social participation [34]. Social participation is also limited in disabled stroke patients and it is diminished in elderly caregivers of stroke survivors.

Strategies to Improve Social Participation

Good health is a major resource for social, economic and personal development, and an important dimension of quality of life. So, adequate social, economic and cultural factors can all favour health [35].

A) Children Strategies

Pre-school socialisation, learning and education are important factors for attainment in the formal educational system. Strategies that prepare children to enter school ready and motivated to learn have greater effect than additional investment in school resources such as reduction on class size. Children's learning and socialisation in high quality day care institutions are the most effective way to combat negative social heritage from the family [23].

Promotion of children's and adolescents' social participation can be considered a form of social intervention in which adults construct and treat children as citizens entitled to be involved in decision-making processes. According to this new paradigm, children are considered as agents of their own lives, competent social actors and citizens entitled to take part in decisions affecting their lives. Promoting social participation means promoting social processes that make children's actions visible in public contexts and influential in decision-making [36].

B) Adult Life Strategies

Main areas for mental health promotion in adult life include social participation and inclusion, personal factors and lifestyle, living spaces, environment and neighbourhood, occupational issues and retirement policies [37,38]. Community awareness campaigns may be useful to promote positive mental health and increase help-seeking behaviours. Prevention strategies targeting vulnerable and at risk groups, including children and adolescents should also be implemented [39].

Participation-based mental health promotion has practical implications. Strategies to increase participation include sign up for a course, undertaking physical activity on a regular basis, and link in with local services, family and friends [40]. Social network can be expanded by taking a dance class, joining a book club or volunteering for a social cause. Getting involved in community groups is a useful way to build social connections and learning. Schedule in regular times with close relationships may be helpful in disabled patients with movement restrictions.

Close and strong friendship-based ties are important network resources for people's health. Measures aiming at strengthening these types of social connections for socially disadvantaged groups might reduce social inequalities in health [41]. These strategies should also be performed to prevent social isolation and loneliness among older people [42].

Raising levels of community participation has been advocated as a mental health promotion strategy and may be valuable for rural locations. Community participation can be improved by means of relatively efficient and inexpensive services such as favouring public transportation in rural areas.

Conclusion

Mental health promotion actions aim at making socio-economic conditions favourable through advocacy for health. Promotion and protection strategies of mental health and social participation should be encouraged. Health care professionals and social service teams should take a leading role in raising awareness of social determinants of health. Specific health targets to improve mental health status among disadvantaged groups should be performed.

Several lines of action should be recommended: 1) the focus on infant mental health; 2) the improvement of working conditions; 3) adding equity to health policy programmes. The concept of social determinants should be central to these policies, with tackling the social influences on health seen as a way to reduce health inequalities [43,44].

Appropriate forms of community participation should be promoted, and tailored to the characteristics of different groups and communities. Strategies to encourage participation in disabled people to connect with and participate in their community are also needed.

Accurate information about target groups (disabled patients, mental illness people) is required. Involvement of social and health researchers, and government agencies that assess mental health in general and mental health and chronic disability are needed in the policy-making process.

References

[1] World Health Organization, International classification of functioning, disability and health, *WHO, Geneva*, 2001.

[2] Kwachi I, Berkman LF. Social ties and mental health. *J Urban Health* 2001; 78: 458-67.

[3] Berry HL. Social capital elite, excluded participators, busy working parents and aging, participating less: types of community participators and their mental health. *Soc Psychiatry Psychiatr Epidemiol* 2008; 43:527-37.

[4] Lindstrom M, Merlo J, Ostergren PO. Individual and neighbourhood determinants of social participation and social capital: A multilevel analysis of the city of Malmo, Sweden. *Soc Sci Med* 2002; 54: 1779-91.

[5] Berkman LF, Melchior M, Chastang JF, Niedhammer I, Leclerc A, Goldberg M. Social integration and mortality: A prospective study of French employees of electricity of France-gas of France: The GAZEL Cohort. *Am J Epidemiol* 2004; 159: 167-74.

[6] Bond L, Glover S, Godfrey C, Butler H, Patton GC. Building capacity for system-level change in schools: lessons from the Gatehouse Project. *Health Educ Behav* 2001; 28: 368-83.

[7] Michael YL, Berkman LF, Colditz GA, Kawachi I. Living arrangements, social integration, and change in functional health status. *Am J Epidemiol* 2001; 153:123-31.

[8] Gautam R, Saito T, Kai I. Leisure and religious activity participation and mental health: gender analysis of older adults in Nepal. *BMC Public Health* 2007; 7:299.

[9] Miller KE, Hoffman JH. Mental well-being and sport-related identities in college students. *Sociol Sport J* 2009; 26:335-56.

[10] Nangle DW, Erdley CA, Newman JE, Mason CA, Carpenter EM. Popularity, friendship quantity, and friendship quality: interactive influences on children's loneliness and depression. *J Clin Child Adolesc Psychol* 2003; 32:546-55.
[11] Hsu HC. Does social participation by the elderly reduce mortality and cognitive impairment? *Aging Ment Health* 2007; 11:699-707.
[12] Morgan C, Burns T, Fitzpatrick R, Pinfold V, Priebe S. Social exclusion and mental health: conceptual and methodological review. *Br J Psychiatry* 2007; 191:477-83.
[13] Jorm AF, Oh E. Desire for social distance from people with mental disorders. *Aust N Z J Psychiatry* 2009; 43:183-200.
[14] Kermode M, Bowen K, Arole S, Pathare S, Jorm AF. Attitudes to people with mental disorders: a mental health literacy survey in a rural area of Maharashtra, India. *Soc Psychiatry Psychiatr Epidemiol* 2009; 44:1087-96.
[15] Salomé F, Petitjean F, Germain C, Demant JC. The subjective quality of life of patients with schizophrenia: influence of psychopathology and patients' expectations. A comparative study. *Encephale* 2004; 30: 60-8.
[16] Putnam RD. Making democracy work. Princeton: Princeton University Press, 1993.
[17] De Silva MJ, McKenzie K, Harpham T, Huttly SR. Social capital and mental illness: a systematic review. *J Epidemiol Community Health* 2005; 59: 619-27.
[18] Loforsa J, Sundquist K. Low-linking social capital as a predictor of mental disorders: A cohort study of 4.5 million Swedes. *Soc Sci Med* 2007; 64: 21-34.
[19] Ferlander S, Mäkinen IH. Social capital, gender and self-rated health. Evidence from the Moscow Health Survey 2004. *Soc Sci Med* 2009; 69:1323-32.
[20] Marmot M. Social determinants of health inequalities. *Lancet* 2005; 365: 1099-104.
[21] Andersen J, Larsen JE. A broader social capital perspective. Measuring the effects of education on health and civic engagement: proceedings of the Copenhagen symposium. Organisation for economic co-operation and development. 2006. Available from: URL: *http://www.oecd.org/dataoecd/15/21/37425723.pdf.*
[22] Emerson E, Hatton C. Poverty, socio-economic position, social capital and the health of children and adolescents with intellectual disabilities in Britain: a replication. *J Intellect Disabil Res* 2007; 51:866-74.
[23] Walsh PN. Health indicators and intellectual disability. *Curr Opin Psychiatry* 2008; 21:474-8.
[24] Robertson J, Emerson E, Gregory N, Hatto C, Turner S, Kessissoglou S, et al. Lifestyle related risk factors for poor health in residential settings for people with intellectual disabilities. *Res Developmental Disabil* 2000; 21:469-86.
[25] Henderson CM, Rosasco M, Robinson LM, Meccarello J, Janicki MP, Turk MA, et al. Functional impairment severity is associated with health status among older persons with intellectual disability and cerebral palsy. *J Intellect Disabil Res* 2009; 53:887-97.
[26] Mansyur C, Amick BC, Harrist RB, Franzini L. Social capital, income inequality, and self-rated health in 45 countries. *Soc Sci Med* 2008; 66:43-56.
[27] Berry HL, Rodgers B, Dear KB. Preliminary development and validation of an Australian community participation questionnaire: types of participation and associations with distress in a coastal community. *Soc Sci Med* 2007; 64:1719-37.
[28] Putnam RD. *Bowling alone: The collapse and revival of American community*, New York: Simon & Schuster, 2000.

[29] Guimarães JM, Jorge MS, Maia RC, de Oliveira LC, Morais AP, Lima MP, Assis MM, dos Santos AM. Social participation in mental health: space of construction of citizenship, policy formulation and decision making. *Cien Saude Colet* 2010; 15: 2113-22.

[30] Truelle JL, Koskinen S, Hawthorne G, Sarajuuri J, Formisano R, Von Wild K, et al. The Qolibri Task Force. Quality of life after traumatic brain injury: The clinical use of the QOLIBRI, a novel disease-specific instrument. *Brain Inj* 2010; 24: 1272-91.

[31] Jette AM, Keysor J, Coster W, Ni P, Haley S. Beyond function: predicting participation in a rehabilitation cohort. *Arch Phys Med Rehab* 2005; 86: 2087-94.

[32] Carod-Artal J, Egido JA, González JL, Varela de Seijas E. Quality of life among stroke survivors evaluated 1 year after stroke: experience of a stroke unit. *Stroke* 2000; 3:2995-3000.

[33] Carod-Artal FJ, Ferreira Coral L, Trizotto DS, Menezes Moreira C. Poststroke depression: prevalence and determinants in Brazilian stroke patients. *Cerebrovasc Dis* 2009; 28:157-65.

[34] Carod-Artal FJ, Ferreira Coral L, Trizotto DS, Menezes Moreira C. Burden and perceived health status among caregivers of stroke patients. *Cerebrovasc Dis* 2009; 28:472-80.

[35] Ottawa Charter for Health Promotion. First International Conference on Health Promotion, Ottawa, 21 November 1986. WHO/HPR/HEP/95.1. Available from: URL: *http://www.who.int/hpr/NPH/docs/ottawa_charter_hp.pdf.*

[36] Rossi E, Baraldi C. The promotion of children's and adolescents' social participation in Italy and Scotland. *Children & Society* 2009; 23: 16-28.

[37] Cattan M. *Mental Health and Well-being in Later Life*. Maidenhead: McGraw-Hill/Open University Press, 2009.

[38] Department of Health. *New Horizons: Confident communities, brighter futures. A framework for developing wellbeing*. London: HMSO, DoH, 2010.

[39] Government of South Australia, SA Health. South Australia's Mental Health and Wellbeing Policy 2010-2015. Available from: URL: *http://www.health.sa.gov.au/mentalhealth/Portals/0/samhwb10-15-mh-sahealth-100531.pdf.*

[40] Mental Health Association NSW. Sign up, Link in, Get involved Factsheet. 2009. Available from: URL: *http://www.mentalhealth.asn.au/wellbeingdocs/3.SignUpFactsheet2009.pdf.*

[41] Gele AA, Harsløf I. Types of social capital resources and self-rated health among the Norwegian adult population. *Int J Equity Health* 2010; 9:8.

[42] Cattan M, White M, Bond J, Learmonth A. Preventing social isolation and Loneliness among older people: a systematic review of health promotion interventions. *Ageing and Society* 2005; 25: 41-67.

[43] Whitehead M, Dahlgren G. What can be done about inequalities in health? *Lancet* 1991; 338:1059-63.

[44] Norheim OF, Asada Y. The ideal of equal health revisited: definitions and measures of inequity in health should be better integrated with theories of distributive justice. *Int J Equity Health* 2009; 8: 40.

In: Social Determinants and Mental Health
Editor: Sabine Bährer-Kohler

ISBN: 978-1-61324-353-4
©2012 Nova Science Publishers, Inc.

Chapter 8

SOCIAL NETWORKS AND MENTAL HEALTH

***Hui-Ching Wu*[1] *and I-Chen Tang*[2]**
[1]National Taiwan University, Department of Social Work, Taipei, Taiwan
[2]Department of Medical Sociology and Social Work, Chung-Shan Medical University
Taichung, Taiwan

THE INTER-RELATIONSHIP BETWEEN SOCIAL NETWORKS AND MENTAL HEALTH

One factor related to mental health is the social network. Since the 1950s, the World Health Organization began to challenge the definition of health as the absence of health, there has been increasingly growing body of literature focusing on discussion of definition and determinants of health (Jacobsen, 2008; Moniz & Gorin, 2010). Mental health is an integral and essential component of health (WHO, 2010). "No health without mental health" say Prince et al. (2007) who believe mental health needs to be recognized as an integrated part of health. According to Hales (2009), the determinants of health can be explored from six dimensions: physical, psychological, social, spiritual, intellectual and environmental health. These factors are not only distinct but also interrelated. Multiple social, psychological, and biological factors were found to determine the level of mental health of a person at any point of time (WHO, 2010).

Individuals have been recognized as social beings living in the ecological environments. Not only individuals have to interact with other people, fulfill social roles effectively but also cope with daily events. WHO (2010) indicated that mental health is a state of well-being in which an individual realizes his or her own abilities, can cope with the normal stresses of life, can work productively and is able to make a contribution to his or her community. People are psychologically affected by the aspects of social environment in which they live such as economic change, poor housing, social status and the financial strain of unemployment (Liem & Liem, 1978; Dooley, et al., 1994; Lin & Peek, 1999; Artazcoz et al., 2004; Brunner & Marmot, 2006; Theodossiou & Zangelidis, 2009). In times of crisis, being in such kind of stressful situations can cause psychological distress, especially when individuals are socially excluded or lack of social connection. All of these problems highlight the level of social integration in the communities and the resources influence the mental health of those individuals (Brugha, 1995; Tuner, 1999).

The network of social connection and interaction provides opportunities through which social support is made available. Networks were viewed as one dynamic element in the process of support and that comprise the properties of social composition, structure and relations. Under the category of structurally focused network composition variables, ties, density and size had generally positive effects, but there were some findings of negative effects on mental health as well as findings of insignificance.

Mental health would be directly affected by ego's access to and use of intimate ties, ties with whom ego can confide and share important and "inner" thoughts (Lin, 1986). The extent to which ego is involved and on the properties of networks. That is, networks may exert effects on a person's mental health indirectly because the social networks, in part, determines whether a person may draw upon a particular tie (node) for intimate and confidential interactions. The psychosocial variables can be concluded have both direct and indirect effects on mental health. Each of the social network's properties may have both significant and insignificant effects on mental health (Lin & Peek, 1999). For instance, people with mental health problems may put demands on their social network without being able to reciprocate when others in the social network need support from them (Kumar & Browne, 2008). This might lead their social network to shrink with an accumulation of negative experience. The negative psychotic symptoms were also found to correlate with smaller, more dysfunctional social networks (Hamilton et al., 1989).

Social Network Functioning

Social networks were defined as individuals or groups with a common bond, shared functions, or geographic of cultural connection (Bowling, 1997). Interest in social networks grew in the 1950s, with attempts to analyze ties common to groups that could go beyond the limitations of conventional construct like kin groups, tribes, and villages (Berkman & Glass, 2000). Wasylenki, et al., (1992) described social networks by using structural and functional terms. Structure refers to network size, density, and kin versus non-kin composition. Functional characteristics include reciprocity, accessibility, homogeneity, multiplexity and others.

Examples of social networks are support system, the natural helping network, self-help groups, and groups of formal organizations that address a common problem (Barker, 1999). The effects of social networks on mental health may be appreciated by focusing on the fact that the utility of network characteristics in providing support (through intimate ties) varies depending on the individual's social position, stage of life course, and composition of role relationships in his or her network. In short, a social network helps people to obtain social resources and supportive behaviors.

Four benefits of social networks on mental health have been identifies. First, it facilitates people social integration in terms of providing a sense of comfort and security to minimize threat or disruption to one's well-being. A well-integrate living environments reduces the likelihood that certain deviant behavior (e.g. community crimes).For instance, minority ethnic groups living in a discriminated society are not only at greater risk from social exclusion and marginalization but also at risk of developing psychological distress and depression (Kelaher et al., 2008; Agudelo-Suárez et al, 2009). Anti-stigma campaign on mental health grounds can also help mental health service users reduce social exclusion. The second, it reinforces one's feeling of social identity, worthiness, and values. Koneru et al. (2007) review existing literature on acculturation and mental health, some evidence indicate that while maintaining one's cultural identity, if individuals can also adopt new ones from the host culture, greater acculturation can help to reduce social alienation and fewer stress symptoms. The third, it provides enduring or intermittent ties that help maintain the psychological and physical integrity of individual (Caplan, 1974). The forth, it helps individuals access from resources when their own resources are limited and may be insufficient to meet certain needs, especially in time of crisis (e.g., death of a loved one, job loss, exposure to political violence or sexual minority) (Pedersen, 2002; Meyer, Schwartz & Frost, 2008; Scutella & Wooden, 2008; Miller & Rasmussen, 2010; Tol et al., 2010).

Social networks may have a protective effect on mental health by buffering individuals from the ill effects of stressful events (Husaini, 1982; Berkman, 1995; Kumar & Browne, 2008) or support treatment (DiMatteo, 2004) for the psychological discomfort. When this buffering is absent or withdrawn due to a fragmented or dysfunctional social network, an individual's vulnerability to mental disorder may increase (Kumar & Browne, 2008).

The Wellness of Mental Health

The wellness of mental health is determined by the degree of social integration. By social integration, it means the level of interaction and cooperation with others in a society. The concept of social integration affects well-being generated from Durkheim's (1987) study of suicide. Durkheim believes suicide rates vary according to the degree of social ties someone has within a community (Stansfeld, 2006; Moniz & Gorin, 2010). He suggested that social relationships such as marriage, parenthood, religious involvement, and employment promote health (i.e., reduce suicide), provide a meaningful and purposeful life, and create a set of social constraints or controls on individual behavior. In other words, the high rates of the mental disorders were attribute to weaker or a lack of social integration (Faris & Dunham, 1939; Leighton, 1959). This suggests that human beings are social, therein, social contact and social interact formulate psychological support. The social integration symbolizes a construction of social networks.

The effects of social networks on mental health are moderate at best. The measuring of social networks depends on numbers, size, frequency or density of contacts individuals interact with a group of persons (Stansfeld, 2006; Eklund & Hansson, 2007). For example, the significance of a spouse is expected to vary depending upon the absence or presence of children, whether both spouses participate in the labor force (Artazcoz et al., 2004), or the extent to which the spouses maintain their own networks. Relations with supervisor or co-worker may be more or less supportive or stressful depending on possibilities for moving to other jobs, offices, or organizations. Likewise, a "significant other" at one time in a person's life may be become less significant at a later phase, when someone who is less significant will assume more significance. Siblings may be important for teenagers, but not as important for the individuals when they form their own marriages, families, and careers (Smith, et al., 2000;

Friedrich, et al., 2008). Yet, as people age, as their children grow up and depart, and as they lose their spouses, siblings may again assume significance as confiding partners. In other words, advantages of certain social compositions in one's network differ over the life course, and the variations may be curvilinear rather than linear over the life-span.

SOCIAL NETWORKS AND SOCIAL SUPPORT

How do social networks work on mental health? There is an emerging trend to view the social network as a construct with several dimensions including the structure of the network, satisfaction with the network and social support (Sandler & Barrera, 1984, Vaux & Harrison, 1985). The social networks and social support are reciprocity. Social networks involve the quantity and structure of a person's relationships, the social support provided by those relationship, and their impact on that person's well-being (O'Reilly, 1988). Perl & Trickett (1988) asserted that social support is one of the functions provided by a social network, and can be viewed as the comfort and support received from other people through various types of relationship.

Social support generally refers to help provided by others that promotes emotional mastery, offers guidance, or provides feedback regarding the individual's identity (Cassel, 1976; Brown & Harris, 1978). Tunder (1999) defined social support as referring to the clarity or certainty with which the individual experience being loved, and it able to count on others should the need arise. The domains of social support include "social bonds" (Henderson, 1977), "social network" (Wellman & Wortley, 1989), "meaningful social contact" (Cassel, 1976), "availability of confidences" (Brown, Bhronchain & Harris, 1975), and "human companionship" (Lynch, 1977, p. 198). Tuner (1999) stressed that social bonds and supportive relationships with others have a significant impact on maintaining mental health and that social support can protect people from the effects of stressors. Social bonds/ties provide the linkage and sources of support system.

To understand the quality and resources of support, social support can be measured according to types of support such as emotional and practical support (Stansfeld, 2006). Cobb (1976) identifies social support as being composed of instrumental (counseling, assisting), active (mothering), and material (providing gods or services) support. Walsh and Connelly (1996) categorized social support as material support, emotional support, and instrumental support. House (1981) defined social support as the form of emotional support, appraisal support, informal support, or instrumental support. He continued to review other studies that examined the value of "social support" for the health and well-being. According to House, emotional support can take the form of esteem affect, trust, and listening to strengthen an individual's ego and that is directly associated with better mental and physical health (Vaux, 1988; Thoits, 1995). Appraisal support is exemplified by affirmation, feedback, and social comparison. Informal social support comes in the form of advice, suggestion, directives, and information. And finally, instrumental support is exemplified by aid in kind, money, labor, time, or modifying the environment in beneficial ways.

Barker (1999) describes social support including formal and informal activities and relationships providing for the needs of humans in their efforts to live in society. These needs include education, income security, health care, and most especially, a network of other individuals and groups who offer encouragement, access, empathy, role models, and social identity (p. 1156).

Social support and mental health are associated. From the positive effects of support, social support has important implications for reducing social strain, protecting health, and enhancing the quality of life for people with mental health difficulties (Eklund & Hansson, 2007; Lischka, et al., 2009). Social support is beneficial for alleviating some of the harmful effects of daily life stress experienced by individuals. Ross and Mirowsky (1989) found that symptoms of depression and anxiety decrease as social support increases. Social support can also minimize the negative effects of stress and bolster coping efforts, decreasing the risk of relapse, and improve social functioning (House, 1981; Etzion, 1984; Beehr, 1985; Ganster et al., 1986). The social support functions act as a stress buffer (Stansfeld, 2006; Wu, 2008) same as social networks. Hence, the more social support a person possess, the less negative impact stressors will have on that person. On the contrary, individuals with a low level of support could increase the risk for depression or for mental health problems generally, whether or not exposure to unusual stressor had occurred (Henderson, 1992; Buchannan, 1995).

El-Bassel, Chen, and Cooper (1998) reviewed two theoretical models to indicate how and why different people seek social support. The Hierarchical-compensatory model suggest that social support is provided in a hierarchical, descending order; beginning with the person whom is closest to, no matter what the task is (Cantor; Shanas as cited in El-Bassel, Chen, & Cooper, 1998). There are optional ties with greater flexibility to change than, for example, original family, work mates or neighbor (Antonucci, 1990). When people face the difficulty, they may go to a spouse, then kin, friends, neighbors, and then formal; organizations. In this model, the choice of whom to ask for support follows an ordered preference according to the degree of intimacy between the receiver and giver. The Task-Specific Model of support developed by Litwak (1985) suggests that the flow of flow of support depends on the match between characteristics of particular tasks and the characteristics of social supports that match those tasks. This model de-emphasizes order of preference and stresses structural and functional properties of the task. In the Task-Specific model, the individual asks: Which group can best help me with my mental health issues and problems?

SOCIAL NETWORKS AND SOCIAL SUPPORT IN COLLECTIVE CULTURES

According to Stansfeld (2006), social support operates both an individual and a societal level. Western cultures strengthen personal independence, encouraging individuals to believe that their decisions are their own and to view longings for depensency as sign of morbidity (Neki, 1973, as cited in Kumar & Browne, 2008). In a collective culture, groups are considered more important than individuals. The social networks should carry more weight in such cultures for maintaining a well-being. Murray (2001) and Loewenthal (2007) suggest culture as a determinant of mental health. Eastern society such as Asian-Chinese society emphasizes collectivistic culture and views the self as an interdependent part of family and community, where group harmony and well-being are more highly values (Wu, 2006). Western culture emphasizes personal independence, self-sufficiency, and the importance and uniqueness of the individual that may be not applicable to an Eastern culture. Consequence, the size, density, ties, and multiplexity might tend to be more limited.

Studies in Taiwan found the social support system as including medical support, family support, and social services support (Zhang, 1988; Lin, 2002). These supportive systems can be viewed as a solid foundation for an individual to use for living in a safe environment and enabling him/her to cope with stressors and hardship in the daily life. Hence, it can be inferred that enhancing social support for people with mental health difficulties both addresses their needs and is psychologically beneficial.

The central structures of authority for most Eastern families are based on kinship (Thornton & Lin, 1994). For instance, when an Asian-Chinese family has a member with mental health difficulties, all the other members tend to look for help from each other and their close friends, relatives or their belief system. Several studies found that people with mental health difficulties had fewer support systems than did healthy people and the majority of their support came from families in both Western and Eastern cultures (Lin, 2002). In a collective culture, the role of informal social support from families and friends placed the greatest impact on quality of life for an individual with mental health difficulties (Wu, 2008).

CONCLUSION

Social networks have the potential to provide individuals with protection and support. The construct of social networks would prevent the negative mental health condition and change unhealthy life style, directly or indirectly. The preventive mechanism aimed at universal (general), selective (at risky) or indicated (mental disorder) population (http://www.euphix.org/object_document/o5484n27411.html) to provide a supportive environment while they encounter the social stress. Through the formation of relationships and/or improved quality of existing relationship would contribute to the mental health conditions. Based on the difference, the effects of social network have to incorporate with the cultural factor to provide the needed social support.

REFERENCES

Agudelo-Suárez, A., Gil-González, D., Ronda-Pérez, E., Porthé, V., Paramio-Pérez,G., Garcia, A.M. & Gari, A. (2009). Discrimination, work, and health in immigrant populations in Spain, *Social Science & Medicine*, 68, 1866-1874.

Artazcoz, L., Benach, J., Borrell, C. & Cortes, I. (2004). Unemployment and Mental Health: Understanding the Interactions Among Gender, Family Roles and Social Class, *American Journal of Public Health*, 94(1), 82-88.

Barker, R. L. (1999). *The social work dictionary*, 4th Ed. Washington, DC: NASW press.

Beehr, T. A. (1985), The role of social support in coping with organizational stress, pp. 375-398 in Beehr & Bhagat (eds), *Human Stress and Cognition in Organizations*, NY; John Wiley & Sons, Inc.

Berkman, L. F. & Glass, T. (2000). A hisotryical framework for social epidemiology. In L. F. Berkman & I. Kawachi (Eds.), *Social epidemiology* (pp.3-12). New York: Oxford Univeristy Press.

Bowling, N. (1997). Measuring social network and social support in measuring health: *Review of quality of life measurement scales* (2nd ed.). Buckingham, UK: Open Univeristy Press.

Brown, G. W., Bhrolchain, M. N. & Harris, T. (1975). Social class and psychiatric disturbance among women in an urban population. *Sociology*, 2:225-54.

Brown, G. W. & Harris, T. O. (1978). *Social origins of depression : A study of psychiatric disorder in women.* New York: Free Press.

Brugha, T. S. (Ed.) (1995). *Social support and psychiatric disorder*. Cambridge, MA: Cambridge University Press.

Brunner, E. & Marmot, M. (2006). Social organization, stress and health. In Marmot, M. & Wilkinson, R.G. (ed.), *Social determinants of health*, (2nd ed., pp.6-30), Oxford, OUP.

Buchanan, J. (1995). Social support and schizophrenia: A review of the literature. *Archives of Psychiatric Nursing*, 9(2), 68-76.

Caplan, G. (1974). *Support system and community mental health: Lectures on concept development*. New York: Behavioral Publications.

Cassel, J. (1976). The contribution of the social environment to host resistance. *American Journal of Epidemiology* 14, 107-23.

Cobb, S. (1976). Social support as a moderator of life stress. Psychosomatic Medicine 38: 300-14. In Horwitz, A.V. & Scheid, T.L. (Eds.) *A handbook for the study of mental health: Social contexts, theories, and systems.* Cambridge, U.K.: Cambridge University Press

DiMatteo, M. R. (2004). Social support and patient adherence to medical treatment: A meta-analysis. *Health psychology*, 23(2). 207-218.

Dooley, D., Catalano, R. & Wilson, G. (1994). Depression and unemployment: Panel findings from the epidemiologic catchment area study. *America Journal Community Psychology*, 22,742-65.

Durkheim, E. (1987). *Suicide: A study in Sociology*. New York: Free Press.

Eklund, M. & Hansson, L. (2007). Social network among people with persistent mental illness: Associations with sociodemographic clinical and health-related factors. *International Journal of Social Pyshicatry*, 55(4), 293-305.

El-Bassel, N., Chen, D. R. & Cooper, D. (1998). Social support and social network profiles among women on methadone. *The Social Service Review*, 72 (3), 379-401.

Etzion, D. (1984). Moderating effect of social suppport on the stress-nurnout relationship. *Journal of Applied Psychology* 69, 615-622.

Faris, R. E.L. & Dunham, H. W. (1939). Mental disorders in urban areas: An ecology study of schizophrenia and other psychoses. University of Chicago Press.

Friedrich, R. M., Lively, S. & Rubenstein, L. M.(2008). Siblings' Coping Strategies and Mental Health Services : *A National Study of Siblings of Persons With Schizophrenia. Psychiatric Services*,(3),261-266.

Ganster, D. C., Fusilier, M. R. & Mayers, B. T. (1986). Role of social upport in the experience of stress at work. *Journal of Applied Psychology* 71, 102-110.

Hales, D. (2009). *An Invitation to Health* (2009-2010 Edition), Belmont: Wadsworth, Cengage.

Hamilton, N. G., Ponzoha, C. A., Cutler, D. L. & Weigel, R. M. (1989). Social networks and schizophrenia. *Schizophrenia Bulletin*, 4,522-545.

Henderson, S. (1977). The social network, support, and neurosis: The functions of attachment in adult life. *Brit. J. Psychiatry*, 131,185-91.

Henderson, A. S. (1992). *Social support and depression.* In Veil & Bauman (1992b: 85-92).

House, J. S. (1981). Work Stress and Social Support. Reading, MA: Addison-Wesley. In Horwitz, A.V. & Scheid, T.L. (1999). In Horwitz, A.V. & Scheid, T.L. (Eds.) *A handbook for the study of mental health: Social contexts, theories, and systems.* Cambridge, U.K.: Cambridge University Press.

Husaini, B. A. (Ed.). (1982). Stress and psychiatric symptoms: Personality and social support as buffers [Special Issue]. *Journal of Community Psychology*, 10, 291-425.

Jacobsen, K.H. (2008). *Introduction to Global Health*, London: Jones and Bartlett.

Kelaher, M., Paul, S., Lambert, H. Ahmad, W. Paradies, Y. & Smith, G. D. (2008). Discrimination and Health in an English Study, *Social Science & Medicine*, 66, 1627-1636.

Kumar, S. & Browne, M. A. O. (2007). Usefulness of the construct of social network to explain mental health service utilization by the Maori population in New Zealand. *Transcultural Psychiatry*, 45(3), 439-454.

Leighton, A. H. (1959). *My name is legion*. New York: Basic Books.

Liem, R. & Liem, J. H. (1978). Social class and mental illness reconsidered: The role of economic stress and social support. *Journal of Health & Social Behavior*, 19, 139-56.

Lin, W. H. (2002). *Employment experience of adults with mental illness living in the community*. Hua Lian: Tziu-Chi University, Masters Dissertation.

Lin, N. & Peek, K. (1999). Social networks and mental health. In Horwitz, A.V. & Scheid, T.L. (Eds.) *A handbook for the study of mental health: Social contexts, theories, and systems*. Cambridge, U.K.: Cambridge University Press.

Litwak, E. (1985*). Helping the elderly: The complimentary roles of Informal networks and formal systems.* NY: The Guilford Press.

Loewenthal, K. (2007). *Religion, culture and mental health*, Cambridge: CUP. Lynch, 1977, p. 198

Meyer, I. H., Schwartz, S. & Frost, D.M. (2008). Social patterning of stress and coping: Does disadvantaged social statuses confer more stress and few coping resources? Social *Science & Medicine,* 67, 368-379.

Miller, K.E. & Rasmussen, A. (2010). War exposure, daily stressors, and mental health in conflict andpost-conflict settings: Beidging the divide between trauma-focused and psychosocial frameworks, *Social Science & Medicine*, 70, 7-16.

Moniz, C. & Gorin, S. (2010). *Health and Mental Health Care Policy: A Biopsychosocial Perspective, 3rd ed.*, London: Allyn & Bacon, pp.244-5.

Murray, C. B. (2001). Culture as a determinant of mental health. In Melser, N.J. & Baltes, P.B. (Ed.), *International Encyclopedia of the Socail & Behavioral Sciences*, pp.3143-3147. Pergamon: Amsterdam.

Neki, J. S. (1973). Guru-chela relationship: The possibility of a therapeutic paradigm. *American Journal of Orthopsychiatry*, 43(5), 755-166.

O'Reilly, P. (1988). Methologicla issues in social support and social network research. *Social Science & Medicine*, 26, 863-73.

Pedersen, D. (2002). Political violence, ethnic conflict, and contemporary wars: broad implications for health and social well-being, *Social Science & Medicine*, 55, 175-190.

Prince, M., Patel, V., Saxena, S., Maj, M., Maselko, J., Phillips, M.R. & Rahman, A. (2007). No Health without Mental Health, *Lancet*, 370, 859-77.

Ross, C.E., & Mirowsky, J. (1989). Explaining the social patterns of depression: control and problem solving - or support and taking? *J. Health & Social Behavior*, 30, 206-19.

Sandler, I. N., & Barrera, M. Jr (1984). Toward a multi-method approach to assessing the effects of social support. *American Journal of Community of Psychology*, 12(1), 37-52.

Scutella, R. & Wooden, M. (2008). The effects of household joblessness on mental health, *Social Science & Medicine*, 67, 88-100.

Smith, G. C., Hatfield, A. B. & Miller, D. C. (2000). Planning by older mothers for the future care of offspring with serious mental illness. *Psychiatric Services*, 51(9), 1162–1166.

Stansfeld, S.A. (2006). Social support and social cohesion. In Marmot, M. & Wilkinson, R.G. (ed.), *Social determinants of health*, (2nd ed., pp.148-71, Oxford, OUP.

Theodossiou, I. & Zangelidis, A. (2009). The social gradient in health: The effect of absolute income and subjective social status assessment on the individual's health in Europe, *Economic and Human Biology*, 7, 229-237.

Thoits, P.A. (1995), Stress, coping, and social support process: where are we? What next? *Journal of Health and Social Behavior*, (extra issue): 53-79.

Thornton, A. & Lin, H.S. (1994). Introduction. In Thornton, A. & Lin, H.S.(ed.), *Social change and the family in Taiwan,* London: University of Chicago.

Tol, W.A., Kohrt, B.A., Jordans, M.J.D., Thapa, S.B., Pettigrew, J. Upadhaya, N. de Jong,J. T. V. M. (2010). Political violence and mental health: A multi-disciplinary review of the literature on Nepal, *Social Science & Medicine*, 70, 35-44.

Turner, S. J. (1999). Social support and coping. In Horwitz, A.V. & Scheid, T.L. (Eds.) *A handbook for the study of mental health: Social contexts, theories, and systems*, 198-210. Cambridge, U.K.: Cambridge University Press.

Vaux, A. & Harrison, D. (1985). Support network characteristics associated with support satisfaction and perceived support. *American Journal of Community Psychology*, 13(3), 245-268.

Vaux, A. (1988). Social support: Theory, research, and intervention. New York: Praeger.

Walsh, J. & Connelly, P.R. (1996). Supported behaviors in natural support networks of people with serious mental illness. *Health & Social Work,* 21(4), PA Research II Periodicals, 296-303.

Wasylenki, D., James, S., Clark, A., Lewis., Goering, P., & Gillies, L . (1992). Clinical issues in social network therapy for clients with schizophrenia. *Community Mental Health Journal* , 38(5), 427-440.

Wellman, B., & S. Wortley. (1989). Brother's keepers: Situating kin relations in broader networks of social support. Sociological Perspectives 32: 273-306. In Horwitz, A.V. & Scheid, T.L. (Eds.). *A handbook for the study of mental health: Social contexts, theories, and systems*. Cambridge, U.K.: Cambridge University Press.

WHO (2010). *www.who.int/mediacentre/factsheets/fs220/en*

Wu, H. C. (2006). The Effect of Work on People with Severe Mental Illness in Taiwan Using a Stress-Social Support Model: An Exploratory Study. *International Journal of Rehabilitation,* Volume 29(2), pp 145-150

Wu, H. C. (2008). Predicting Subjective Quality of Life in Workers with Psychiatric Disabilities. *Community Mental Health Journa*l, Volume 44(2), pp 135-146

Zhang, Y. C. (1988). *The relationship between social support and rehabilitation for the chronic mentally ill.* Tai Chung: Tung-Hai University, Masters Dissertation.

In: Social Determinants and Mental Health
Editor: Sabine Bährer-Kohler

ISBN: 978-1-61324-353-4

Chapter 9

SOCIAL SUPPORT AND MENTAL HEALTH: SOCIAL SUPPORT AND MENTAL HEALTH IN AGEING AND OLD AGE

Ignat C. Petrov
Bulgarian Association of Ageing, Sofia, Bulgaria

INTRODUCTION

The World Health Organization has proposed a definition of health that includes mental health as an integral component. Health is a state of optimal physical, mental and social well-being, not just the absence of diseases and infirmity. One important factor relating to mental health is social support.

The WHO notices that poor mental health is also associated with rapid social change, stressful work conditions, discrimination, unhealthy lifestyle, risks of violence and physical ill-health, human rights violations and social exclusion (WHO, 2010).

Social support, in turn, is a generic term describing a wide range of experiences from which people of all age groups and different biographical backgrounds draw feelings of security and comfort that protect them from emptiness, loneliness and despair (Angermeyer et al. 1989). Social relationships are defined as social structures of contact bonds among individuals or groups of relatives, colleagues, friends and neighbors. These relationships are based upon reciprocal trust (de Belvis & coll., 2008).

The term social network describes mainly the structure, whereas social support refers to the content of that structure (Klusmann 1989). Social networks differ in composition, number of members, frequency of contacts, and also geographic proximity. Social networks are crucial for individual's way of life and represent a dimension of social capital influencing reciprocal exchanges of support and knowledge (de Belvis & coll., 2008).

Like Dr. Bährer-Kohler has written in her foreword social support is related also to the ability to cope with stress and illness and has been demonstrated by, for example, Klauer et al. (2001) and Wills et al. (2001).

In the next lines we quote some examples which illustrate the importance of social support not only for the mental health of older people but also in relation with other health problems.

A recent Canadian study of 3,834 Canadian-born and 1,495 foreign-born women clearly shows that depression in pregnant minority women deserves more attention, independently of their length of stay in Canada. It also demonstrates unmistakably that social support favoring integration and poverty reduction interventions could reduce this risk of depression (Miszkurka et al. 2010).

In another current study entitled *Marital Loss, Mental Health and the Role of Perceived Social Support: Findings from Six Waves of an Australian Population-based Panel Study*, Hewitt et al. were able to prove that marital loss has a significant impact on mental health. They conclude that increasing, or maintaining, high levels of social support has the potential to improve widowed men's mental health immediately after the death of their spouse (Hewitt et al. 2010).

Writing about *social support and mental health among college students*, Hefner et al. (2009) found that college students with lower-quality social support, as measured by the Multidimensional Scale of Perceived Social Support, were more likely to experience mental health problems.

Furthermore, Lee et al. (2007), in their work on *The Effect of Social Support on Mental and Behavioral Outcomes Among Adolescents With Parents With HIV/AIDS*, underscore the complex relations between social support and mental and behavioral outcomes among adolescents affected by HIV/AIDS. They conclude that future prevention programs must focus on increasing social support to reduce negative outcomes among adolescents affected by HIV/AIDS as well as on the need to reduce the influence of negative role models.

In meta-analyses like that by Stansfeld et al. (2006) entitled *Psychosocial Work Environment and Mental Health* it was documented that low social support, high psychological demands, effort-reward imbalance, and high job insecurity predict common mental disorders.

The WHO also points out that integrated government policies that promote social cohesion through the development and stimulation of social networks and empowerment, and through decreases in material inequalities, will also contribute to the promotion of mental health and reduce the premature death and disability that results from mental ill health (WHO 2004; Patel 2005).

AGING: A PSYCHOSOCIAL VIEW

With respect to the demographic processes we now see increasing proportions of the world population live to experience old age. The great increase in the world old age population comes nowadays from the rapidly developing countries. The prospect of merely living longer presents many problems related with physical and mental health, psychological and social well-being, of the elderly people.

Ageing is a biological, as well as psychic and social phenomenon. With other words, ageing is a bio-psycho-social unity. And, it is a process of individual development and life-long adaptation.

A distinguishing feature of the human from the other living beings is that psychic and social development may not coincide with the biological trajectory of ageing. In individual cases successful ageing could be a time of continued growth, development, and achievement. In the history of the world culture, talented personalities have created their best work at the very end of their lives notwithstanding the obvious signs of biological decline (Petrov, 1981). One of the most brilliant examples is Michelangelo Buonarroti (1475-1564). Dying at the age of 89 years, he intended to continue to work on his fourth and most profound Pieta - Pieta Rondanini. At his death he headed as architect the construction of the cathedral of San Pietro in Rome and finished off its cupola. And, after the age of 70 he wrote his best verses.

Aside from the examples of genial creators, in all historical periods there were a proportion of people who developed with their ageing an expertise called wisdom enabling them to give good advices in matters of the practical life (Baltes, 1993; Baltes & Staudinger, 2000). And, for the majority of people, the late-life period could also be successful and meaningful in the terms of simply "being in life" (Coleman & O'Hanlon, 2004).

Mental Health and Social Gerontology Approaches

According the World Health Organization definition of health, it is a state of optimal physical, mental and social well-being, not just the absence of diseases and infirmity. Such a comprehensive integrative view of physical, mental and social well-being is often encountered in the multidimensional assessments of older persons in gerontology and geriatrics (Busse, 1987).

The social dimensions of the mental health are often studied in gerontology using different, but close of meaning concepts, like: successful ageing, adjustment to ageing, active ageing, contentment, life satisfaction, self-esteem, morale, subjective well-being, and quality of life in ageing and old age.

A number of gerontological studies on various populations interpret the role of social factors for mental health in ageing. One example is the Handbook of Mental Health and Aging (co-eds. J.E. Birren and R.B. Sloane) (1980) with diverse chapters on the subject, and another example is the comprehensive review of Alan Walker on Quality of life in old age in Europe, a part of the book *Quality of life in old age* (Eds. H. Mollencopf & A. Walker), Springer, 2007.

In most cases, the preconditions for having a successful and active life include relatively good health, economic security, and family and social support. Studies on Bulgarian rural elderly population revealed that value orientations at the age 70 years and over were focused on few vital themes: the own health and the health of the partner, the family relations in a narrow circle, and economic security (Petrov, 1975; 1976).

Health of the Aged in Social Context

A relatively good health is a condition for psychological well-being in older ages. Not only the full absence of diseases. In older age almost every person has a number of diseases and/or functional limitations. In most cases they are chronic and well compensated disorders, with a slow progression. The cardiovascular and the musculoskeletal diseases affect more than the half of the older people (Bourliere and Vallery-Masson, 1985). Common are also the diseases of respiratory system, of the eyes, and other disorders. In very old age, where the limitations are more expressed, the person learns "to live with a disease" (Senin, 1999). The prevalence of mental disorders in the age 60 or 65 and over is about 20-30%. Only one third of them are dementias or psychoses. The majority are mild disorders (Slater and Roth, 1969; Blazer, 1980; Petrov and coll., 2007). Cognitive decline is the main mental health problem in older age. Moderate and severe dementias affect 5-7% of the population aged 65 and over. Dementias are age-dependent: at the age of 65-69 their prevalence is 1.4%, but it doubles every 5 years and reaches 23,6% at the age of 85 and over (Jorm, 1987). Currently around 35.6 million people worldwide are living with dementia. (ADI, 2010). The second main mental health problem in older age is depression, mostly minor depressions.

While older adults are at increased risk for mental illness, most of them can be characterized as mentally healthy (Busse, 1987; Petrov and coll., 2007).

According to various population studies the level of general health in older age correlates with the scores of life satisfaction at 0.2 – 0.5 (Edwards and Klemmack, 1973; Larsson, 1978; Bourne, Morris and Eldemire-Shearer, 2010). The data from the National Survey on the State of Life and the Desire for Welfare of the Elderly in South Korea on 3 278 people aged 65 and over revealed that the life satisfaction was influenced mostly by the economic condition and health status (Jung, Muntaner & Choi, 2010).

The theme of the health takes up a cardinal place in the value orientations of the older people and it is a common reason of concern and worries (I. Petrov, 1975; 1976; 1978a). It is interesting to know what aspects of the polimorbidity of older people mostly influence their self-esteem? The study on the Bulgarian rural population shows that the self-evaluations of health and happiness were affected mostly by diseases (arthroses, fractures, stroke, severe impairment of vision, and others) which impede directly the mobility and independent mode of life (Petrov, 1976; 1978a). The self-rated overall health is related to the life satisfaction, especially of older women (Berg, 2008).

The Role of Economic Security

The correlation between the amount of income and the life satisfaction of older people is about 0.1 and 0.4 according to various studies. The link is more expressed at the lower rates of income. After passing some level of income, its influence on the life satisfaction become more weak (Larsson, 1978, and others). According to the classical New York study of Kutner, differences determined by the income were greater among the still working than among retired elderly people (Kutner et al., 1956). These data confirm that work activity has an influence on the self-esteem not only through the income but also with other, more complex characteristics. According to the same study of Kutner, the ill health influences less the life satisfaction of the elderly with higher financial status (minimal differences between people with better and worse health) than the life satisfaction of the poor elderly people (the corresponding differences were greater). Moreover, two thirds of the people from the group with lower incomes have been at the same time partly or fully socially isolated. Hence, ill health, poor financial security and social isolation could be regarded as three social factors mutually aggravating each other. According to the study of Arnaudova and coll. (1984) 42% of the elderly from Bulgarian rural population and 34% in the cities have specified that their incomes were insufficient. After the study on the rural population aged 70 years and over from 46 Bulgarian villages (Petrov, 1975, 1976) the concern about financial security was presented at 35% in the content of the values of happiness and at 29% in the motives of dissatisfaction; and, the correlation between the amount of income and the self-evaluation of social prestige was 0.23. According to the recent ISTAT cross-sectional survey on 33 744 people aged 60 years and over in Italy, those who reported a lower household income tended to have lower life satisfaction and worse mental state (de Belvis & coll., 2008). Uhde (2009) also founds that concern about the economic situation has a negative impact on the personal life satisfaction of the German population. We quoted above the data from the National Survey on the State of Life and the Desire for Welfare of the Elderly in South Korea on 3 278 people aged 65 and over. According to that study the most influential factor to the life satisfaction in both men and women was the economic condition (Jung, Muntaner & Choi, 2010).

Another important aspect closely linked with the financial security and well-being is the housing of the older people. The every-day life of these people is almost entirely bound with their homes. The significance of the own home for the personality increases with ageing. Its role for the life satisfaction is confirmed by a series of cross-sectional and some longitudinal studies – before and after moving to a better housing (Larson, 1978). According to the study of Arnaudova and coll. (1984) 20% of the people in the age after retirement have shared housing problems – inadequacy of floorage and/or of supplying with utilities; 17% of them (single or couple) didn't dispose with a separate room, and they used one room with others, mostly with children and/or grandchildren. In the villages the lack of flowing water and of lavatory inside the home created some problems (for 89% of the examined households); and in the cities the higher storey was uncomfortable for the older people with difficulties of moving – every one from eleven elderly had three or more floors to climb. A part of the households of the older people were not furnished with cardinal appliances easing the domestic work like washing machine or refrigerator (Arnaudova and coll., 1984).

Providing convenient transport and communications also has certain importance for the mental health of older people. American studies e.g. of Carp (after Larson, 1978) have found a correlation between good transport and life satisfaction about 0.1-0.2. The relation was higher at elderly people who had lower incomes, worse health and lived far from the centre of the city.

Another important question is whether living in rural areas is better for mental health of the older people or living in urban setting? The question is complicated, and many elements are essential to give a global answer. The mode of life varies in diverse countries and social conditions. One serious investigation in England on 12 962 adults revealed a better overall mental health when living in rural areas (Mylene Riva & coll., 2009), but in other countries the answer could be diverse.

THE ROLE OF FAMILY

Family has a first-rate importance for the mental balance in older ages. With ageing the family relations - between the spouses and between the parents and their grown yet children –

undergo transformations. On the other hand, family life attains with ageing major affective significance. The "relative weight" of the family roles increases in contrast to the most out-of-family roles. We said that old people are mostly bound with the home. The concern about family relations – with the partner and with the children – took the first place in the content of the values and motives of dissatisfaction of the rural people over 70. This first place was shared with the concerns about health and economic security (Petrov, 1975, 1976).

In many cases ageing strengthens the ties between the spouses. According to our observations, older people, especially older men, are more vulnerable to becoming widowed, than people in earlier age groups. The death of the partner has multilateral consequences, beginning with economic difficulties that it may engender, and completing with possibly increasing feelings of loneliness and uselessness. How far the older person will adapt to the widowhood depends on many circumstances; one of the most important is the support offered by the children. A series of studies found lower life satisfaction, higher anxiousness, increased amount of sedative drugs and tranquilizers taken, increased rates of depressive states and suicides after becoming widowed.

Psychological consequences of widowhood are more pronounced in combination with inadequate income and ill- health. In most countries the widowhood is a serious problem first and foremost for women. The widows surpass widowers three or more times. In most psychological investigations the correlation between the presence of live partner and the life satisfaction is between 0.1 and 0.3. The Bulgarian-Hungarian study on a group of citizens of Sofia and Budapest in the age 55-88 years revealed a coefficient of correlation of the family state with the self-evaluation of health at 0.05 and with the self-evaluation of happiness at 0.39. The significance of the marital life experience appeared in the following range: the higher self-evaluation of happiness had the married elderly, followed by the widows/widowers; next were the divorced; and the lowest self-evaluation had the never married persons (Petrov, Kolozhi, Dumeva and Bartok, 1982).

Recent data from a national psychiatric morbidity survey in England confirmed, on the basis of 7399 people living in private homes that living with a partner strongly predicted happiness in the people in their 70's, compared with younger people (Cooper, Bebbington, King & coll., 2010). The doctoral dissertation work of Berg (2008) on 80+ years old people in Sweden revealed that widowhood was significantly associated with low life satisfaction especially among men. Berg concluded that the loss of spouse particularly in men is a predictor of decrease of life satisfaction.

Byrne and Rafael (1994) studied and described longitudinally the grief phenomena in older Australian widowers at different times after the bereavement. Some symptoms, such as intrusive thoughts of the deceased, a sense of sadness, and yearning for the lost person were almost universal at six weeks after bereavement. Grief symptom scores tended to diminish over time, but 8.8% of widowers were still achieving grief scores at six and thirteen months after the loss similar to the total groups' mean score at six weeks after the loss. This group is experiencing what is commonly termed "chronic" or "delayed" or "complicated" grief (Harwood, 2001). The syndrome of chronic grief is rare and approaches 9.2% of a mixed age sample (Middleton & coll., 1996).

Bereavement is a major risk factor for depression in old age. The cohort population study of Turvey & coll. (1999) showed the rate of "syndromal depression" to be nine times higher in newly-widowed older community people compared with married subjects in the same cohort. A study of 328 widows and widowers using a self-rating scale of Zisook & coll.

(1997) found 31% suffered "minor" and "subsyndromal" depression in addition to the 20% with "major depression" at two months after bereavement. The rates of depressions declined to the point that 70% were not longer depressed at 25 months after the bereavement, but rates of "subsyndromal" depression remained stable.

A study from the Netherlands showed that the association between widowhood and depression was greater for men than women (Van Grootheest & coll., 1999). Women also seemed to adapt to widowhood more successfully than men in the longer term. In contrast, a longitudinal US study found that older widows had higher levels of depressive symptoms than widowers (Chen & coll., 1999).

There is a modest, but definite excess mortality in the year after bereavement (Woof & Carrer, 1997; Schaefer & coll., 1995). Mendes de Leon & coll. (1993) found a small increased mortality in both sexes between seven and twelve months after bereavement. Harwood (2001) thought that increased risk of death was short-lived and affected mostly widowed men aged 75 years and over. An examination of a large Belgian sample showed that higher educational levels, although associated with a lower mortality in general, do not alleviate the effects of bereavement (Lusyne & coll., 2001). In fact, for reasons, which were unclear, the more highly educated appeared to have a greater excess mortality in the period immediately after the spousal loss. The causes of the higher mortality rates after bereavement are likely to be complex. The increased rates of depression may contribute for greater mortality after bereavement. Another factor could be that recently bereaved people lead less healthy lifestyles, as found Williams (2004).

The recent loss of a partner and female gender were associated with increased suicidal ideation (Stroebe & coll., 2005). But there is a real small increase of completed suicides, and it is higher in bereaved older men. A US study on a cohort of older people showed that there is an increased risk of suicide in the widowed persons, mostly men (Li, 1995). The risk of suicide for widowed men was over three times as high as for married men whereas the risk of suicide for the widowed women was the same as that for married women. A study based on Danish population statistics found a significant increase in suicide risk during the first year after bereavement for the oldest old and especially for men (Erlangsen & coll., 2004)

A number of studies show that different aspects of the quality of marital relationship do influence the adjustment to bereavement (Carr & coll., 2000; Harwood, 2005). A recent study of Hewitt & coll. (2010) confirmed that marital loss decreased mental health of elderly men and women. Social support improved mental health (only of men) immediately after the death of their spouse.

Usually, social participation levels decrease before the death of a spouse, but increases following the loss. The majority of widowed persons (87%) said that they actively tried to keep busy as a way to cope with feelings of grief and loneliness.

Widowed persons have higher levels of informal participation, not formal. Usually, they prefer to maintain relationships and activities that have been meaningful to them prior to the bereavement, rather to engage in new activities after their bereavement (Utz & coll., 2002; Harwood, 2005).

In the age after retirement often appears a shift of the roles in the sense that the week in the past child gradually has become an independent and financially and socially more important member of the family and the parent has turned to be more powerless and dependent. All this may be a source of stress and dissatisfaction. After the age of 70-75 years other reasons of dissatisfaction stand out: the inadequate care and consideration on the part of their children, often with the feeling to be abandoned and lonely (Petrov, 1975, 1976). With the advance of ageing increases the dependence from physical and emotional support, which the older people, especially after becoming widowed, do expect principally from their children.

The demographic processes lead to the fact that a substantial part of older people live separately from their children. But some of them live together with other relatives, or with other persons. In 1980 in the USA only 28% of the people aged 65 and over lived alone (U.S.Bureau of Census, 1981). In other countries, like Bulgaria, the really living alone elderly people were a smaller proportion. The homes of one part of the older people who live alone are situated not far from the homes of their children. In Bulgarian villages the old parents often live in one home but on separate floors with the family of some of their children or in annex building in the same yard. In these cases the households are separated but the contacts are direct and natural. According to Arnaudova and coll. (1984) the majority of older people preferred to live together with their children, but one third preferred to live separately and not far from the homes of their children. The study in Bulgarian villages revealed a positive correlation of the self-evaluation with living together with some one (Petrov, 1975, 1976). Many other investigations confirm that the majority of older people live together with their children and grandchildren or (if living alone) keep regular contacts with them. Another question is about the quality of the relations. In the group of 707 Bulgarian rural elderly studied 13% shared some conflicts within their families (Petrov, 1976). Recently Prema & coll. (2009) found in a sample of Indian population a positive and significant relationship between family solidarity and life satisfaction of the elderly i.e. good family solidarity improved the life satisfaction and poor family solidarity reduced the life satisfaction of the elderly.

Experience (Petrov, 1996) suggests that communication between older people and their offspring do enrich both sides. Younger people acquired from their parents and grandparents models of behaviour, crystallized views and values, worldly wisdom and professional experience. The older also learn from the younger in the family; the communication with them enriches them and brings a moral support. Many elderly suffer if they are deprived from younger people around.

The majority of older people e.g. in Bulgaria still has live siblings. With the ageing of the young nowadays people (bearing in mind the low birth rate in last decades) the number of the children, grandchildren, brothers and sisters will diminish, and the portion of older people without children and close relatives will increase.

The recent ISTAT study on 33 744 non-institutionalized Italian older people revealed that those who lived too far from their relatives and had few relationships with relatives and friends – they had lower life satisfaction (de Belvis & coll., 2008). The authors summarized that family support in Italy has been declined in Italy in recent years.

In late life appears one new social role, which brings much enjoyment and satisfaction. The care of grandchildren helps in many cases the subjective well-being of older people also in situations after retirement or bereavement. The extent in which the elderly people engage themselves with carrying their grandchildren varies considerably in different societies and cultures. The health, social support characteristics, and stressors in the life of the grandparents are important (Leder & coll., 2007).

THE ROLE OF SOCIAL ACTIVITY

It goes without saying that majority of people reduces with ageing the level of their activity and social contacts. The question is if the disengagement is natural and desired from the ageing persons. What is its essence? Based on their work in Kansas City in the 1950's Cumming and Henry theorized that the turning inward typical of ageing people produces a natural and normal withdrawal from social roles and activities, an increasing preoccupation with self, and decreasing involvement with others. According to the disengagement theory, optimum ageing is the result of acceptance and desire for disengagement from active life (Cumming and Henry, 1961; Atchley, 1987b). Individual disengagement was conceived as primarily a psychological process involving withdrawal of interest and commitment. Social withdrawal was seen as a consequence of individual withdrawal, coupled with society's withdrawal of opportunities and interest in older people's contributions. Human ageing could be viewed as is an inevitable process of individuals and social structures mutually disengaging and adaptively withdrawing from each other in anticipation of the person's inevitable death. Discussing the problem of theory in today's gerontology, Bengtson, Putney & Johnson (2005) found that disengagement theory was the most explicitly developed social gerontology theory, elegant, multidisciplinary, parsimonious and intuitively provocative, but its validity and generalizability claims could not be supported.

Activity theory is arguing with the disengagement theory. Activity theory was coined by Havighurst and his colleagues (Havighurst, Newgarten and Tobin, 1963) to refer to one point of view with regard to optimum or successful ageing. According to this view,

- except for the inevitable changes in biology and health, older people are the same as middle-aged people, with essentially the same psychological and social needs. In this view the decreased social interaction that characterizes old age results from the withdrawal by society from the aging person; and the decrease in interaction proceeds against the desires of most aging men and women.
- The older person who ages optimally is the person who stays active and manages to resist to shrinkage of his social world. He maintains the activities of middle age as long as possible, and then finds substitutes for those activities he is forced to relinquish – substitutes for work when he is forced to retire; substitutes for friends and loved ones whom he losses by death (Havighurst, Newgarten and Tobin, 1963, p. 419).

After many years of psychogerontological research it is now clear that disengagement is neither natural nor inevitable and that most cases of disengagement result from a lack of opportunities for continued involvement (Roman et al. 1967; Carp, 1968; Atchley, 1971; 1987b). Withdrawal may be result of illness, loss of close persons, forced retirement, perceived rejection or underestimation from society and younger persons, and in consequence decreased self-confidence (Petrov, 1978b).

Streib and Schneider (1971) suggested that differential disengagement was more likely than total disengagement. That is, people may withdraw from some activities but increase or maintain their involvement in others. Troll (1980) supported this notion when he talked of disengagement *into* the family, meaning that older people cope with lost roles by increasing their involvement with their families. In most cases with ageing the trend is towards less formal and more personal (not group) activities.

Activity theory served as a focus for early research, but the field has long since outgrowing the simplistic approaches. How feasible activity is for dealing with lost roles or activities depends on a number of factors. Substitutes must be available and the person must have the physical and mental capacities to perform in a substitute role or activity. However, substitutes are often not available. Widows often cannot find new mates; people who have been forced to relinquish certain activities often cannot develop new ones without inordinate investments of time and energy to develop new skills. Age discrimination limits opportunities not only in job roles but in many other roles as well (Atchley, 1987a).

On the other hand, some older people do not want to find substitute roles or activities. Some retired people do not want to find a substitute job. To the extent that the person sees himself or herself as having been previously too active, he or she may not want to replace lost activity (Atchley, 1987a). We will repeat that such attitudes are diverse in different social conditions and that they depend also from the level of economic security of retired persons.

Attempts to test activity theory have shown that the relation between activity and well-being is not a simple one. Lemon, Bengtson and Peterson (1972), Longino and Kart (1982) as well Harwood (2005) found that involvement in rather informal types of activities promoted well-being whereas involvement in formal, structural roles had just the opposite effect.

All things considered there is no one and only mode of combining social activity and satisfaction. Optimal for the age balance could be achieved in some cases through partial withdrawal and in other cases through continuing activity (Bengtson, Putney & Johnson, 2005).

Social Contacts and Networks

The social coherence in a broader context has been studied through the medium of quantitative appraisal of the contacts or of social roles carried out. In a number of investigations these have been compared with the indices of life satisfaction, and the coefficient of correlation found was from 0.1 to 0.3 (Larson, 1978 – bibliography).

Social contacts and networks in that older people live exert strong influence on their psychological well being. In her classical research on the population of New York, Christine Morgan (after Kuhlen, 1959, p. 886) has compared the feeling of happiness of older adults with a number of social contacts. In the next table the comparison has been between the happiest respondents (the upper third of the range) and the least happy (the lowest third).

The importance of the out-of-family interpersonal contacts in the late life emerges from the next table of Cutner which we reproduce from Kuhlen (1959). One could see from the table that the relation between the interpersonal contacts and psychological well-being is more expressed in case of worse economic state i.e. when the unfavourabe living situation of the elderly is formed by several adverse factors.

Percentage of some activities and social contacts of the happiest and the least happy older people

Activities and Social contacts	Percentage		
	happiest	least happy	difference
Living with her/his children since they want this	72.7	31.5	41.2
Every day has a lot of things to do	84.5	47.5	37.0
Satisfied with her/his children being proud of them	79.3	46.9	32.4
Having special interests or hobby	61.3	38.8	22.5
Having friends near by	62.7	41.8	20.9
Being able to visit the friends	64.8	47.8	17.0
Taking part in social activities, clubs, etc.	62.7	13.1	49.6

Relations between rates of contacts with friends and morale state of older people

Economic Security	Contacts with friends – more - or less once a week	Number of the-persons	Morale state in percents		
			high	medial	low
high	frequent	88	49	29	2
	rare	77	48	27	25
	no friends	36	47	33	20
low	frequent	102	35	37	28
	rare	100	29	33	20
	no friends	87	23	20	57

Informal out-of-family social contacts, like visiting friends and neighbors have strong relation with the life satisfaction of older people (Edwards and Klemmack, 1973; Larson, 1978 - bibliography). We suppose that a lack of social contacts could have negative impact not only on mental health status but also on the physical aspects of ageing. In a longitudinal study of approximately 5 years on 906 autonomous older people Buchman & coll. (2009) found that less frequent participation in social activities is associated with a more rapid rate of motor function decline in old age.

Participation in voluntary organizations does not usually decline among healthy older persons. Several studies have shown that, when the effects of socioeconomic differences and health are controlled, age bears little or no relationship in later life (Cutler, 1977, 1987). However, declining health does tend to decrease participation (Palmore, 1988). Voluntary participation in organized forms of meetings, like in church for the religious older people, has positive relationship with higher life satisfaction in samples of the rural American population (Edwards and Klemmack, 1973; R. Larson, 1978). By older people from the American urban population such relation has not been found (Bull and Aucoin, 1975). And, when socio-economic and health factors are controlled, the relationship between informal social contacts or participation in voluntary meetings with life satisfaction decreases (Bull and Aucoin, 1975; Cutler, 1976, 1977). Larson (1978) sees a gap in the research on the relationship social activity – psychological well-being, resulting from the lack of longitudinal studies. Still few studies, have found an increase of the life satisfaction after increasing the social contacts or social roles. Maddox (1963) has found an increase of the well-being for those elderly who had an essential increase of the social activity for three years. On small sample of older people Graney (1975) has found a moderate correlation between both variables in a four years longitudinal study. Higher correlation link has found Bultena (after Larson, 1978), but his results have been based on a retrospective analysis.

The role of social activity should be appraised in the large context of the whole social network at which older people live. The recent study of Litwin (2009) on more than 9000 older people living in five Mediterranean and seven Non-Mediterranean European countries showed that social networks of older people should be seen within their unique regional milieu and in relation to the values and social norms that prevail in different sets of societies. The results of that research revealed differences in each of realms of social network, above and beyond the differences that existed in background characteristics and health status. The findings also showed that the social network variables had different effects on the well-being outcomes in the respective settings (Litwin, 2009).

LONELINESS

Loneliness is often discussed in relation with mental health of older people. Social isolation and loneliness have long been identified as problems associated with old age. Social isolation refers to the objective state of having minimal contacts with other people, while loneliness refers to the subjective state of negative feelings associated with perceived social isolation (Wenger & coll., 1996).

While social isolation and loneliness are seen as common problems of old age, the prevalence of these problems is likely to have been overestimated (Freeman, 1988; Wenger and coll., 1996). Many observations revealed that few older people live alone and have not contacts with others. For example around 4% of the respondents in the age after retirement from Bulgarian population asserted that they have not been visited at all by close persons, relatives and/or neighbors and 10% have themselves visited no one; 38% have been visited seldom and 46% have themselves visited seldom someone; but 58% respectively 44% considered to have frequent contacts (Arnaudova and colleagues, 1984). Freeman (1988) found that social isolation is not widespread except along the very old.

Another question is that the quality of family and social contacts may not satisfy the older person and she/he may feel alone. The work of Lowenthal and Haven of 1968 is the first which indicated clearly that the psychological well-being in older age depends not only on the quantity of social contacts, but first of all on the presence of one confidant. According to the quoted study of Arnaudova and coll. each fifth older person in older age feels lonely; this is each fourth person over 80. The study of Gierveld, Groenou, Hoogendoorn and Smit (2008) on older Amsterdam citizens, who were married, revealed that 1 in 4 elderly exhibited moderate or strong emotional or social loneliness. The impairment of health and mobility increases the feeling of loneliness. It was found that older people with limitations in mobility have been visited most rarely (Arnaudova and coll., 1984). A number of American studies generalized by Larson (1978) indicated that the correlation link between social support and satisfaction was greater when populations studied included older people with various health and financial status, and decreased when ill-health and poor persons have been excluded from the study. Studying all residents over the age of 65 years of one district of London, Prince, Harwood, Blizard, Thomas and Mann (1997) found a relationship between social support, personal illness, life events over the previous year like bereavement, loneliness, handicap and depression. In their comprehensive work on social isolation and loneliness in old age Wenger and coll. (1996) concluded that the critical factors for isolation were: marital status, network type and social class; and for loneliness: network type, household composition and health.

Beeng alone influences not only the life satisfaction, psychological well-being and mood, but also the physical functioning of older people. Buchman, Boyle & coll. studied the relationship between psychosocial factors and motor functions in old age. In a longitudinal study on 985 community-dwelling older persons they found that both feeling alone and being alone were associated with more rapid motor decline (Buchman & coll., 2010)

The Role of Religious and Spiritual Belief

The interaction between religion and mental health remains complex. In certain circumstances religion can heighten feelings of guilt and anxiety (Coleman, 2010). Empirical evidence indicates that religious belief and practice has, in general, a positive influence on mental health. Religious faith prevents depression by both promoting positive mood and counteracting despair. Religion encourages healthy behaviour, cultivating an attitude of respect to the body and against attitudes of despair (Coleman, 2010). Persons aged 50 and over who engage in religious activity are less likely to commit suicide (Nisbet, Duberstein, Conwell, et al., 2000). The study of Coleman and colleagues on samples of rural elderly aged 60 and over in Bulgaria and Romania revealed lower levels of spiritual belief but significantly higher levels of depression in the Bulgarian compared with Romanian sample. Analyses of the data do suggest that spiritual belief may both influence and reflect physical and mental illness (Coleman, Carare, Petrov, Forbes, Saigal, Spreadbury, Yap & Kendrick, 2010). Religious faith and practices have a social importance. Church participation and membership of a religious organization both encourage activity and provide a potential support network. We still quoted data (p.8) that voluntary participation in organized forms of meetings, like in church, had positive relationship with higher life satisfaction in samples of the rural American population (Edwards and Klemmack, 1973; R. Larson, 1978). By older people from the American urban population such relation has not been found (Bull and Aucoin, 1975). The recent data from the English national psychiatric morbidity survey (Cooper, Bebbington, King & coll., 2010) revealed that attendance at religious services and places is an important predictors of happiness mostly in the oldest old.

It is supposed that religious belief can increase the resilience and help older persons to cope more effectively with stresses and losses of later life (Levin, Markides & Ray, 1996; Coleman, 2010). The attitudes that are learned from religiously committed peers may benefit ones health through encouragement of healthy behaviours and lifestyles lowering the risk of disease (Levin & Chatters, 1998). The most striking findings relevant to health and ageing come in studies of longevity. An extensive cross-state study in the USA has found a life expectancy difference of more than 7 years between those never attending religious services and those attending more than once weekly (Hummer et al., after Coleman, 2010).

Necessity of Social Support for Mental Health

The notion of health integrates mental health issues. It is a state of optimal physical, mental and social well-being. Older people are diverse, and old age is heterogeneous. Along with this, the needs of social and family support, of relatively good health and economic security, of independent and harmonious mode of life is essential for subjective well-being and successful ageing. Gerontology research and practice evidences give a good basis and approaches to further work at that direction.

A movement of knowledge transfer of scientists, public officials, advocacy and individuals is necessary to establish a new knowledge about the importance of social support and on the interpersonal and cultural context of mental disorder and mental wellbeing for everyone during the life cycle. It is necessary that everyone and everything concerned, from individuals to integrated government policies, should be aware of the importance of social networks and social support for all people and generations.

References

ADI (2010). *http://www.alz.org/documents/national/World_Alzheimer_Report_2010.pdf.*

Angermeyer, M. C., Klusmann, D. (1989*). Soziales Netzwerk. Ein neues Konzept für die Psychiatrie.* Berlin, p. 17 - 63.

Arnaudova Z. and colleagues (1984). *A study on life conditions and social problems of the population in the age after retirement in Bulgaria.* Sofia, National Statistics Institute.

Atchley R.C. (1987a). Activity Theory. In: G. L. Maddox (Editor-in-Chief) *Encyclopedia of Aging*. New York, Springer, p. 5.

Atchley R. (1987b). Disengagement. In: G. L. Maddox (Editor-in-Chief) *Encyclopedia of Aging*. New York, Springer, 186-187

Atchley R.C. (1971). Disengagement among professors. *J. Gerontol.*, 26, 476-480.

Baltes P.B. (1993). The aging mind: potentials and limits. *The Gerontologist*, 33, 580-594.

Baltes P.B. & U.M. Staudinger (2000). Wisdom: a metaheuristic (pragmatic) to orchestrate mind and virtue towards excellence. *Am. Psychol.*, 55, 122-136

Bengtson V.L., Morella M. Putney & M.L. Johnson (2005). The problem of theory in gerontology today. In M.L. Johnson (ed.) *The Cambridge Handbook of Age and Ageing.* Cambridge University Press, 3-20

Berg Anne Ingeborg (2008). Life satisfaction in late life: markers and predictors of level and change among 80+ year olds. Doctoral dissertation at University if Gothenburg. Geson, Gothenburg.

Birren J.E. & R.B. Sloane (co-eds.) (1980). *Handbook of Mental Health and Aging* (1980). Englewood Cliffs, N.J., Prentice-Hall, Inc.

Blazer D (1980). The epidemiology of mental illness in later life. In E.W. Busse & D.G. Blazer (Eds), *Handbook of Geriatric Psychiatry*, Van Nostrand Reinhold, 1980, 249-281.

Boback M. & M. Marmot (1996). East-West mortality divide and its potential explanations: Proposed research agenda. *British Medical Journal*, 312, 421-425.

Boback M. & J. Powles (2001). Poverty and non-communicable diseases in Central and Eastern Europe and the Former Soviet Union. *A report for the non-communicable diseases and mental health cluster. WHO Geneva.* University College, London.

Bourliere F., J. Vallery-Masson (1985). Epidemiology and sociology of aging. In J.C.

Brocklehurst (Ed), *Textbook of Geriatric Medicine and Gerontology*. 3-d edition. Edinburgh etc., Churchill Livingstone, 3-28

Bourne P.A., C. Morris & D. Eldemire-Shearer (2010). Re-testing theories on the correlations of health status, life satisfaction and happiness. *North American Journal of Medical Sciences*, 2, 313-315.

Busse E.W. (1987). Mental health. In: G. L. Maddox (Editor-in-Chief) *Encyclopedia of Aging*.. New York, Springer, 438-439.

Buchman A.S., P.A. Boyle, R.S. Wilson, D.A. Fleischman, S. Leurgans & D.A. Bennett (2009a). Association between late-life social activity and motor decline in older adults. *Arch. Intern. Med,* 2009 Nov. 9, 169, 12, 1149-1146.

Buchman A.S., P.A. Boyle, R.S. Wilson, B.D. James, S.E. Leurgans, S.E. Arnold & D.A. Benett (2009b). Loneliness and the rate of motor decline in old age: the Rush Memory and Aging Projact, a community based cohort study. *BMC Geriatr.*, Oct. 29

Busse E.W. & E. Pfeiffer (1977). Functional psychiatric disorders in old age. In: E.W. Busse, E. Pfeiffer (Eds), *Behavior and Adaptation in Late Life*. 2nd ed. Boston, Little-Brown, 158-211.

Byrne G.J.A. & B. Raphael (1994). A longitudinal study of bereavement phenomena in recently widowed elderly men. *Psychol. Med*, 24, 411-421.

Byrne G.J.A. & B. Raphael (1997). The psychological symptoms of conjugal bereavement in elderly men over the first 13 months. Int. J. Geriatr. Psychiatry, 12, 241-251.

Carp, F. M. (1968). Some components of disengagement. *J. Gerontol.*, 23, 382-386.

Carr D., J.S. House, R.C. Kessler, R.M. Nesse, J. Sonnega & C. Wortman (2000). Marital quality and psychological adjustment to withoudhood among older adults: a longitudinal analysis. *J. Gerontol., B Psychol. Sci. Soc. Sci.* 55, S197-207.

Chen J.H., A.J. Bierhals, H.G. Prigerson, S.V. Kasl, C. M. Mazure & S. Jacobs (1999). *Psychol. Med.* 29, 367-380.

Coleman P.G. & A. O'Hanlon (2004). *Ageing and development. Theories and research.* Oxford Univesity Press.

Coleman P.G. (2010). Religion and age. In *The Sage handbook of social gerontology* (in press)

Coleman P.G., R.O. Carare, I.C. Petrov, E. Forbes, A. Saigal, J.H. Spreadbury, A.Yap & T. Kendrick (2010). Spiritual belief, social support, physical functioning and depression among older people in Bulgaria and Romania. *Aging and mental health*, 1-7

Cooper C., P. Bebbington, M. King & coll. (2010). Happiness across age groups: Results from the 2007 National Psychiatric Morbidity Survey. *Int. J. Geriat. Psychiatry*, 2010, Dec. 9.

Cumming E. & W. E. Henry (1961). *Growing Old.* New York, Basic Books.

Cutler S. (1975). Transportation and changes in life satisfaction. *The Gerontologist*, 15, 155-179.

Cutler S. (1976). Membership in different type of voluntary associations and psychological well-being. *The Gerontologist*, 16, 335-339.

Cutler S. (1977). Aging and voluntary association participation. *Journal of Gerontology*, 32, 470-479.

Cutler S. (1987). Attitudes. Group membership. In G. L. Maddox (Editor-in-Chief) *Encyclopedia of Aging*.. New York, Springer, 43-45; 297-298.

De Belvis A.G., Maria Avolio, Lorella Sicuro, A. Rosano, Elide Latini, G. Damiani, W. Ricciardi (2008). Social relationships and HRQL: A cross-sectional survey among older Italian adults. *BMC Public Health*, 8, 348.

Edwards J.N. & D.L. Klemmack (1973). Correlates of life satisfaction: A re-examination. *J. Gerontol., 28,* 4, 297-302.

Erlangsen A., B. Jeune, U. Bille-Brahe & J.W. Vaupel (2004). Loss of partner and suicide risks amongst oldest old: a population-based register study. *Age Ageing,* 33, 478-383.

Freeman H. (1988). Psychosocial effects of social isolation in the elderly. *Danish Medical Bulletin: Journal of Health Sciences, Gerontology: Special Supplement Series*, 6, 13-23.

Gierveld J, M. van Groenou, A. Hoogendoorn & J.M. Smit (2008). Quality in marriages in later life and emotional and social loneliness. *The Journals of Gerontology*, Series B, 4, 497-506.

Harwood D. (2001). Grief in old age. *Reviews in Clinical Gerontology*, 11, 167-175.

Harwood D. (2005). Grief in old age. *Reviews in Clinical Gerontology,* 15, 281-287.

Havighurst J. E., B. Neugarten & S. S. Tobin (1963). Disengagement, personality and life satisfaction in the later years. In P. From Hansen (Ed.) *Age with a Future*. Copenhagen, Munksgaard, 419-425.

Hefner J, Eisenberg D. (2009). Social support and mental health among college students. *Am J Orthopsychiatry.* Oct;79(4):491-9.

Hewitt B, Turrell G, Giskes K. (2010). Marital loss, mental health and the role of perceived social support: findings from six waves of an Australian population based panel study. *J Epidemiol Community Health*. p.1-7.

Jorm A.F. (1987). A guide to understanding of Alzheimer's disease and related disorders. New York, New York University Press.

Jung M., C. Muntaner & M. Choi (2010). Factors related to perceived life satisfaction among the elderly in South Korea. *Journal of Preventive Medicine and Public Health*, 43, 4 292-300.

Kiemo K. (2003). *Towards a socio-economic and demographic theory of elderly suicide: A comparison of 49 countries at various stages of development.* PhD dissertation. Uppsala, Repro Economicum.

Klauer, T., Schwarzer, R. (2001). Soziale Unterstützung und Depression [Social support and depression]. *Verhaltenstherapie und Verhaltensmedizin. Themenheft: Soziales Netz und psychische Störungen, 22*, 333-352.

Klusmann, D. (1989). Methoden zur Untersuchung sozialer Unterstützung und persönlicher Netzwerke. In: Angermeyer, M.C., Klusmann, D. (Eds.) : *Soziales Netzwerk. Ein neues Konzept für die Psychiatrie.* Berlin, p. 17 - 63.

Kuhlen R.G. (1959). Aging and life adjustment. In J.E. Birren (ed.) *Handbook of aging and the individual*. Chicago, University of Chicago Press, 852-900.

Kutner B., D. Fanshel, A. M. Togo & T.S. Langner (1956). *Five hundred over sixty: A community survey on aging*. New York, Russel Sage Foundation.

Larson R. (1978). Thirty years of research on the subjective well-being of older Americans. *J. Gerontol.*, 33, 109-125.

Leder, S., Grinstead, LN., Torres, E. (2007). Grandparents raising grandchildren: stressors, social support, and health outcomes. *J Fam Nurs*. Aug;13(3):333-52.

Lee, S. J., Detels, R. , Rotheram-Borus, M.J., Duan, N. (2007). The Effect of Social Support on Mental and Behavioral Outcomes Among Adolescents With Parents With HIV/AIDS. *American Journal of Public Health*. Vol 97, No. 10:1820-1826.

Lemon B. W., V. L. Bengtson & J.A. Peterson (1972). An exploration of the activity theory of aging: activity types and life satisfaction among inmovers to a retirement community. *J. Gerontol*., 27, 511-523.

Levin J., K.S. Markides & L.A. Ray (1996). Religious attendance and psychological well-being in Mexican Americans. *The Gerontologist*, 36, 454-463.

Levin J. & L.M. Chatters (1998). Religion, health, and psychological well-being in older adults: finding from three national surveys. *Journal of Aging and Health*, W(4), 504-531.

Li G. (1995). The interaction effect of bereavement and sex on the risk of suicide in the elderly: an historical cohort study. *Soc. Sci. Med*., 40, 825-828.

Litwin H. (2009). Social networks and well-being: a comparison of older people in Mediteranean and Non-Mediteranean countries. The *Journals of Gerontology*, Series B, Oct 28, 2009.

Longino C.F., Jr. & C. S. Kart (1982). Explicating activity theory: A formal replication. *J. Gerontol*., 37, 713-722.

Lowenthal M. F. & C. Haven (1968). Interaction and adaptation: Intimacy as a critical variable. *American Sociological Review*, 33, 20-30.

Lusyne P., H. Page & J. Lievens (2001). Mortality following conjugal bereavement, Belgium 1991-96: the unexpected effect of education. Popul. Stud. (Camb) 55, 281-289.

Mendes de Leon C. E., S. V. Kasl & S.C. Jacobs (1993). Widowhood and mortality risk in a community sample of the elderly: a prospective study. *J. Clin. Epidemiol*., 46, 519-527.

Middleton W., P. Burnett, B. Raphael & N. Martinek (1996). The bereavement response: a cluster analysis. *Bri. J. Psychiatry*, 169, 167-171.

Miszkurka, M., Goulet, L., Zunzunegui, MV. (2010). Contributions of immigration to depressive symptoms among pregnant women in Canada. *Can J Public Health*. Sep-Oct;101(5):358-64.

Mollencopf, H. & Walker, A. (Eds.) (2007). Quality of life in old age. Springer, 2007.

Nisbet P.A., P.R. Duberstein, P.R. Conwell (2000). The effect of participation in religious activities on suicide versus natural death in adults 50 and older. *Journal of nerve disorders*, 188, 543-546.

Palmore, E. (1988). *The facts on Aging Quiz*. New York, Springer. 1988.

Patel, V. (2005). Poverty, gender and mental health promotion in a global society, Promotion and Education, Supplement 2. www.iuhpe.org.

Petrov I.C. (1975). Medical-psychological problems in older people according to their self-evaluation of happiness. *Nevrol., psihiat. i nevrohirurg. – Sofia,* 14, 306-313 (In Bulgarian; summary in English).

Petrov I.C. (1976). *Self-evaluation of some personality aspects of the aged by the Dembo-Rubinstein test. Experimental-psychologic and clinical psychopathologic investigation*. Ph.D. Dissertation. Sofia, Meditsinska Akademija (In Bulgarian; abstract in English).

Petrov I.C. (1978a). Self-evaluation of health and illness in elderly persons. *Nevrol., psihiat. i nevrohirurg. – Sofia,* 17, 238-244 (In Bulgarian; summary in English).

Petrov I.C. (1978b). *Mental ageing*. Meditsinska akademiya - Centar za nauchna informatsia po meditsina i zdraveopazvane, Sofia (in Bulgarian).

Petrov I.C. (1981). Age and creation. *Nauchen jivot*, 1981, 3, 8-11 (in Bulgarian).

Petrov I. C. (1996). Feelings and attitudes toward the changes during social and economic transition: A study of Sofia autonomous elderly subjects. *Rom. J. Gerontol. Geriatr*. 17, 73-82.

Petrov I.C., Vl. Denev, Iv. Petkov, Z. Arnaudova, D. Petrov (2007). Correlates of active and healthy ageing over seventy in a rural setting in Bulgaria. *Advances in gerontology*. Abstract book, 20, 330.

Petrov I. C., B. Kolozhi, N. Dumeva, J. Bartok (1982). Social-psychological investigations of dispensarized elderly volunteers – inhabitants of Sofia and Budapest. Part II: Analysis of the self-evaluation. *Nevrol., psihiat. i nevrohirurg. – Sofia,* 21, 188-197 (In Bulgarian; summary in English).

Prema P.B., V. S. Vadav & V. Gaonka (2009): Influence of family solidarity on life satisfaction of the elderly. Journap of Dairying, Foods and Home Sciences, 28, 2.

Prince M.J., R.H. Harwood, R.A. Blizard, A. Thomas & A. Mann (1997). Social support deficit, loneliness and life events as risk factors for depression in old age. *Psychological Medicine*, 27, 323-332.

Riva, M., Bambra, C. Curtis, S., Gauvin, L. (2010). Collective resources or local social inequalities? Examining the social determinants of mental health in rural areas. *European Journal of Public Health.* April 19.

Roman P., Taietz, P. (1967). Organizational structure and disengagement: The emeritus professor. *The Gerontologist,* 7, 147-152.

Schaefer C., C.P. Quensbury & S. Wi (1995): Mortality following conjugal bereavement and the effects of a shared environment. Am. J. Epidemiol., 141, 1142-1152.

Senin B. (1999). *Paziente anziano e paziente geriatrico. Fondamenti di gerontologia e geriatria*. Napoli, EdiSES.

Slater E., Roth, M. (1969). *Clinical Psychiatry*, 3-d ed. London, Balliere, Tindall and Cassell.

Stansfeld, S., Candy B. (2006). Psychosocial work environment and mental health-a meta-analytic review. *Scand J Work Environ Health*. Dec;32(6):443-62.

Streib G & C. Schneider (1971). *Retirement in American Society*. Ithaca, New York, Cornel University Press,

Stroebe W., E. Zech, M.S. Stroebe, & G. Abakoumkin (2005). Does social support help in bereavement? *J. Soc. Clin. Psychol.*, 24. 1030-1050

Tobin S. S. & M. A. Lieberman (1976). *Last home for the aged*. San Francisco, Jossey-Bass.

Troll L.E. (1980). Intergenerational relations in later life; A family approach. In N. Datan & N. Lohmann (Eds.), *Transitions of Aging*. New York, Academic Press.

Turvey, C.L., C. Carney, S. Arndt, R. B. Wallace & Herzog, R. (1999). Conjugal loss and syndromal depression in a sample of elders aged 70 years and older. *Am. J. Psychiatry*, 156, 1596-1601.

Uhde N. (2009). Social seurity and life satisfaction. Evidence from the German socio-economic panel. Presentation at the Conference: "*From GDP to Well-Being: Economics on the Road to Sustainability*", Ancona, 3-5 December 2009.

Utz R.L., D. Carr, R. Nesse & C. Wortman (2002). The effect of widowhood on older adults' social participation: a an valution of activity, disengagement, and social theories. *Gerontologist*, 42, 522-533.

US Bureau of Census (1981). *Current Population Reports* (Series P-20, No 372). Washington, DC: US. Government Printing Office.

Van Grootheest D.S., A.T.F. Beekman, M. I. Broese van Groenou & D.J.H. Deeg (1999). Sex differences in depression after widowhood. Do men suffer more? *Soc. Psychiatry Psychiatr. Epidemiol.*, 34, 391-398.

Wenger G., Clare., R. Davies, S. Shahtahmasebi & Scott, A. (1996). Social isolation and loneliness in old age: review and model refinement. *Ageing and Society.* 16, 333-358.

World Health Organization (2004). *Promoting Mental Health: Concepts, Emerging Evidence, Practice*. A report from the World Health Organization, Department of Mental Health and Substance Abuse in collaboration with the Victorian Health Promotion Foundationand the University of Melbourne. Geneva: WHO.

WHO (2010). *http://www.who.int/mediacentre/factsheets/fs220/en/index.html.*

Williams K. (2004):. The transition to widowhood and the social regulation of health: consequences for health and health risk behaviour. *J. Gerontol. B Psychol. Sci. Soc. Sci.*, 59, 5343-5349.

Wills T. A., Filer, M. (2001). Social networks and social support. In A. Baum, T. A. Revenson, & J. E. Singer (Eds.). *Handbook of health psychology* (p. 209-234). Mahwah, NJ: Erlbaum.

Woof W. R. & Y. H. Carter (1997). The grieving adult and the general practitioner: a literature review in two parts (Part 1). *Brit.J. Gen. Pract.*,47, 443-448.

Zisook S. M. Paulus, S.R. Shuchter & L.L. Judd (1997). The many faces ofof depression following spousal bereavement. *J. Affect. Disord.* 45, 85-95.

In: Social Determinants and Mental Health
Editor: Sabine Bährer-Kohler
ISBN: 978-1-61324-353-4

Chapter 10

SERVICE UTILIZATION AND MENTAL HEALTH: THE FACTS

Richard Uwakwe
Faculty of Medicine, College of Health Sciences, Nnmadi Azikiwe University Awka-Nnewi Campus, Awka, Nigeria

INTRODUCTION

Many studies in all parts of the world indicate that the rate of mental health service utilization is low. In one of the early pioneering epidemiological investigations of mental disorders in the US, Regier et al [14] reported that in the five site ECA study the rate of mental health service use was only 14.7%. Studies in Australia have consistently reported mental health service use in the range of 8.6% to 14.5% [15-17]. Other studies have reported much lower current and one year rates of mental health service utilization [16-18]. In the UK, Bebbington et al reported that less than 14% of persons with neurotic disorders utilized mental health service [19]. In the US, Kessler et al [20, 21] consistently reported much lower rates of mental health service use compared to the ECA study. Only 13.3% of respondents used some type of outpatient service for a psychiatric problem in the previous 12 months—3.9% accessed the general medical sector, 5.8% the specialty sector, 5.1% the human services sector, and 3.2% the self-help sector. The authors cited methodological differences as responsible for the previous higher estimates of mental health service use reported in the ECA study [20, 21].

Population based studies have consistently shown that in both developed and developing countries about 12.2%- 48.6% suffer from mental disorders [1, 2]. The WHO Global Burden of Diseases report indicates that mental health problems contribute about 13% of the disease burden. [3]. Mental disorders are of public health importance with huge social, psychological, physical and financial implications especially when mental health services are not utilized. [68] Promotion of mental health, prevention and treatment of mental disorders, including rehabilitation are the key issues in mental health service provision.

MENTAL HEALTH SERVICE PROVIDERS

There are various professionals that serve as mental health service providers. Psychiatrists, psychologists, psychiatric nurses, community mental health nurses, psychiatric social workers, occupational therapists, counsellors [including pastoral counsellors] are primarily involved in mental health service provision. Also primary health care workers, general practitioners, traditional and faith healers may contribute to mental health care provision or some times be the sole providers of mental health care in some locations. Mental health service utilization may involve the service use of any of these professional groups.

Mental health service utilization has been variously defined as one mental health visit in the past year, talking to health care provider about personal health, total services over a period of time [4, 5]. Besides other numerous socioeconomic and psychological or physical factors – "external factors", the prime driver of mental health service utilization is need –"internal factor" [4, 5, 7]. Therefore, any individual who is in need [whether the need is defined by an expert assessment or perceived as such by the individual concerned] of mental health service, should use it irrespective of whether it is once or over any given period of time depending on the nature of the mental health problem. An ideal situation is an optimal intersection between mental health needs and service provision and utilization. In practice however, this does not happen as need has often been found to outstrip utilization.

THEORETICAL FRAME WORK OF MENTAL HEALTH SERVICE UTILIZATION

Health behaviour and health seeking are inseparably linked with health service use. A number of conceptual models have been proposed to understand the complex phenomenon of health care service use. While these models were not primarily developed for mental health, they apply by extension to all forms of health services use, although some details may differ with peculiarities in different health conditions and services.

One of the most popular models is the *Anderson's behavioural model* [6]. According to this model, three principal factors determine the visit to a physician or use of health care service. The predisposing factors are internally located in the potential health care service utilizer, such as age, gender, and social status. The enabling factors are factors that will either enhance or limit the use of a health care service such as distance to the place of care, type of municipality, family size and working time. The need variables include presence of [chronic] diseases, disability days, psychological well being and new illness conditions [6].

The *health belief model*, based on sociocogntive theory was initially conceptualized by Becker [8]. In this model, the person's reactions to symptoms of illness are modified or determined by various factors, including motivation, the experienced threat of illness and coping factors. The model groups these factors into "perceived" experiences. The hypothesis is that people are likely to take a particular health action if the following conditions exist: 1. perceived susceptibility if the individual perceives that he/she could get the illness in question or is susceptible to the illness of interest. 2. Perceived severity if individual is of the view that the illness has serious consequences or will interfere with daily functioning. 3. Perceived benefits if individual believes that the expected action or intervention will be effective in addressing the health problem. 4. Perceived barriers if there will be only few barriers to taking action. 5. Cues to action are incidents that serve as a reminder of the severity or threat of an ill health and may include [internal] personal experiences or external cues such as a discussion with an expert [physician]. Leavitt [9] called this, *final stimulus to action.* 6. Perceived self efficacy later proposed by Becker and colleagues implies that one's expectations about the ability to influence outcome is an important component in understanding health behaviour outcomes [10].

In *Purola"s model,* three important factors are proposed as basic to health care service use: the disease [in the medical sense of the word] and the perceived illness as an originator of behavioural reaction. The predisposing and enabling factor then act as modulators of the individual's behavioural reactions [11].

In *Antonovsky's model* of utilization there is a consideration that medical care constitutes a small social system, which may be used to deal with diffuse social and psychological needs when the system is available, when its use is socially encouraged, and when it is receptive to peoples' needs and orientation. The model includes host characteristics, characteristics of the medical institutions and characteristics of the larger sociocultural environment [12].

The *Biopsychosocial model* initially proposed by Engels [13] was based on the general systems theory which implies that all levels of an organization or system, beginning from molecules and cells and ending up with society or biosphere, are linked to each other in a hierarchical relationship, so that a change in one affects changes in the others. The model is used in health care service utilization in an attempt to understand the relationships between various explanatory factors [such as somatic diseases, psychological factors and social environment, such as family] of health care utilization.

*The Theory of Planned Behaviour.*Ajzen [64] hypothesizes that intentions are influenced by attitudes toward the usefulness of engaging in behaviour, perceived expectations of important others such as family or friends, and perceived ability to engage in the behaviour if desired. This theory has been applied to a variety of health behaviours and has received support for its utility in predicting health behaviours.

The Self-Regulation Model focuses on an individual's personal representation of his or her illness as a predictor of mental health treatment use [65]. The model proposes that individuals' representation of their illness is comprised of how the individual labels the symptoms he or she is experiencing, the perceived consequences and causes of the symptoms for the individual, the expected time in which the individual would expect to be relieved of symptoms, and the perceived control or cure of the illness.

Mental Health Service Use Across the World

An Ontario study reported a one year mental health service use of 7.8% [18]. In the recent World Mental Health Survey [WMH], a WHO initiative that investigated mental health disorders and service use in over thirty countries of the world, the proportion of respondents who received health care treatment for emotional or substance-use problems in the previous 12 months varied widely across surveys from a low of 0.8% in Nigeria to a high of 15.3% in the United States. In all the surveys, mental health service use was low [2]. In the ECA study, Regier et al reported that of the subjects with affective disorders, only 37.8% had used health services [general medical or specialist services] and only 45.7% had used any type of service [including health care services, other professional human services or voluntary support networks] for their depression in the previous year [14]. Of all 1348 subjects identified with depression in Edmonton, du Fort et al [41] reported that only about 64% had ever sought treatment.

Wang et al [42] estimated proportions of respondents with 12-month *DSM-IV* anxiety, mood, impulse control, and substance disorders who received treatment in the 12 months before the interview in any of 4 service sectors (specialty mental health, general medical, human services, and complementary and alternative medicine). The result showed that of 12-month cases, 41.1% received some treatment in the past 12 months, including 12.3% treated by a psychiatrist, 16.0% treated by a non-psychiatrist mental health specialist, 22.8% treated by a general medical provider, 8.1% treated by a human services provider, and 6.8% treated by a complementary and alternative medical provider [treatment could be received by more than one source]. The authors concluded that mental health problems continue to remain untreated in the US and unmet need for treatment is greatest in traditionally underserved groups, including elderly persons, racial-ethnic minorities, those with low incomes, those without insurance, and residents of rural areas.

Karan et al reported that in Lebanon only a minor proportion of those with mental disorders ever received any treatment [43]. In the Mexico National Comorbidity survey Borges et al reported that fewer than one in five respondents with any psychiatric disorder during the previous 12 months used any service during the prior year [44]. Only 13.2% of those with any anxiety disorder had had any health care service [14.1% for generalized anxiety disorder, 25.1% for panic, agoraphobia 16%, social phobia 15.3% and specific phobia 11. %]. On the other hand, only 22.2% of those with any mood disorder had had health care service [22.1% for any major depressive disorder and 23.1% for any bipolar disorder]. For the subjects with substance/ alcohol abuse, 18.8% had had any health care; the figures were 19.8% and 17.1% respectively for alcohol dependence and any substance disorder.

A WHO European report [45] indicated that throughout Europe many of those with depression, dysthymia, panic, bipolar disorder, generalized anxiety disorder, obsessive compulsive disorder and other mental disorders do not receive any treatment. The ESEMeD study, the first largest European population based study to investigate the epidemiology of mental disorders and mental health service use in Europe showed that the mental health service use by persons with mental disorders in the previous twelve months was as follows: any disorder 25.7 %, any mood 36.5% any anxiety 26.1%, any alcohol disorder 8.3%. About two thirds of those with mental disorders who had contacted the health services had done so with mental health professionals, and 21.2% of those with mental disorders who had consulted formal health service received no form of treatment at all [46]. Other reports indicate that 76%-85% of persons with mental health problems did not receive any treatment and those who did, were not appropriately treated [47]. In the Canadian Community Health survey, only few individuals with mental disorders, less than 10% received any treatment, one reason being that self perceived need for mental health care did not always match the actual presence of mental disorder [48]. Analyzing data from Australian surveys and WHO Reports, Andrews, Issakidis and Carter reported that only about a third of persons with mental disorders sought or received treatment [49]. The probability of seeking or receiving treatment varied by diagnosis, age, gender, marital status and disability. In a study to ascertain the extent of the community's preference, needs for and utilization of mental health services in

Singapore, Ng, Fones and Kua [51] reported that an estimated 37% of the general population indicated they would seek professional help if they experienced a serious emotional or mental problem. The authors reported that even though 16.9% were determined by their high general health questionnaire [GHQ] score to need mental health services, only 2.6% in the population used the services of any professional caregiver. Among persons with high GHQ scores, only 5.9% sought any professional help. Among those with a high GHQ score and who were receptive to professional help, only 10.4% actually sought professional help. General practitioners were the most commonly preferred caregiver [49.3%], and were used by 41.1% of those who sought help. Malays used mental health services more than Chinese, but they did not show a significantly greater prevalence of high GHQ scores, or a greater preference to seek professional help. Receptivity to professional help, high GHQ score, and Malay ethnicity were independent significant predictors of use of mental health service. Studies in Israel concluded that as in western countries, mental health service use was low (33, 34). In a later Israeli study using the WMH survey method, Levinson et al reported that only about 10.3% of the Israeli adult population utilized the mental health and general health services for mental health reasons in any one year [35]. In a similar study in Nigeria, Gureje and Lasebikan reported that only 9.0% of those with any 12-month DSM-IV disorder had received treatment [36]. According to the authors, while 11% of those with a mood disorder had received some treatment, none of those with substance use disorders had used a mental health service. The study further reported that most treatments were received from general medical settings, rather than specialist mental health services where only about 1% of those with DSM-IV disorders received treatment. Complementary or alternative health providers were also consulted by only about 4% of those with mental disorders. Irrespective of the disorders or the sector where treatment was received, virtually no treatment was adjudged minimally adequate [36]. Using a somewhat novel method, Kohn et al [37] reviewed community-based psychiatric epidemiology studies that used standardized diagnostic instruments and included data on the percentage of individuals receiving care for schizophrenia and other non-affective psychotic disorders, major depression, dysthymia, bipolar disorder, generalized anxiety disorder, panic disorder, obsessive–compulsive disorder , and alcohol abuse or dependence. The authors calculated the median rates of untreated cases of these disorders and presented examples of the estimation of the treatment gap for WHO regions.

In all, thirty-seven studies had information on service utilization. The median treatment gap for schizophrenia, including other non-affective psychosis, was 32.2%. For other disorders the gap was: depression, 56.3%; dysthymia, 56.0%; bipolar disorder, 50.2%; panic disorder, 55.9%; Generalized Anxiety Disorder [GAD], 57.5%; and Obsessive Compulsive Disorder [OCD] 57.3%. Alcohol abuse and dependence had the widest treatment gap at 78.1%. The treatment gap for major depression in the WHO European Region was 45.4%, and for the Americas it was 56.9%. It was estimated that the average 12-month prevalence for major depression, weighting for the proportion of the population over the age of 15 years were: 4.7% for the WHO European Region and 6.2% for the Americas which suggests that in these regions there were about 31 million people and 35 million people, respectively, with major depression during a 12-month period out of whom, about 14 million in the European Region were untreated and about 20 million in the Americas were untreated. The authors were of the opinion that these treatment gaps were obvious under estimations [37]. The authors cited a Belize study which reported that about 63% of individuals with schizophrenia,

89% of those with affective disorders and 99% of those with an anxiety disorder had not been treated [38].

Mental Health Service Use in Immigrants

In population-based survey of first generation Turkish and Moroccan migrants and ethnic Dutch in Netherlands Fassaert et al [52] recruited 580 participants in structured interviews using their own languages. The authors measured uptake of mental health services by self-report. Of the subjects with a common mental disorder during six months preceding the interview, 50.9% reported care for mental problems in that period; 35.0% contacted specialised services. In relation to common mental disorder, ethnic groups were equally likely to access specialised mental health services. In relation to psychological distress, however, Moroccan migrants reported fewer uptakes of primary care services [OR = 0.37; 95% CI = 0.15 to 0.88]

Studies of mental health service use among Mexicans in the US have been consistent in reporting minimal rates [22-27]. Although Asian Americans are reported to be a highly heterogeneous group, in general they share the common feature of under utilization of mental health service [28].

Mental Health Service Use by Children

Most studies [apart from Garland et al) report that among children and adolescents, mental health service use is very low, accentuated by ethnic differences [29-32].

In Oman, Al Riyami et al [39] reported the mental health service use of school going children. Only between 6 to 12% of those having some form of mental disorder used any treatment facility. The proportions of lifetime cases having ever made treatment contact were very low, being 5.2% for any anxiety disorder and 13.2% for any mood disorder category. Those with anxiety disorders were mainly treated by the general medical system while more of those with mood disorders were treated by the specialist mental health service providers. In general, males and younger participants with social phobia were less likely to receive any treatment. Wu et al [40] reported that in a sample of American children, 36% of those with depression never received treatment from any professionals. In a rural African American Community, Angold et al [50] reported a 21.1% rate of mental disorders among the studied young people [similar in African American and Whites, though there was excess depression in white youths with a rate of 4.6% as against 1.4% for African American youths]. Only 36% of those with mental disorders had received any treatment in the previous three months.

In summary, it seems evident that every where mental health service has been studied, there is no doubt that there is under use.

All over the world the majority of people who have mental health problems do not receive any form of treatment. Some of the theoretical frame works of health service use [which ever one considers] help us to understand how a gap exists between need and use. We now turn attention to some of the barriers to mental health service use.

BARRIERS TO MENTAL HEALTH SERVICE USE

In a study of service use for neurotic disorders, Bebbington et al reported that treatment access was affected by employment status, marital status, and age, but the major determinant was symptom severity [19]. Neither sex nor social class influenced which people received treatment. In the US National Comorbidity Survey, Kessler et al also showed that illness severity and co- morbidity affected utilization of mental health service use. Similarly, Saren et al, in the Canadian study [48] indicated that severity of distress, social support and the presence of comorbid physical illness raised the likelihood of seeking and receiving mental health service. In the Israel mental health survey, the authors concluded that those with more severe illness were more likely to have sought help; respondents with milder degrees of mental ill health consulted religious and alternative mental health service providers more than allopathic health professionals [35].

The Anderson model gives broad and inter-related determinants of health service utilization. Enabling factors include cognitive, financial, cultural and linguistic issues. Some studies report that immigrants are less likely to use mental health service compared to the indigenous source population [53].

For example, cultural factors such as differences in explanatory models of beliefs and cultural idioms or modalities that are used to describe distress [e.g. "somatization"] can influence the type of care sought [53]. Personal and family perceptions of mental health problems as highly stigmatizing may discourage immigrants from using the mental health care system. For many minority groups, the family is the primary source of treatment especially for mental health problems and outside help is sought only after all family resources have been exhausted [53]. Preferences for alternative remedies and modes of treatment seeking, including religious leaders, elders and folk healers have been documented [53].

In reviewing some mental health service utilization studies, Mechanic [54] argued that very many factors including stigma about the label of mental disorder, having co-morbid mental disorders, insurance cover etc determined whether people would use mental health service or not. He concluded that overall, the magnitude and severity of distress and disability are the most important determinants of perceiving a need for care. Help seekers with greater distress are more likely to use mental health specialty care than are those with less distress. The author further stated that social selection, however, occurs across the range of distress and impairment, and factors independent of psychopathology and disability help to explain who enters treatment and the varying trajectories of care.

Fredrick et al [55] argued that cognitive, affective and value orientation factors may act as barriers to mental health service use. *Cognitive Barriers*: Culturally informed conceptions of mental illness are an important barrier to mental health service use. The notions of the nature, causes, and cures of mental illness and of well-being, labelling process of mental disorders all determine whether a mental health service will be used. *Affective Barriers*: Feelings of shame and stigma may prevent the seeking or receiving of mental health service. *Value Orientation Barriers*: Cultural value orientations may influence mental health service utilization. For example, Atkinson and Gim [56] argue that the conflict between cultural values of Asian Americans and the values inherent in the Western mental health system may be the cause of lack of initial contact with the system, whereas the inappropriateness of services may account for the high dropout rate among Asian Americans who do enter the system. Differences in value orientation can present barriers to acceptance of mental health services as a legitimate source of assistance.

Socioeconomic Factors are Associated with Service Use

In children and adolescents, multiple youth-, family-, and system-level factors have been shown to predict youth mental health service use, and many of these factors are associated with race/ethnicity. For example, one of the most consistent predictors of child mental health service use is the caregiver's perception of the strain of caring for the child [57, 58]. Recent evidence has identified significant and robust racial/ethnic differences in caregiver strain. Caregiver is comparable to level of distress and perceived need for care. Song, Sands and Wong [59] examined mental health service use among publicly insured white and African-American pregnant and postpartum women who live in a metropolitan area of Pennsylvania. The authors wanted to know the extent to which ethnicity, physical health problems, and behavioural health risk factors were associated with the probability of service use during the prenatal- postpartum period. Women were more likely to use services if they were Caucasian, had a number of chronic diseases, had a number of pregnancy complications, and smoked.

Scheppers et al [60] reviewed 54 articles published between 1990 and 2003 on health service use by ethnic minorities. They summarized the findings indicating that potential barriers occurred at three different levels: patient level, provider level and system level. The barriers at patient level were related to the patient characteristics: demographic variables, social structure variables, health beliefs and attitudes, personal enabling resources, community enabling resources, perceived illness and personal health practices. The barriers at provider level were related to the provider characteristics: skills and attitudes. The barriers at system level were related to the system characteristics: the organisation of the health care system, policy, structural factors etc. Although many of the cited studies concerned either general health care or ethnic minorities, there are nevertheless both universal and specific applications; for example, low income, lack of transport may act as barrier at any place and for any people. In the Singaporean survey of older adults mental health service use, Nyunt and colleagues [61] reported that poor or fair self rated mental health [O.R = 2.63 versus excellent or very good] and disability from mental illness [OR = 79.9] were positively associated with service use. Among non-need variables, female gender [OR = 2.25] and formal education [OR = 2.40] were independently associated with greater mental health service use. Higher household income was associated with less mental health service use [OR = 0.31] but a self-report of financial resource limitation for medical care was associated with less mental health service use [OR = 0.38)]. Reported availability of caregiver was also associated with less use of mental health services [OR = 0.20]. Among health beliefs, a belief that 'mental illnesses can be cured' was significantly associated with more mental health service use ['to a great extent', OR = 6.89; to some extent', OR = 4.01; versus not at all].

In a recent discourse on the health belief model in understanding mental health service use, Henshaw and Freedman –Doe [62] observed that several demographic variables have been found to consistently predict utilization of mental health services. Despite similar levels of distress, some groups are less likely to seek professional treatment than others, creating a gap between need and actual use of outpatient mental health services. Groups identified as consistently underutilizing services include men, adults aged 65 and older and ethnic minority groups in the United States. Within the health belief model framework, these demographic variables are hypothesized to influence clients' perceptions of severity, benefits, and barriers to seeking professional mental health services. The authors provided suggestions on how to improve mental health service use by working on the barriers based on the health belief model.

In a study of mental health service use in Chile, Saldivia et al (63) reported that financial problems, time constraints, lack of available service, not knowing where to go for treatment, stigma, belief that mental disorders have no treatment or are self limiting, low income, low levels of education, limit the use of mental health service use.

Mental Health Resources and Barriers to Care Use

In 2001, the WHO World Health Report advocated for and had as an objective a way to ensure adequate access to effective and humane treatment for all those who suffer from a mental disorder [68]. However, mental health care services can only be used if they are available.

In most parts of the world, mental health resources are poor. For example, in the World Health Organization Project Atlas, mental health policies were reported to be present in only 59.5% of the countries in the world. A mental health policy was found to be present in only 47.8% and 48.1% of countries of the African and Western Pacific Regions, respectively. More than 30% of countries do not have a national mental health programme [66]. In every part of the developing countries, mental health services are poor, have very low priority with grossly inadequate human and other resources. Report from Nigeria using the WHO-AIMS showed that the entire country of about 150 million people have fewer than 100 psychiatrists, few psychiatric nurses and other mental health professionals; at the same time these mental health professionals are densely concentrated only in the urban areas where minority of the country population dwells [67]. In a review of mental health resources, Saxena et al concluded that there is world wide paucity in terms of human, community, policy, infrastructure and financial resources [69]. The authors contended that the poor mental health resources invariably mean scarcity, inequity of distribution and inefficiency of resource use. Especially lacking in most low and middle income countries are community based mental health care services which are known to enhance services. This has led to calls for scaling up of mental health services [70].

The World Health Organization launched the Mental Health Gap Action Programme [mhGAP], and the Movement for Global Mental Health in October 2008. The goal and intent of mhGAP is to scale up care for mental, neurological, and substance use disorders, with strategies identified particularly for resource-constrained settings and countries. On the other hand, the Movement for Global Mental Health [MGMH] aims to improve services for people with mental disorders worldwide through the coordinated action of a global network of individuals and institutions [71].

Bridging the Gap

No illness can be treated unless it is recognized as an illness either by those who experience it or by health care professionals or even by policy makers who allocate resources for such care. To receive mental health service patients, mental health and general health professionals, governments at all levels all have a role to play. Despite much effort, the public is still only vaguely aware of most types of mental disorders and the availability of effective treatments. In many parts of the world, much effort has gone into increasing awareness of some common mental disorders such as clinical depression by non-psychiatrists. The knowledge of the general public about mental disorders is undoubtedly low. There is need for creating awareness both among non-psychiatric health care professionals and the lay public. [54].

Mechanic [54 has argued that behavioural research makes clear that knowledge by itself is not a sufficient inducement to bring people into needed care. He posits that distress and impairment and awareness of treatment potential provide motivation, but a range of other enabling factors make it more probable that perceived need will translate into treatment. These include the implementation of an action plan with such steps as specifically knowing how to call for help or where to go and overcoming barriers of payment, transportation, embarrassments, and other disincentives to action. Involvement in social circles supportive of treatment helps some to overcome barriers of what to do and how to do it and makes taking some action more acceptable. Public information campaigns have to more clearly include and explain action plans.

In the US, Clark [72] has argued that insurance coverage for everybody does not look feasible. Instead she advocated providing care to the low-income uninsured, such as using public funds to support safety-net institutions offering direct access to free and reduced-cost services. This seems to have worked reasonably well in the State of Louisiana. It is possible to extend this kind of design to mental health service.

Mental disorders are common and have enormous consequences when untreated. Many people who suffer from mental disorders are unrecognized and untreated. This is mainly due to multiple barriers at personal and various other levels. A multi-pronged approach is needed to bridge the gap between mental health need and use.

References

[1] Kessler RC, Chiu WT, Denler O etc Prevalence, severity, and comorbidity of twelve month DSM-IV disorders in the National Comorbidity Survey Replication (NCS-R). *Archives of General Psychiatry* 2005; 62: 612-617.

[2] WHO World Mental Health Consortium: Prevalence, severity and unmet need for treatment of mental disorders in the World Health Organization World Mental Health Surveys. *Journal of American Medical Association* 2004; 291: 2581-2590.

[3] World Health Organization. *The World Health Report 2004*. Geneva, Switzerland. WHO, 2004.

[4] Lemming MR, Calsyn RJ. Utility of the behavioural model in predicting service utilization by individuals suffering from severe mental illness and homelessness. *Community Mental Health Journal* 2004; 40: 347-364.
[5] Spencer MS, Chen J. Effects of discrimination on mental health service utilization among Chinese Americans. *American Journal of Public Health* 2004; 94: 809-814.
[6] Andersen AS, Laake P. A model for physician utilization within 2 weeks. *Analysis of Norwegian data. Med Care* 1987; 25: 300–310.
[7] Phillips KA, Morrison KR, Andersen R, Aday LA. Understanding the context of healthcare utilization: assessing environmental and provider-related variables in the behavioural model of utilization. *Health Services Research* 1998; 33: 571–596.
[8] Janz NK, Becker MH. The Health Belief Model: a decade later. *Health Education Quarterly 1984.* 11: 1–47.
[9] Leavitt F. The health belief model and utilization of ambulatory care services. *Social Sciences and Medicine* 1979; 13A: 105–112.
[10] Rosenmastock SM, Stretcher WJ, Becker MH. Social learning theory and the health Belief Model. *Health Education and Behaviour* 1988; 15: 173-183.
[11] Purola T. A systems approach to health and health policy. *Medical 1972; Care* 10: 373–379.
[12] Antonovsky A. A model to explain visits to doctor: With specific reference to the case of Israel. *Journal of Health and Social Behaviour* 1972; 13: 446–454.
[13] Engel GL. The need for a new medical model: A challenge for biomedicine. *Science* 1977; 196: 129–136.
[14] Regier DA, Narrow WH, Rae DS, Manderscheid RW, Locke BZ, Goodwin F. The de facto US mental health and addictive service system. Epidemiologic Catchment Area 1-year prospective prevalence rates of disorders and services. *Archives of General Psychiatry* 1993; 50: 85-94.
[15] Bland RC, Newman SC, Orn H. Health care service utilization for emotional problems: Results from a community survey. *Canadian Journal of Psychiatry* 1990; 35: 397-400.
[16] Fournier L, Lesage AD, Toupin J, Cyr M. Telephone surveys as an alternative for estimating prevalence of mental disorders and service utilization: a Montreal catchment area study. *Can J Psychiatry* 1997; 42:737–43.
[17] Vasiliadis HM, Lesage, A, Adair C, Boyer R. Service Use for Mental Health Reasons: Cross-Provincial Differences in Rates, Determinants, and Equity of Access *Canadian Journal of Psychiatry* 2005; 50:614–619.
[18] Lin E. Goering P, Offord DR, Campbell D, Boyle MH. Use of Mental Health Services in Ontario: Epidemiologic Findings. *Canadian Journal of Psychiatry* 1996; 41:572-577.
[19] Bebbington P, Brugha T, Meltzer H, Jerkins R, Ceresa C, Farrell M Lewis G: Neurotic disorders and the receipt of psychiatric treatment. *Psychological Medicine 2000,* 30:1369- 1376.
[20] Kessler RC, Frank RG, Edlund M, Katz SJ, Lin E, Leaf P: Differences in the use of psychiatric outpatient services between the United States and Ontario. *New England Journal of Medicine* 1997; 8:551–557.
[21] Kessler RC, Zhao S, Katz SJ,. Kouzis AC, Frank RG, Edlund M, Leaf P. Past-Year Use of Outpatient Services for Psychiatric Problems in the National Comorbidity Survey *American Journal of Psychiatry* 1999; 156:115–123.

[22] Vega, W, Kolody B, Valle R: Depressive symptoms and their correlation among immigrant Mexican women in the United States. *Social Science and Medicine* 1986; 22:645–651.

[23] Shrout PE, Canino GJ, Bird HR, et al: Mental health status among Puerto Ricans, Mexican Americans, and non-Hispanic whites. *American Journal of Community Psychology* 1992; 20:729–752.

[24] Moscicki EK, Locke BZ, Rae DS, et al: Depressive symptoms among Mexican Americans: the Hispanic Health and Nutrition Examination Survey. *American Journal of Epidemiology* 1989; 130: 348–360.

[25] Hu TW, Snowden L, Jerrell J, et al: Ethnic populations in public mental health: services choice and level of use. *American Journal of Public Health* 1981; 81:1429–1434.

[26] Hough RL, Landsverk JK, Karno M: Utilization of health and mental health services by Los Angeles Mexican Americans and non-Hispanic whites. *Archives of General Psychiatry* 1987; 44:702–709.

[27] Peifer KL, Hu T, Vega W. Help Seeking by Persons of Mexican Origin with Functional Impairments. *Psychiatric Services* 2000; 51: 1280-1298.

[28] Leong FTL, Lau ASL Barriers to Providing Effective Mental Health Services to Asian Americans. *Mental Health Services Research* 2001; 2:201-214.

[29] Bui KT, Takeuchi DT: Ethnic minority adolescents and the use of community mental health care services. *American Journal of Community Psychology* 1992; 20:403–417.

[30] Kataoka SH, Zhang L, Wells KB: Unmet need for mental health care among US children: variation by ethnicity and insurance status. *American Journal of Psychiatry* 2002; 159:1548–1555.

[31] McCabe K, Yeh M, Hough RL, Landsverk J, Hurlburt MS, Culver SW, Reynolds B: Racial/ethnic representation across five public sectors of care for youth. *Journal of Emotional and Behavioural Disorders* 1999; 7:72–82.

[32] Garland AF, Lau, AS, Yeh M, McCabe KM, Hough RL, Landsverk JA. Racial and Ethnic Differences in Utilization of Mental Health Services Among High-Risk Youths. *American Journal of Psychiatry* 2005; 162:733.

[33] Levinson D, Popper M. Ambulatory mental health treatment under universal coverage: *Policy insights from Israel*, Milbank Q 1997; 75: 235–260.

[34] Aviram U, Zilber N, Lerner Y, Popper M. Chronically mentally ill persons in Israel: Estimations of their number and characteristics. *Social Security* 1998; 53: 92– 105.

[35] Levinson D, Lerner Y, Zilber, N, Grinshpoon A, Levav I Twelve-Month Service Utilization Rates for Mental Health Reasons: Data from the Israel National Health Survey. *Israel Journal of Psychiatry and Related Sciences* 2007; 44: 114-125.

[36] Gureje O, Lsebikan VO. Use of mental health services in a developing country. Results from the Nigerian survey of mental health and well-being. *Social psychiatry and Psychiatric Epidemiology* 2006; 41(1):44-9.

[37] Kohn R, Saxen S, Levav I, Saraceno B. The treatment gap in mental health care. *Bulletin of the World Health Organization 2004*; 82:858-866.

[38] Bonander J, Kohn R, Arana B, Levav I. An anthropological and epidemiological overview of mental health in Belize. *Transcultural Psychiatry* 2000; 37:57-72.

[39] Al Riyami AS, Al Adawi SH, Al Kharusi HA , Morsi MM, Jaju SS. Health services utilization by school going Omani adolescents and youths with DSM IV mental

disorders and barriers to service use. *International Journal of Mental Health Systems* 2009; 3:22.
[40] Wu P, Hoven CW, Cohen P, Liu X, Moore RE, Tiet Q, Okezie N, Wicks J, Bird HR. Factors Associated With Use of Mental Health Services for Depression by Children and Adolescents. *Psychiatric Services* 2001; 52:189–195.
[41] du Fort GG, Newman SC, Boothroyd LJ, *et al.*: Treatment seeking for depression: role of depressive symptoms and comorbid psychiatric diagnoses. *Journal of Affective Disorders* 1999, 52:31-40.
[42] Wang PS, Lane M, Olfson M, Pincus HA, Wells KB, Kessler RC. Twelvemonth use of mental health services in the United States: results from the National Comorbidity Survey Replication. *Archives of General Psychiatry* 2005, 2005; 62:629-640.
[43] Karam EG, Mneimneh ZN, Dimassi H, Fayyad JA, Aimee N. Karam AN,. Nasser SC, Chatterji S, Kessler RC. Lifetime Prevalence of Mental Disorders in Lebanon: First Onset, Treatment, and Exposureto War. *PLoS Medicine* 2008; 5: 580-586.
[44] Borges G, Medina-Mora ME, Wang PS, Lara C, Berglund P, Walters E. Treatment and Adequacy of Treatment of Mental Disorders among Respondents to the Mexico National Comorbidity Survey. *American Journal of Psychiatry* 2006; 163: 1371-1378.
[45] WHO. *Mental health services in Europe: the treatment gap.* WHO European Ministerial Conference on mental health. EUR/04/5047810/B13. Nov 2004.
[46] The ESEMed/MHEDEA 2000 investigators. Use of mental health services in Europe: results from the European study of the Epidemiology of Mental Disorders [ESEMed] project. *Acta Psychiatrica Scandinavica* 2004; 109 [Supplement 420]: 47-54.
[47] Chisoholm D, Flisher A, Lund C, Patel V, Saxena S, Thornicroft G, Tomlinson M. Scale up services for mental disorders: a call for action. *Lancet* 2007; 370: 1241-1252.
[48] Sareen J, Cox, BJ, Afifi TO, Clara I, Yu BN. Perceived Need for .Mental Health Treatment in a Nationally Representative Canadian Sample. *Canadian Journal of Psychiatry* 2005; 50: 643-651.
[49] Andrews G, Issakidis C, Carter G. Shortfall in mental health service utilization. *British Journal of Psychiatry* 2001; 179: 417-425.
[50] Angold A, Erkanli A, Farmer EMZ, Fairbank JA, Burns BJ, Keeler G, Costello EJ. Psychiatric disorder, impairment and service use in rural African and White youth. *Archives of General Psychiatry* 2002, 59: 893-901.
[51] Ng TP, Fones CSL, Kua EH. Preference, need and utilization of mental health services, Singapore National Mental Health Survey. Australian and New Zealand *Journal of Psychiatry* 2003; 37:613–619.
[52] Fassaert T, de Wit MAS, Verhoeff AP, Tuinebreijer WC, Beekman ATF, Jack Dekker J. Uptake of health services for common mental disorders by first-generation Turkish and Moroccan migrants in the Netherlands. *BMC Public Health* 2009, 9:307.
[53] Fenta H, Hyman I, Noh S. Health Service Utilization by Ethiopian immigrants and refugees in Toronto. Journal of immigrant and minority health. 2007; 9: 349-357.
[54] Mechanic D. Emerging trends in mental health policy and practice. *Health Affairs 2002*; 21:137-147.
[55] Frederick T. L. Leong FTL, Lau ASL. Barriers to Providing Effective Mental Health Services to Asian Americans. *Mental Health Services Research* 2001; 3: 201-214.
[56] Atkinson, D. R, Gim, R. H. Asian American cultural identity and attitudes toward mental health services. *Journal of Counselling Psychology* 1989; 36: 209–212.

[57] Angold A, Messer SC, Stangl D, Farmer EMZ, Costello EJ, Burns BJ: Perceived parental burden and service use for child and adolescent Psychiatric disorders. *Am J Public Health* 1998; 88:75–80.

[58] Brannan AM, Heflinger GA, Bickman L: The Caregiver Strain Questionnaire: measuring the impact on the family of living with a child with serious emotional disturbance. *Journal of Emotional and Behavioral Disorders* 1997; 5:212–222.

[59] Song D, Sands RG, Wong I. Utilization of Mental Health Services by Low-Income Pregnant and Postpartum Women on Medical Assistance. *Women and Health* 2004; 39: 1-24.

[60] Scheppers E, van Dongen E, Dekker J, Geertzen J , Dekker J. Potential barriers to the use of health services among ethnic minorities: a review. *Family Practice* 2006; 23: 325–348.

[61] Nyunt MSZ, Chiam PC, Kua EH, Ng TP. Determinants of mental health service use in the national mental health survey of the elderly in Singapore. *Clinical Practice and Epidemiology in Mental Health,* 2009, 5:2.

[62] Henshaw EJ, Freedman-Doan CR. Conceptualizing Mental Health Care Utilization Using the Health Belief Model. *Clinical Psychology in social practice* 2009; 16: 420-439.

[63] Saldivia S, Vicente B, Kohn R, Pedro Rioseco P, Torres. Use of Mental Health Services in Chile. *Psychiatric Services* 2004; 55: 71–76.

[64] Ajzen, I. The theory of planned behaviour. *Organizational Behaviour and Human Decision Processes* 1991; 50: 179–211.

[65] Lau, R. R., & Hartman, K. A. 1983. Commonsense representations of common illnesses. *Health Psychology* 1983; 2: 167–185.

[66] Saraceno B, Saxena S. Mental health resources in the world: results from Project Atlas of the WHO. *World Psychiatry* 2002; 1:40-44.

[67] WHO & Ministry of Health, Ibadan Nigeria. *WHO-AIMS Report on Mental Health System in Nigeria.* WHO & Ministry of Health, Ibadan Nigeria, 2006.

[68] WHO. World Health Report 2001. *Mental Health: New Understanding, New Hope.* Geneva, Switzerland. World Health Orgaanization 2001.

[69] Saxena S, Thornictoft G, Knapp M, Whiteford H. Resources for mental health: scarcity, inequity and inefficiency. *The Lancet 2007*; Published online Sept 4, 2007. DOI: 10.1016/501406736(07)612446; PP32-43.

[70] Lancet Global Mental Health Group. Scale up services for mental disorders; a call for action. *The Lancet 2007*; Published online Sept 4, 2007. DOI: 10.1016/501406736 (07)612446; PP87-98.

[71] World Health Organization: mhGAP: *Mental Health Gap Action Programme: Scaling up care mental, neurological, and substance use disorders Geneva:* World Health Organization; 2008.

[72] Clark, M. A. Access to Care versus Access to Coverage: What Can We Learn from the Louisiana State Hospital Model? *World Medical and Health Policy* 2010: Vol. 2: Issue. 1, Article 10.

In: Social Determinants and Mental Health
Editor: Sabine Bährer-Kohler

ISBN: 978-1-61324-353-4

Chapter 11

HOUSING, HOMELESSNESS AND MENTAL HEALTH

Sabine Bährer-Kohler
Behavioral Disorders, Switzerland
Bern University of Applied Science, Bern, Switzerland
Representative to the WHO Advisory Group for the Revision of the *ICD-10* Mental and
Director of the International Psychogeriatric Association, US

INTRODUCTION: HOUSING AND HEALTH

The Universal Declaration of Human Rights (1948) of the United Nations states in Article 25: (1) Everyone has the right to a standard of living adequate for the health and well-being of himself and of his family, including food, clothing, *housing* and medical care and necessary social services, and the right to security in the event of unemployment, sickness, disability, widowhood, old age or other lack of livelihood in circumstances beyond his control.

The article highlights as important the right to an adequate standard of living, including *adequate housing*, reiterating the importance of, inter alia, infrastructure and services, particularly those related to water, sanitation, health, transportation and energy, as well as security of tenure and the principle of non-discrimination in the context of housing (Commission on Human Rights 2004).

The WHO (2010a) postulates that national mental health policies should not be solely concerned with mental disorders but should also recognize and address the broader issues which promote mental health. This includes mainstreaming mental health promotion into policies and developing related programs in government and business sectors including education, labor, justice, transport, environment, *housing*, and welfare as well as the health sector.

Forms of residence differ widely, but good-quality, affordable, safe housing is essential to wellbeing and health (Johnson et al. 2005), keeping in mind that housing conditions influence people's health in positive and negative ways (WHO, Regional Office for Europe, 2011a) and that substandard housing is a major public health issue (Sharfstein et al. 1998).

Healthy living calls for functional and adequate physical, social and mental conditions in terms of health, security, hygiene, comfort and privacy (WHO Regional Office for Europe, 2004). The declaration of the UN Habitat Conference (Istanbul 1996) specifies additional characteristics, such as giving priority consideration to the tendency towards excessive lack of basic infrastructure and services; lack of adequate planning; growing insecurity and violence; environmental degradation; and increased vulnerability to disasters.

It is important in this context that adequate standards may vary from country to country, being dependent on specific cultural, social, environmental and economic factors. Gender- and age-specific aspects should also be taken into account in this context (WHO Regional Office for Europe, 2004).

In contrast to desirable living conditions, the National Housing Federation (NHF) defined poor housing in 2010 as dwellings that are cold and damp, overcrowded, or badly designed and built. Currently, the WHO is calling for international guidance on "healthy housing" which should be developed to help prevent a wide range of diseases and unintentional injuries that can be effectively addressed through better housing. This was a key message emerging from an international consultation hosted by the WHO in Geneva in 2010 (WHO, 2010b).

Aspects of Housing and Mental Health

There are connections between housing and mental health. What is important is that the vast majority of people with a mental illness is living in the community, and therefore is in need of a place to live (Knapp et al. 2007).

Evans et al. (2000) found that studies, including a prospective longitudinal design, demonstrate that physical housing quality predicates mental health. In another analysis concerning poor housing and mental health, Hopton et al. 1996 examined 114 men and 333 women aged between 17 and 65 from 451 households in Scotland. They found that reporting a problem with dampness was significantly and independently associated with scores of > or = 5 on the GHQ30 (General Health Questionnaire) after checking for possible confounding variables.

In a structured review of published evaluations of interventions to improve health by modifying housing in the United States that were conducted between 1990 and 2001, Saegert et al. (2003) stated that the literature demonstrates repeatedly that poor housing can contribute to infectious disease transmission, injuries, asthma symptoms, lead poisoning, and mental health problems.

In a systematic review of studies that investigated the relationship between housing-related independent variables and health-related dependent variables in the self-perception of the people concerned, Kyle et al. (2008) found that individuals with severe and persistent mental illness (SPMI) identify housing as an important factor in achieving and maintaining their health. Kyle et. al. analyzed twenty-nine studies of which 14 reported healthcare utilization outcomes; 12 mental status outcomes; and 9 quality-of-life outcomes. Moreover, Meltzer et al. 2002 document that people with mental health problems are four times as likely to believe that their accommodation is aggravating their health problems.

One prominent finding on housing as an input and an outcome was that living in independent housing was associated with greater satisfaction with housing and neighborhood (Newman, 2001).

The issue will have to be studied at greater depth before we can say more precisely what aspects of housing do or do not affect mental health, for which group of persons, and to what extent. Only a few years after the aforementioned publication, Evans et al. documented that research on housing and mental health is remarkably underdeveloped in general (Evans et al. 2003), that analyses of the effect of poor housing on psychological well-being and health are missing, and that besides a deeper understanding of the relationship between mental health problems and housing provision was necessary (Page, 2002). A few years after Evans, Knapp et al. also documented that in general, there is a profound lack of systematic information on the housing situation of people with mental illness (Knapp et al. 2007), and that there is a dearth of research

- concerning housing programs and serious mental illness as well as
- rural populations, which heightens the relevance of research findings for health service planning (Montgomery et al. 2008).

Mental disorder in combination with substance abuse represents an extended challenge. The need for supported housing for people with dual diagnosis is important and represents a challenge for communities as well as psychiatric services. (Kielland, 2002).

What might be helpful in the context of mental health is Shaw's explanatory model with its factor analysis. In 2004, Shaw developed a model which describes the manifold interactions between living conditions and health. Among other things, she distinguishes between hard factors such as furnishings and soft factors such as personal judgments of living quality, deriving from her model potential direct and indirect effects on the inhabitant's mental and physical health.

Aspects of Homelessness and Mental Health

Next to individual accounts, structural explanations locate the reasons for homelessness in social and economic structures, highlighting factors like poverty, a negative labor market, inadequate social service coverage, cuts and restrictions of social welfare payments and a lack of accessible and affordable housing. (Busch-Geertsema et al. 2010).

All in all, homelessness is an increasing public health problem and a significant public health concern (Matte et al. 2000), representing an extreme form of poverty and marginalization (Study Group on Homelessness, 1993).

The global prevalence of homeless families has dramatically increased in recent years (Badiaga et al. 2008; Parks et al. 2007), despite the diversity of the homeless population and the fact that the homeless population has contributed to the methodological difficulties (Busch-Geertsema et al. 2010; Harvey, 1999). Homeless people constitute a heterogeneous population (WHO, Regional Office for Europe, 2005). According to the ethos typology, homelessness is defined by exclusion from several or all three domains which constitute a home: the social, the legal and the physical domain. (Busch-Geertsema et al. 2010).

An estimated 100 million persons worldwide experience homelessness (Badiaga et al. 2008/ Burt et al. 2001). In its annual Homeless Assessment Report to Congress (2009), the US Department of Housing and Urban Development documented that around 650,000 sheltered or unsheltered homeless people were living in the US in January 2009. In 2004, India posted much greater numbers of homeless people and runaway adolescents roaming the streets of the country (Khurana et al. 2004). For Germany, the Protestant homeless relief charity estimates (for there is no nationwide statistic) that more than 250,000 people are homeless.

People who are homeless have

- poor living conditions,
- often limited access to healthcare systems (Badiaga et al. 2008) and
- often problems with obtaining suitable healthcare (WHO Regional Office for Europe, 2011b).

The WHO states that homeless people have poorer physical and mental health than the general population (WHO Regional Office for Europe, 2011b; WHO Regional Office for Europe, 2005). Other studies indicate a high prevalence of mental health problems among homeless people (Odell et al. 2000, Timms et al. 1997). These statements jibe with those made by the Pathways Project. The Pathways Project in Canada collected data over an 18-month period in order to "estimate the prevalence of mental illness among people who are homeless" (Riordan, 2004) in the City of Toronto. They found that approximately 66% of homeless persons have a lifetime diagnosis of mental illness. This is 2-3 times the rate in the general population. The WHO's statements also agree with a study by the US National Survey of Homeless Assistance Providers and Clients 1996 (published 1999) on lifetime self-reported alcohol, drug and mental health problems of homeless people, which found that 57% have problems with mental health (lifetime), 62% have problems with alcohol (lifetime) and 58% have problems with drugs (table 2.4). Accumulations of mental health problems among the homeless were also reported by Fazel et al.. They documented in 2008 that homeless people in Western countries are substantially more likely to have alcohol and drug dependence than the age-matched general population in those countries, and that the prevalence of psychotic illnesses and personality disorders is higher. Grinman et al. 2010 analyzed 603 homeless single men, 304 homeless single women, and 284 homeless adults with dependent children in Canada. Forty percent of the study sample had drug problems in the last 30 days. The substances used within the past 2 years were marijuana (40%), cocaine (27%), and opiate analgesics other than heroin or methadone (i.e., oxycodone, hydromorphone, meperidine, codeine, and pentazocine) (8%). Drug problems are common among homeless individuals and drug problems can be associated with poorer mental health and represent an extended challenge.

Although it is known that many homeless people have limited access to healthcare systems McNiel and Binder found that homeless individuals with mental disorders may have frequently received psychiatric emergency treatment. In 2005, they examined relationships between homelessness, mental disorder, violence, and the use of psychiatric emergency services. They examined data of 2,294 individuals who were treated in the county hospital's psychiatric emergency ward in San Francisco, California, and documented that homeless individuals with mental disorders accounted for a large proportion of rthose who received psychiatric emergency treatment in the community mental health system.

Even though it is known that mental illnesses occur more frequently among the homeless there is still, as mentioned above, some debate about, for instance, measuring the prevalence of homelessness and the personal characteristics of homeless persons (Begin, 1999).

Busch-Geertsema et al. (2010) wrote that the diversity of the homeless population has contributed to the methodological difficulties associated with estimating the prevalence of homelessness.

Added to this there are structural and systemic factors contributing to homelessness. Thus, for example, Buckland et al. (2001) commented that, due to the lack of good data, most researchers have been understandably reluctant to provide estimates of the total number of Canadians experiencing homelessness.

The debate over whether homelessness is a "pathway" to mental illness and substance abuse, or mental illness and substance abuse are "pathways" to homelessness could not be settled by this study (Riordan, 2004). By way of contrast, a new Canadian study documents that British Columbia's homeless suffered from severe mental health challenges long before they lost their homes (Krausz, 2010). In it, 500 homeless British Columbians living in Vancouver, Victoria and Prince George were examined. It found that health challenges and especially traumatic experiences start much earlier among homeless individuals than among those living in substandard housing, very often in childhood or critical developmental periods.

Housing, Socioeconomic Status and Mental Health

Housing is a concrete manifestation of socioeconomic status (Dunn, 2002) which has an important part to play in the development of explanations of the social context of health inequalities.

The lower the socioeconomic status (SES) of an indivudual is, the higher is the risk of mental illness (Hudson, 2005). One of the first studies to identify the relationship between SES and schizophrenia and other psychoses was the study of Faris and Dunham (1939). They found disproporationate rates of mental disease in the poorest parts of Chicago (Hudson, 2005). Poverty and housing are mutually dependent. A current systematic review by Lund et al. (2010) of 115 studies on poverty in low- and middle-income countries found that most reported positive associations between a range of poverty indicators and common mental disorders. While variables such as education, food insecurity, *housing*, social class, socioeconomic status and financial stress exhibit a relatively consistent and strong association with CMD (common mental disease), others such as income, employment and particularly consumption are more equivocal. 73% and 79% of studies reported positive associations between a variety of poverty measures and CMD.

Poverty is not measured by consistent standards, and the European Commission's Eurostat agency points out that, as multi-dimensional concepts, poverty and social exclusion cannot easily be measured through statistics. As a result, both monetary and non-monetary indicators have been developed, such as the at-risk-of-poverty rate, the at-risk-of-poverty threshold, the income quintile ratio and the material deprivation rate. (Eurostat, 2009). At the same time, the agency stated that in 2007, approximately 79 million people (16%) in the EU lived below the poverty threshold, a state of affairs which also affects forms of residence. And according to an EU report, 38% of the people who are at risk of poverty spend more than 40% of their disposable income on housing – more than twice the average for the overall population (EU news, 2010).

A longitudinal study of the population of Massachusetts examined patients with psychiatric hospitalizations during 1994-2000, correlating unemployment, poverty and housing unaffordability with the risk of mental illness (Hudson, 2005). The results of the study suggest that SES (socioeconomic status) impacts the development of mental illness directly as well as indirectly through its association with adverse economic stressful conditions among low- and middle-income groups. The conclusion was that mental illness prevention efforts and early intervention strategies should pay attention to the impact of unemployment, economic displacement, and housing dislocation (including homelessness).

The results of another study done in Australia indicate that people with mental illness want housing similar to that of Australians in general (Lambert et al. 2000). However, unemployment or very low incomes may affect the ability not only of people with mental illness to realize their housing choice (Lambert et al. 2000; Edgar et al. 2002). Edgar et al. analyzed the European housing market, the provision of housing and their impact on homelessness. The rising cost of housing was quoted as another unfavorable condition. These macroeconomic conditions cannot be neglected. (McQuistion et al. 2003).

One consequence for the promotion of mental health within the public health system is that that the financial situation of individuals should be sufficient to acquire suitable accommodation.

In addition, there is a clear need and opportunity for governments and others to promote health in the course of making investments in housing (WHO, 2010b).

As far as housing availability and access to social and health services are concerned, both urban and rural factors should be taken into account. Writing about people with a mental illness living in rural and regional areas, Grigg et al. (2008) documented that while there was a wide variety of housing options in the region under investigation, housing availability was not evenly distributed. In this context, access to services should be included, concerning which the WHO published the report "Hidden cities: unmasking and overcoming health inequities in urban settings" together with the United Nations Human Settlements Program (UN-HABITAT). The report was launched at the Global Forum on Urbanization and Health in Kobe, Japan, as part of the WHO's 2010 World Health Day campaign. It revealed that urban residents tend to have greater access to social and health services than their rural counterparts (WHO Regional Office for Europe, 2010f; WHO, 2010e).

The Need for Good Housing

Recognizing that adequate housing is a key element in fostering family integration, contributing to social equity and strengthening the feeling of belonging, security and human solidarity (Office of the high commissioner for human rights 2004), and that housing should be seen as a place for growth and a foundation for the fulfillment of life objectives that provides for good physical and mental health and personal well-being (Ambrose, 1997), it must be admitted that the priority of the housing needs of people with a mental illness has been relatively low in both mental health and housing policies (Knapp et al. 2007). This should be changed.

For it is an acknowledged fact that in the field of housing and health, legal housing and construction regulations offer governments and local authorities a wide range of options to improve the housing conditions and thus the health of European citizens (WHO Regional Office for Europe 2010c). Moreover, the fourth Ministerial Conference on Environment and Health (Budapest, 2004) called for initiatives and programs that facilitate the integration of health and environmental concerns into housing policies (WHO Regional Office for Europe, 2010d).

Policymakers and housing practitioners should consider refocusing improvement schemes from predominantly physiological health gains to include enhancing mental health (Page, 2002).

Inter alia, good housing in the context of mental health calls for

1. Adequate and affordable accommodation
2. Decision-makers who are well informed about the social determinant of housing and its relation to mental health components
3. Additional scientific surveys and studies on the subject
4. Programs that represent people's interests both nationally and internationally in the spirit of equity in health and the principles of health for all (WHO Regional Office for Europe, 2009)
5. The integration of global health priorities
6. The integration of aspects of prevention
7. The promotion of mental health.

Especially mental illness prevention efforts and early intervention strategies should pay special attention to the impact of housing dislocation, including homelessness (Hudson, 2005).

Further important concerns include countering the social exclusion and marginalization of people who suffer from discrimination on multiple grounds, in particular by ensuring non-discriminatory access to adequate housing for indigenous people and persons belonging to minorities (Office of the high commissioner for human rights, 2004). We also need to promote participation in decision-making processes and include relevant stakeholders in the planning stage when developing an adequate standard of living and housing. (Office of the high commissioner for human rights, 2004).

REFERENCES

Ambrose, P. (1997). Better Housing as Preventative Medicine. *Housing Review.* 46 (3).

Badiaga, S., Raoult, D., Brouqui, P. (2008). Preventing and controlling emerging and reemerging transmissible diseases in the homeless. *Emerg Infect Dis.*14 (9).

Begin, P., Casavant, L., Miller Chenier, N. & Dupuis, J. (1999). Homelessness. *Library of Parliament document, Parliamentary Research Branch*, PRB 99-1E, pp. 10-16.

Buckland, L., Jackson, A., Roberts, P., Smith, P. (2001). Structural and Systemic Factors Contributing to Homelessness in Canada: An Analysis of Research Gaps and Proposed Research Directions, Canadian Council on Social Development, Ottawa. In: Riordan, T. (2004). Exploring the Circle: Mental Illness, Homelessness and the Criminal Justice System in Canada. Political and Social Affairs Division. PRB 04-02E. *http://www2.parl.gc.ca.*

Burt, M.R., Aron, L.Y. (2001). Helping America's homeless. Washington: Urban Institute.

Busch-Geertsema, V., William, E., O`Sullivan, E., Pleace, N. (2010). Homelessness and Homeless Policies in Europe: Lesson from Research. FEANTSA. Brussels, Directorate-General for Employment, *Social Affairs and Equal Opportunities*. 1, 88.

Dunn, J. R. (2002). Housing and inequalities in health: a study of socioeconomic dimensions of housing and self reported health from a survey of Vancouver residents. *Epidemiol Community Health*. Sep; 56(9): 671-81.

Edgar, B., Doherty, J. (2002). Access to housing: homelessness and vulnerability in Europe. *The Policy Press*.

EU News (2010). Homelessness– a major challenge for Europe 29/06/2010. *http://ec.europa.eu.*

Eurostat (2009). Social inclusion statistics. *http://epp.eurostat.ec.europa.eu.*

Evans, G.W., Wells, N.M., Chan, H.Y., Saltzman, H. (2000). Housing quality and mental health. *J Consult Clin Psychol*. Jun;68(3): 526-30.

Evans, G.W., Wells, N.M., Moch, A. (2003). Housing and Mental Health: A Review of the Evidence and a Methodological and Conceptual Critique. *Journal of Social Issues*. 59, 3, 475-500.

Faris, R.E., Dunham, W. (1939). Mental Disorders in Urban Areas: An ecological study of Schizophrenia and other psychoses. Chicago, IL: *University of Chicago Press*.

Fazel, S., Khosla, V., Doll, H., Geddes, J. (2008). The Prevalence of Mental Disorders among the Homeless in Western Countries: Systematic Review and Meta-Regression Analysis. *PLoS Med* 5(12): e225. *http://www.plosmedicine.org*.

Grigg, M., Judd, F., Ryan, L., Komiti, A. (2005). Identifying marginal housing for people with a mental illness living in rural and regional areas. *Aust N Z J Psychiatry*. Nov-Dec; 39(11-12): 995-1000.

Grinman, M.N., Chiu, S., Redelmeier, D.A., Levinson, W., Kiss, A.,Tolomiczenko, G., Cowan, L., Hwang, St. W. (2010). Drug problems among homeless individuals in Toronto, Canada: prevalence, drugs of choice, and relation to health status. *BMC Public Health*. 10: 94.

Harvey, B. (1999). The problem of the homelessness: A European Perspective, in: Hutson, S., Clapham, D. (eds.) *Homelessness: Pubic Policies and Private Troubles*. Cassell.

Hopton, J. L., Hunt, S. M. (1996). Housing conditions and mental health in a disadvantaged area in Scotland. *J Epidemiol Community Health*. 50 (1): 56-61.

Hudson, C.G. (2005). Socioeconomic Status and Mental Illness: Tests of the Social Causation and Selection Hypotheses. *American Journal of Orthopsychiatry*. 75 (1): 3-18.

Johnson, R., Griffiths, C. (2005). At Home? A study of mental health issues arising in social housing. Report published on NSIP website: p. 10. *http://www.robinjohnson-associates.org.uk*.

Khurana, S., Sharma, N., Jena, S., Saha, R., Ingle, G. K. (2004). Mental health status of runaway adolescents. *Indian Journal of Pediatrics*. 71, 5: 405-409.

Kielland, K.B. (2002). Shortage of supported housing for patients with mental disorder and substance abuse. *Tidsskr Nor Laegeforen*. 122(25): 2458-60.

Knapp, M., McDaid, D., Mossialos, E., Thornicroft, G. (Edit.) (2007). Mental Health Policy and Practice across Europe. The future direction of mental health care. *Open University Press*.

Krausz, M. (2010). Health of the Homeless. Health of the Homeless, summit in Vancouver. *http://thetyee.ca*.

Kyle, T., Dunn, J.R. (2008). Effects of housing circumstances on health, quality of life and healthcare use for people with severe mental illness: a review. *Health Soc Care Community*. 16(1): 1-15.

Lambert, G., Ricci, P., Harris, R., Deane, F. (2000). Housing Needs of Consumers of Mental Health Services in Rural New South Wales, Australia. Int J Soc Psychiatry.46 (1): 57-66.

Lund, C., Breen, A., Fisher, A.J., Kakuma, R., Corrigall, J., Joska, J., Swartz, L., Patel, V. (2010). Poverty and common mental disorders in low and middle income countries: A systematic review. *Social Science and Medicine*. 71(3): 517-28.

Matte, T., Jacobs, D. (2000). Housing and health- current issues and implications for research and programs. *J Urban Health*. 77: 7–25.

McNiel, D.E., Binder, R.L. (2005). Psychiatric emergency service use and homelessness, mental disorder, and violence. *Psychiatr Serv*. Jun; 56(6): 699-704.

McQuistion, H.L., Finnerty, M., Hirschowitz, J., Susser, E.S. (2003). Challenges for psychiatry in serving homeless people with psychiatric disorders. *Psych Serv*. 54(5): 669-676.

Meltzer, H., Singleton, N., Lee, A., Bebbington, P., Brugha, T. and Jenkins, R. (2002). The social and economic circumstances of adults with mental disorders. London: *The Stationery Office*.

Montgomery, P., Forchuk, C., Duncan, C., Rose, D., Bailey, P.H., Veluri, R. (2008). Supported housing programs for persons with serious mental illness in rural northern communities: A mixed method evaluation. *BMC Health Services Research*. 8:156.

National Housing Federation (2010). Housing and Mental Health. London, NHF. *http://www.housing.org.uk*.

Newman, S.J. (2001). Housing Attributes and Serious Mental Illness: Implications for Research and Practice. *Psychiatr Serv*. 52:1309-131.

Odell, S.M., Commander, M.J. (2000). Risk factors for homelessness among people with psychotic disorders. *Social Psychiatry and Psychiatric Epidemiology*. 35 (9): 396-401.

Office of the high commissioner for human rights, Commission on Human Rights resolution (2004). Adequate housing as a component of the right to an adequate standard of living. *www.unhabitat.org*.

Page, A. (2002). Poor Housing and Mental Health in the United Kingdom: Changing the Focus for Intervention. *JEHR Journal of Environmental Health Research*. Volume:1, Issue:1.

Parks, R.W., Stevens, R.J., Spence, S.A. (2007). A systematic review of cognition in homeless children and adolescents. *Journal of the Royal Society of Medicine*. 100: 46-50.

Protestant/Evangelische Obdachlosenhilfe in Deutschland e.V. (2010). Willkommen auf unserer Webseite. *www.evangelische-obdachlosenhilfe.de/*, retrieved from the Evangelische Obdachlosenhilfe in Deutschland e.V. website 01 February 2011.

Riordan, T. (2004). Exploring the Circle: Mental Illness, Homelessness and the Criminal Justice System in Canada. *Political and Social Affairs Division*. PRB 04-02E. *http://www2.parl.gc.ca.*

Saegert, S.C., Klitzman, S., Freudenberg, N. J., Cooperman-Mroczek, J., Salwa Nassar, B.S (2003). Healthy Housing: A Structured Review of Published Evaluations of US Interventions to Improve Health by Modifying Housing in the United States, 1990–2001. *Am J Public Health*. September; 93(9): 1471–147.

Sharfstein, J., Sandel, M., eds. (1998). Not Safe at Home: How America's Housing Crisis Threatens the Health of Its Children. Boston, Mass: *Boston University Medical Center*.

Shaw, A. (2004). Housing and Public Health. *Annual Review of Public Health.* 25: 397-418.

Study Group on Homelessness (1993). Homelessness-Report. Prepared by the Study Group on Homelessness (Strasbourg: Council of *Europe Press*).

Timms, Ph., Balázs, J. (1997). ABC of mental health: Mental health on the margins. BMJ. 315: 536.

U.S. Department of Housing and Urban Development HUD (1999). Homelessness: Programs and the People They Serve. *http://www.huduser.org.*

U.S. Department of Housing and Urban Development HUD (2009). The Annual Homeless Assessment Report (*AHAR*).

United Nations (1948). The Universal Declaration of Human Rights. *http://www.un.org.*

United Nations (1996). UN-HABITAT- United Nations Human Settlements Programme. Habitat II Conference. Istanbul.

WHO Regional Office for Europe Europe (2004). Housing and Health. *http://test.cp.euro.who.int.*

WHO Regional Office for Europe (2005). How can health care systems effectively deal with the major health care needs of homeless people? *http://www.euro.who.int.*

WHO Regional Office for Europe (2009). Phase V (2009–2013) of the WHO European Healthy Cities Network: goals and requirements. *http://www.euro.who.int/en/what-we-do/health-topics/environmental-health/urban-health/publications.*

WHO (2010a). Mental health: strengthening our response. Fact sheet N°220 *http://www.who.int/mediacentre/factsheets/fs220/en/.*

WHO (2010b). Housing and Health. 'Healthy housing' - Experts call for international guidelines *http://www.who.int/hia/housing/en,* retrieved from the WHO website 26 January 2011.

WHO Regional Office for Europe (2010c). Housing and health. Risk management and policy options. *http://www.euro.who.int/en/what-we-do/health-topics/environmental-health/Housing-and-health/country-work/local-housing-and-health-action-plans,* retrieved from the WHO Regional Office for Europe website 25 January 2011.

WHO Regional Office for Europe (2010d). Housing and health. Local Housing and Health Action Plans. *http://www.euro.who.int/en/what-we-do/health-topics/environmental-health,* retrieved from the WHO Regional Office for Europe website 25 January 2011.

WHO (2010e). Hidden cities: new report shows how poverty and ill-health are linked in urban area. *http://www.who.int/mediacentre/news,* retrieved from the WHO website 26 January 2011.

WHO Regional Office for Europe (2010f). Urban health. *http://www.euro.who.int/en/what-we-do/health-topics,* retrieved from the WHO Regional Office for Europe website 26 January 2011.

WHO Regional Office for Europe (2011a). Housing and health. *http://www.euro.who.int/en/what-we-do/health-topics/environmental-health/Housing-and-health,* retrieved from the WHO Regional Office for Europe website 25 January 2011.

WHO Regional Office for Europe (2011b). Health Evidence Network (HEN). How can health care systems effectively deal with the major health care needs of homeless people? *http://www.euro.who.int/en/what-we-do/data-and-evidence,* retrieved from the WHO Regional Office for Europe website 26 January 2011.

In: Social Determinants and Mental Health
Editor: Sabine Bährer-Kohler

ISBN: 978-1-61324-353-4

Chapter 12

Residential Situations and Mental Health: Mental Health Issues in Nursing Homes

David K. Conn
University of Toronto Department of Psychiatry, and Baycrest Centre for Geriatric Care
Toronto-Ontario, Canada

Introduction

One of the social determinants of mental health is place of residence, in particular the quality of housing conditions. Good-quality, affordable, safe housing is essential to wellbeing (Johnson et al. 2006).The WHO (2010) points out that *national mental health policies* should not be solely concerned with mental disorders, but should also recognize and address the broader issues which promote mental health. This includes incorporating mental health promotion into policies and programs across government and business sectors including education, labour, justice, transport, environment, housing, and welfare, as well as the health sector. Housing is a concrete manifestation of socioeconomic status, which has an important part to play in the development of explanations of the social production of health inequalities (Dunn, 2002). Unfortunally research on housing and mental health is remarkably underdeveloped (Evans et al. 2003). In a literature review on this subject the strongest finding on housing as an input and an outcome was that living in independent housing was associated with greater satisfaction with both housing and neighborhood (Newman, 2001). In addition three studies found better outcomes for settings that have fewer occupants and another study suggested that individuals who live in small-scale, good-quality, noninstitutional environments are less likely to engage in disruptive behavior when a significant proportion of other tenants also have serious mental illness.

This chapter addresses a different but somewhat related subject, providing an overview of mental health issues in nursing homes, also referred to as long-term care (LTC) homes. The profile of nursing homes for older adults has changed dramatically over the past century. Until the twentieth century, most facilities were primitive, badly run and offered only custodial care. Institutions for the disabled and infirm initially developed in the Middle East in the third or fourth century AD and over many years the concept subsequently spread to

Western Europe (Forbes et al. 1987). By medieval times it was common that the aged and sick were cared for by a variety of religious orders, often in remote locations. As the number of monasteries declined in the 1500s, "poorhouses" were established for individuals who were mentally or physically ill, blind or disabled as well as for the destitute. By the nineteenth century, between one third and one half of the occupants in a typical poorhouse were elderly or disabled persons. In the nineteenth century as the modern concept of the hospital developed, the primary emphasis was placed on treatment of the acutely ill, although some special homes for the elderly were established. In other institutions the elderly, the poor, the chronically sick, the mentally ill and the disabled were crowded together often in dreadful conditions. Early in the twentieth century there was clearly a need for convalescent and chronic care beds and it was only at this point that the modern concept of the nursing home was firmly established.

With the dramatic growth of the elderly population around the world, particularly those 80 years and over, there will be a rapidly growing need for nursing home beds over the next 30 years. The rate of growth of this population is now rapidly accelerating as the baby boom generation enters old age. In recent years, nursing home residents are more likely to be of low income with poor social supports and reduced levels of social engagement and to have a more complex array of physical and mental disabilities (Gillespie and Katz, 2009)

Characteristics of Nursing Home Residents

There are significant differences around the world in how older disabled individuals are cared for. A recent review of seventeen countries noted that the lowest rates for the population aged 65 and over and living in care homes was in Italy (2%) and Japan (2.9%) and the highest rates were in Norway (11.8%) and Denmark (9.1%) (Knapp et al, 2007). In the United States there are approximately 1.43 million residents receiving care in almost 16,000 nursing homes. There has been an overall increase in the size of facilities in the United States, from an average of 79 beds per facility in 1977 to 107 beds in 2004. Eighty percent of the nursing home population over the age of 65 are long-stay residents (with length of stay of 90 days or more) (Kasper and O'Malley, 2007). There has been an increase in the number of residents with short length of stay coinciding with increased funding of post-acute care in nursing homes. Each year there are approximately 2.5 million discharges. Only nine percent of nursing home residents are younger than 65 years of age. They represent a growing, but little recognized, population. In a recent study, a majority of younger residents were men with significant physical and mental health problems. The mental health problems include chronic serious mental illnesses such as schizophrenia as well as early onset dementia and traumatic brain injury. Younger residents want a greater variety of recreational activities and more meaningful relationships with family, staff and other residents as compared to older residents (Persson and Ostwald, 2009).

Over two-thirds of long-stay residents in American skilled nursing home facilities have multiple medical conditions (Gillespie and Katz, 2010). Almost 40% of older adults are diagnosed with heart failure or ischemic heart disease. Diabetes is reported in 22% of new admissions and stroke in 26%. Other prevalent health conditions include chronic obstructive pulmonary disease, hypertension, arthritis and hip fractures. More than half of long-stay nursing home residents require supervision or hands-on assistance in five different activities of daily living (such as eating, bathing, dressing, transferring and toileting). About 75% of nursing home residents require assistance in three or more ADLs (Gillespie and Katz, 2009). Problems with bladder or bowel control are reported in almost 60% of newly admitted and 40% of long-stay nursing home residents. Only 59% of older long-stay residents are fully ambulatory and hearing and visual impairments are found in 36% and 39% of residents respectively. Approximately 76% of long-stay residents are female and more than half of the older adults who are long-stay or permanent residents are over 85 years of age.

Trends in Nursing Home Care

There are many important trends in nursing home care which have been influenced by the aging population. These trends which will have a critical impact on the future of LTC include: a) a greater focus on the need to optimize the environment (physical space and activities); b) experimentation with new models of LTC involving smaller homes and less institutional environments; c) an increase in the availability of multiple levels of care; d) a significantly greater percentage of residents with dementia and severe cognitive impairment; e) more residents with psychiatric and behavioural disorders; f) greater interest in involvement of university programs in nursing homes with the development of "teaching nursing homes" and; g) increased legislation such as OBRA 1987 in the United States to ensure higher standards of care focused on quality and the development of Best Practices.

Overview and Prevalence of Mental Disorders

Care of nursing home residents with mental disorders has been an issue of significant concern for many years. Rovner and Katz (1993) described nursing homes as the modern mental institutions for the elderly and noted that care and training of staff is often deficient. Given these concerns, the International Psychogeriatric Association formed a Task Force in 2005 to focus on mental health issues in long-term care homes. The goals were: a) to gather information and share views from diverse countries and settings about how best to restore or ensure good mental health in LTC settings and; b) to support and strengthen mental health services in the LTC sector. Following several meetings of the task force, a one-day expert meeting was held during the IPA Congress in Montreal in September 2009. A variety of papers were presented, most of which were recently published in *International Psychogeriatrics* (November 2010). The main conclusions from a number of these papers will be described in this chapter.

The prevalence of psychiatric disorders among older adults in LTC homes was described by Seitz et al. (2010). The systematic review included 74 studies which met criteria for inclusion. These studies included 30 on the prevalence of dementia, nine on behavioural symptoms associated with dementia and 26 studies on depression. Most of these studies were of small scale and were conducted in developed countries. The median prevalence of dementia in these studies was 58% while the prevalence of the behavioural and psychological symptoms of dementia (BPSD) was 78% among individuals with dementia. The median prevalence of major depressive disorder was ten percent while the median prevalence of depressive symptoms was 29%. Anxiety disorders were also prevalent, for example, in a study from the Netherlands (Smalbrugge et al, 2005) the prevalence of anxiety disorders was 5.7% with 4.2% having sub-threshold anxiety disorders and 29.7% having symptoms of anxiety. In 1996, a study suggested that 5.9% of nursing home residents suffer from schizophrenia (Mechanic and McAlpine, 2000) and another study found a 3% prevalence rate for bipolar disorder. Studies of delirium show rates that range from 6% to 14% (Cacchione et al, 2003).

PRINCIPLES GUIDING THE CARE OF RESIDENTS IN NURSING HOMES

Canadian guidelines for the assessment and treatment of mental health issues in long-term care homes were published in 2006 (Canadian Coalition for Seniors' Mental Health, 2006). Basic principles guiding the care of residents in LTC homes are described with a plea that these should underpin the caregiving milieu in LTC homes.

- Residents should receive care that is individualized, person-centred, and, to the extent desired and possible, self-directed.
- Families should be respected as part of the resident's ongoing social support system and integrated within the LTC setting in mutually acceptable and supportive roles.
- Care should reflect an integrated consideration of biological, psychological and social needs. A biopsychosocial model expands the focus from individual pathology to a consideration of the whole person, including both strengths and limitations, within the context of their social and physical environment.
- A culture of caring that includes principles of psychosocial rehabilitation to maximize quality of life should be established. Psychosocial rehabilitation emphasizes the importance of involvement in developing and realizing one's own personal care and life goals. The need for health promotion and treatment services that assist residents to manage their symptoms and build on their strengths is integral to this approach.
- An increasingly supportive and assistive social and physical environment, responsive to residents' changing needs, should be created to maintain function and compensate for functional decline (e.g., in individuals with dementia). This includes shifting the primary focus from tasks to relationships.
- Preventative interventions, including strategies for maintaining wellness, and early interventions for mental health problems and disorders, should be developed, implemented and incorporated into specific training programs for both informal and formal caregivers.
- All staff, regardless of their discipline or role, should be supported in maintaining the knowledge and skills necessary to provide informed and competent care.

Optimizing the Environment in Nursing Homes

As noted above, there has been a movement to find new models of care for residential homes. A variety of models designed to humanize LTC homes with the creation of a homelike environment have been developed. The goals include optimizing the residents' quality of life at the same time as raising the quality of care. These models include the Eden Alternative (http://www.edenalt.com), the Greenhouse Project (www.thegreenhouseproject.org), and the Wellspring Program (www.WellspringProgram.org).

A number of countries such as Japan, the Netherlands and Sweden have also developed alternative living arrangements for seniors with dementia such as small group homes (Verbeek et al, 2009). Marshall (2001) recommended that residential facilities for people with dementia should:

- control stimuli, especially noise
- enhance visual access
- include unobtrusive safety features
- have rooms for different functions with furniture and fittings familiar to the age and generation of the residents
- have single rooms big enough for a reasonable amount of personal belongings
- be domestic and homelike
- have scope for ordinary activities
- provide a safe outside space
- provide good signage and multiple cues where possible
- use objects rather than color for orientation

Fleming and Purandare (2010) have provided a detailed analysis of environmental design studies for LTC of individuals with dementia. After careful screening of articles, 57 papers were identified as being sufficiently strong to be reviewed. The authors concluded that designers may confidently use unobtrusive safety measures, vary ambience, size and shape of spaces, provide single rooms, maximize visual access and control levels of stimulation. They note that there is less agreement on the usefulness of signage, a homelike environment, provision for engagement in ordinary activities, small size and the provision of outside space. They concluded that there is sufficient evidence available to come to a consensus on guiding principles for the design of LTC environments for people with dementia.

Screening and Assessment of Mental Disorders

The issue of screening for mental disorders in nursing homes was reviewed by Pachana et al (2010). The literature on measurement development, testing standards, psychometric considerations and the nursing home environment were considered. Rather than recommend specific screening instruments, issues surrounding the selection, administration, interpretation and use of screening instruments are discussed. The authors recommend that screening should be undertaken in the context of a comprehensive assessment and that humane care and the particular circumstances of the nursing home be considered. They note that screening for the sake of screening not only serves no purpose but any assessment is a strain on the individual, uses resources and requires ethical use of assessment instruments. Screening programs should be adequately resourced so that the clinical utility can be properly evaluated and demonstrated. The authors report that a common complaint in nursing homes is the limited amount of time available for tasks, and screening is no exception and must be properly supported. They note that part of the support is the training of staff in the use of specific screening instruments. This may have indirect gains of an increased sense of efficacy on the part of the staff member and increased meaningful communication between staff, residents and their family members. The authors also recommend the development of a resource bank to support screening tool selection and implementation. They suggest that a public domain resource bank would help developing countries to provide a higher standard of care and that screening measures should be periodically reviewed to take advantage of new knowledge and developments in the field.

Koopmans et al (2010) reviewed the need for comprehensive assessment of depression and behavioural problems in LTC settings. They reviewed guidelines from the United States, Canada, Germany and the Netherlands. The authors recommend that comprehensive assessment of depression in LTC homes is a multidisciplinary process with all members of the team being involved. The authors recommend that an assessment procedure should consist of a two-step screening process, an investigation to identify factors that influence the symptoms, followed by a formal diagnosis. They also recommended a full medical evaluation as part of the assessment procedure which should consist of a diagnostic interview, history taking, physical examination and laboratory and diagnostic testing as needed. They recommend cognitive screening to rule out dementia as well as a variety of screening instruments for depression including the Hammond Scale or the Depression Rating Scale for initial screening as well as the eight-item Geriatric Depression Scale (GDS) or the GDS (Residential). For patients who are cognitively impaired or who have difficulty communicating, they recommend the Cornell Scale for Depression in Dementia. For behavioural problems, they also recommend a comprehensive multidisciplinary assessment. They note that the assessment procedure should consist of three consecutive steps: description and clarification of the behaviour, additional investigation and assessment of probable causes of the behaviour. They suggest that it is important to establish whether a patient has dementia or not and, if possible, what type of dementia. It is recommended that when a resident exhibits new onset or changes in behavioural symptoms, a full person-centered and tailor-made comprehensive assessment is carried out. The Neuropsychiatric Inventory for Nursing Homes (NPI-NH) is recommended for screening of behavioural symptoms. When there is a need for specific screening for agitation or aggression, the Cohen-Mansfield Agitation Inventory is recommended. It is also recommended that delirium should be ruled out first as a possible cause for the behavioural problems. Finally, it is recommended that residents with new onset or changes in behavioural symptoms should be initially evaluated for possible physical conditions, medication changes, psychiatric conditions and personal or environmental factors that are possibly contributing to the cause of the behaviour.

Psychosocial Interventions

The expression of mental illness in the nursing home population is extremely multidimensional. The available evidence suggests psychiatric signs and symptoms reflect biological (e.g., neurodegeneration, neurotransmitter changes and medical illnesses) and psychological vulnerabilities as well other significant environmental and social factors (Reichman and Conn, 2010). These factors include the physical environment, as described above, limited social relationships and family involvement, the processes of care and the behaviour of care providers and other residents. These multiple contributors may interact significantly with the vulnerabilities of the nursing home population to precipitate or significantly affect the expression of mental illness in this setting.

There has been considerable research over the last 20 years examining psychosocial interventions in nursing home settings. Although few of these studies use randomized controlled trial conditions, numerous studies do appear to demonstrate that a variety of interventions such as social contact, sensory enhancement, modifications to the environment and a large number of structured recreational activities can have a significantly positive effect on the overall levels of challenging behaviours in this environment. Much of this work is based on behavioural theory,the unmet needs model, the environmental vulnerability model and models of depressed affect (Cohen-Mansfield et al, 2007). A recent review of psychosocial interventions in dementia care specific to nursing homes concluded that the most effective interventions utilized cognitive stimulation, behaviour management techniques or physical activity interventions (Vernooij-Dassen et al, 2010). For depression and related symptoms, there is also evidence that psychotherapies such as cognitive behaviour therapy and reminiscence therapy can lead to improvements (Bharucha et al, 2006).

Use of Psychotropic Medication

Although some residents can benefit from psychotropic medications, numerous studies have raised concern about the quality of prescribing to elderly nursing home residents (Conn et al, 2007). The nursing home is a unique setting for drug prescription for a number of reasons including the extreme frailty of the residents, the complexity of the social institution, limited physician input, non-physicians' contribution to treatment decisions, limited staffing levels and staff education. Studies have shown that there is often a failure to document reasons for prescribing medications in nursing homes. It is certainly important to describe and document the target problem being treated, to consider alternatives to medications and to review potential side effects. Most international studies suggest that between 50% and 75% of nursing home residents have at least one prescription for a psychotropic medication. Nevertheless, the patterns and rates of use of these medications vary widely from institution to institution and from country to country. Factors which might explain these variations include differences in the prevalence and severity of disorders, levels of physical disability, prescribing patterns of physicians, involvement by pharmacists, the number of untrained staff, size and design of institutions, funding and type of institutions, socioeconomic background of the residents and policies regarding admissions. Particular concerns have been raised regarding the use of antipsychotic medications and benzodiazepines. A recent report found that in a cross sectional analysis of antipsychotic and benzodiazepine use from the 2004 United States National Nursing Home Survey, 26% of residents were prescribed an antipsychotic medication and 13% received a benzodiazepine (Stevenson et al. 2010). Although it is difficult to agree on an ideal target for rates of use, it is clear that prescribing rates remain high. Long-term care facilities must ensure optimal prescribing practices through active training of personnel and practice monitoring programs.

Providing Mental Health Services

Numerous studies from different countries document the lack of adequate mental health services in nursing homes. One review of nine controlled trials concluded that liaison-style services utilizing educational approaches, treatment guidelines and ongoing involvement of mental health staff are more effective than a purely case-based consultation model (Draper and Low, 2005). Snowdon (2010) reviewed a variety of models of mental health service provision which include solo practitioners, multidisciplinary teams and both internal and external consultants. He suggested a series of recommendations including adequate screening, designation of staff members who take responsibility for identification and, if necessary, referral to a specialist, active involvement of the primary care physician and effective liaison between the facility and mental health teams or consultants. A number of reports have also highlighted the benefits of having nurse specialists provide significant front-line consultation and care.

Staff Education and Training

Moyle et al (2010) recently reviewed the literature on the vital role and benefits of staff education in the nursing home. Core training and mental health care of older residents should be developed for all healthcare professionals. They recommend that nursing homes should have an established staff development program related to resident mental healthcare needs. They suggest that a process of staff evaluation should be in place and homes should facilitate staff attendance at education and training sessions with a reward system for staff who undertake educational programs. They note that it is particularly important to support unregulated staff to achieve competency in mental healthcare and that curriculum designers must take into account the special needs and schedules of LTC staff. Stolee et al (2005) studied factors associated with the effectiveness of continuing education in long-term care. They utilized focus groups to identify staff perceptions of factors that promote the transfer of learning into practice. Interestingly, support from management was identified as the most important factor impacting the effectiveness of continuing education. Other factors included staff funding, space resources and the need for ongoing expert support.

Conclusion

In summary, there has been a trend in many countries for nursing home residents to be more frail and more likely to suffer from dementia or other mental disorders. Many concerns have been raised about the care of residents with mental health problems. Solutions should include improved design of the environment, careful screening and assessment, provision of mental health services including optimal psychosocial and, when necessary, pharmacological interventions, staff education and the implementation of best practice guidelines.

References

Bharucha AJ, Dew MA, Miller MD, Borson S, Reynolds C 3rd (2006). Psychotherapy in Long-Term Care: a Review. *J Am Med Dir Assoc.* 7(9): 568-80.

Cacchione PZ, Culp K, Laing J, Tripp-Reimer T (2003). Clinical Profile of Acute Confusion in the Long-Term Care Setting. *Clin Nurs Res.* 12(2):145-58.

Canadian Coalition for Seniors' Mental Health (2006). *National Guidelines for Seniors' Mental Health: The Assessment and Treatment of Mental Health Issues in Long Term Care Homes.* Toronto: Canadian Coalition for Seniors' Mental Health. Available at www.ccsmh.ca.

Cohen-Mansfield J, Laje RP. (2009). Environmental and Milieu Interventions. In: *Psychiatry in Long-Term Care*, Reichman WE, Katz PR (eds.); New York: Oxford University Press; pp 391-413.

Conn DK . Optimizing the use of psychotropic medications. (2007) In*: Practical Psychiatry in the Long-Term Care Home: A Handbook for Staff*, Conn DK et al (eds.); Cambridge, MA : Hogrefe and Huber. pp 203-16.

Draper BM, Low L-F. (2005). Evidence-Based Psychogeriatric Service Delivery; In: *Psychogeriatric Service Delivery*, Draper BW, Brodaty H (eds.); Oxford University Press: Oxford, pp 75-123.

Dunn, J. (2002). Housing and inequalities in health: a study of socioeconomic dimensions of housing and self reported health from a survey of Vancouver residents. *J Epidemiol Community Health.* 56(9): 671–681.

Evans, G.W., Wells, N.M., Moch, A. (2003). Housing and Mental Health: A Review of the Evidence and a Methodological and Conceptual Critique. *Journal of Social Issues.* 59(3): 475–500.

Forbes WF, Jackson JA, Kraus AS. (1987).Institutionalization of the Elderly in Canada. Toronto: Butterworth.

Fleming R, Purandare N (2010). Long-Term Care for People with Dementia: Environmental Design Guidelines. *Intl Psychogeriatr*, 22(7):1084-1096.

Gibson MC, Carter MW, Helmes E, Edberg A-K (2010). Principles of Good Care for Long-Term Care Facilities. *Intl Psychogeriatr*, 22(7):1072-1083.

Gillespie SM, Katz PR (2009). An overview of residents, care providers, and regulation of medical practice in the long-term-care continuum, in Psychiatry in Long-Term Care. Edited by Reichman WE, Katz PR. New York: Oxford University Press, pp. 449–464

Gillespie SM, Katz PR . (2010). Nursing Home Care. In: *Geriatrics Review Syllabus: A Core Curriculum in Geriatric Medicine*, Pacala JT, Sullivan GM (eds.); New York: American Geriatrics Society.

Johnson, R. et al. (2006). Housing and community care. *Mental Health Today*, November, pp. 25-28.

Kasper J, O'Malley M. (2007). *Changes in Characteristics, Needs and Payments for Care of Elderly Nursing Home Residents:* 1999-2004. Henry J. Kaiser Family Foundation.

Knapp M, Comas-Herrera A, Somani A, Banerjee S (2007). *Dementia: International Comparisons*. London, UK: Personal Social Service Research Unit.

Koopmans RT, Zuidema SU, Leontjevas R, Gerritsen DL (2010). Comprehensive Assessment of Depression and Behavioral Problems in Long-Term Care. *Intl Psychogeriatr*, 22(7):1054-1062.

Marshall M (2001). Environment: How it helps to see dementia as a disability. *Care of Homes and Dementia: Journal of Dementia Care*, 6:15-17.

Mechanic D, McAlpine DD (2000). Use of Nursing Homes in the Care of Persons with Severe Mental Illness: 1985-1995. *Psychiatr Serv*, 51(3):354-8.

Moyle W, Hsu MC, Lieff S, Vernooij-Dassen M (2010). Recommendations for Staff Education and Training for Older People with Mental Illness in Long-Term Aged Care. *Intl Psychogeriatr*, 22(7):1097-1106.

Newman, S. J. (2001). Housing Attributes and Serious Mental Illness: Implications for Research and Practice. *Psychiatr Serv*. 52:1309-1317.

Pachana NA, Helmes E, Byrne GJ, Edelstein BA, Konnert CA, Pot AM (2010). Screening for Mental Disorders in Residental Aged Care Facilities. *Intl Psychogeriatr*, 22(7):1107-1120.

Persson DI, Ostwald SK (2009). Younger Residents in Nursing Homes. *J Gerontol Nurs*. 35(10): 22-31.

Reichman W, Conn DK (2010). Nursing Home Psychiatry: Is it time for a reappraisal? *Am J Geriatr Psychiatry*, 18:1049-53.

Rovner BW, Katz IR (1993). Psychiatric Disorders in the Nursing Home: A selective review of studies related to clinical care. *Int J Geriatr Psychiatry*, 8(1):75-87.

Seitz D, Purandare N, Conn D (2010). Prevalence of Psychiatric Disorders Among Older Adults in Long-Term Care Homes: A systematic review. *Intl Psychogeriatr*, 22(7):1025-1039.

Smalbrugge M, Pot AM, Jongenelis K, Beekman AT, Eefsting JA.(2005). Prevalence and Correlates of Anxiety Among Nursing Home Patients. *J Affect Disord*, 88(2):145-53.

Snowdon J (1993). Mental Health in Nursing Homes: Perspectives on the use of Medications. *Drugs and Aging*, 3(2): 122-30.

Snowdon J (2010). Mental Health Service Delivery in Long-Term Care Homes. *Intl Psychogeriatr*, 22(7):1063-1071.

Stevenson DG, Decker SL, Dwyer LL, Huskamp HA, Grabowski DC, Metzger ED, Mitchell SL. (2010). Antipsychotic and benzodiazepine use among nursing home residents: findings from the 2004 National Nursing Home Survey. *Am J Geriatr Psychiatry*, 18(12): 1078-92.

Stolee P, Esbaugh J, Aylward S, Cathers T, Harvey DP, Hillier LM, Keat N, Feightner JW. (2005). Factors associated with the effectiveness of continuing education in long-term care. *Gerontologist.*, 45(3): 399-409.

Verbeek H, van Rossum E, Zwakhalen SM, Kempen GI, Hamers JP (2009). Small, Homelike Care Enviroments for Older People with Dementia: A literature review. *Int Psychogeriatr*, 21(2):252-64.

Vernooij-Dassen M, Vasse E, Zuidema S, Cohen-Mansfield J, Moyle W (2010). Psychosocial Interventions for Dementia Patients in Long-Term Care. *Intl Psychogeriatr*, 22(7):1121-1128.

WHO (2010). *http://www.who.int/mediacentre/factsheets/fs220/en/*.

In: Social Determinants and Mental Health
Editor: Sabine Bährer-Kohler
ISBN: 978-1-61324-353-4

Chapter 13

SOCIOECONOMIC FACTORS AND MENTAL HEALTHCARE

Patryk Piotrowski
University Wroclaw, Wroclaw Medical University, Department of Psychiatry
Wroclaw, Poland

INTRODUCTION

One of the social determinants of mental health is the socioeconmomic factor. Mental health comes at a price. One important aspect is to prevent mental diseases in order to keep everyone's share in the cost of health to the lowest necessary minimum.

The relationship between socioeconomic status and prevalence of mental disorders has been widely discussed. Subjects with lower socioeconomic status (SES) are more prone to mental disorders, as confirmed in many national research projects. As estimated prevalence of mental disorders is about twice as frequent among people form poorer populations as among the rich [1]. Individuals with the lowest SES have approximately eighth times more RR (relative risk) of developing schizophrenia in comparison to wealthier populations [2]. People suffering form this severe mental disorder are one third more likely not to graduated from high school and three times more likely to get divorced [2]. Moreover, their access to mental services and treatment is often restricted, mostly due to inadequate financing. Among 101 countries which have provided information in WHO's survey referring to mental health budgeting 20.9 % covering population of more than 1 billion spend less than 1 % of total health expenditures on psychiatric services [3]. Since mental disorders tend to be regarded as persistent health status rather than temporary symptoms, more importance should be attached to future consequences of current decisions. Such groups, therefore, need to be provided with mental health care in order to decrease overall costs of subsequent treatment, social support or society's outgoings spent on prison system. The main goal of the publication is to give an overview of the current situation in countries of different developmental status, varied health insurance systems and national public policy towards groups of citizens at risk of social exclusion.

Historical Perspective and Current Aspects of Mental Healthcare

Proper consideration of the issue presented in this article requires discussion on primary events that have brought today's psychiatry to the current model of service provision.

Mental health care has been subjected to extensive modifications over the years. From the historical perspective three periods might be distinguished, time frames of which differ when it comes to particular countries [4]. In its general principle the process consisted of three main components:

- transfer of residents to community settings,
- redirection of potential admissions to alternative forms of care and
- development of services network for patients living outside the hospital walls [5]

A shift in care from large locally separated hospitals towards community settings not always went according to guidelines. The idea of closing down large hospital units did not escape criticism. Community care, which supported this idea, was generally underdeveloped and that often led to dramatic social situation of discharged patients [6, 7].

Modification of American system of mental health care provision revealed the existence of a certain "trap" resulting from idealistic concepts devoid of thorough systemic preparations, backed by the realistic, economic estimations. A considerable number of Americans received either medical care of low level or none, as the access to services was significantly limited [7] Thousands of people with severe mental disorders were left on their own, living on the streets. An indefinite number of individuals ended up in care homes and penitentiaries, lacking in care on an acceptable level [6, 7]. Worse still is that a large population of patients discharged from hospitals and swelling the group of homeless Americans, were in fact young patients, staying relatively short in the stationary health care institutions [8]. According to Lamb, sudden shift of care from long-term wards to an "open model" not necessarily improves quality of patients' life. Long-term patients, who gained "trained passivity", due to living for years in the structuralized environment and being used to external aid, after discharge facilitated contact with care providers, even though such care was offered in entirely unlike environment [9]. However, at the early stages of care reforms the existent but deficient support system was disadvantageous for younger patients, not used to formal support; thus considerably restricting their possibility of social functioning [9]. Similar processes previously observed in the US, with a slight delay and on a different scale, appeared locally in the European countries [74]. In the late eighties a growing problem of homelessness was observed in Great Britain. It was a new phenomenon, resulting, to a large degree, from the restrained access to social benefits. A certain part of the homeless population, however, also suffered from long-term mental disorders. Severe disorders were more prevalent among homeless citizens in comparison to general population [10, 11, 12, 13, 14, 15]. Moreover, they seem to be more vulnerable to stressors associated with homelessness with successive exacerbation of psychopathological symptoms, manifestations of which result in involvement in criminal acts [16, 17, 18, 19]. Hence, paradoxically, the reintroduction of the patients to the society, supported by a rather fragmentary community care system, led to both social and communal exclusion. As already mentioned above, "polarized" service provision based on care supplied mostly by hospitals was equally insufficient to that provided predominantly by community settings. Nowadays, the model of care provision in developed countries is becoming a more balanced structure. As observed, some patients benefit form holistic care while others from modern forms of support. Nevertheless according to WHO's report published in 2005 69 % of psychiatric beds are still located in large psychiatric facilities separated from general hospitals and community settings [3].

Mental Healthcare and Economical Issues

Humanistic ideas of charismatic thinkers like Foucault, Laing, Szasz or Basaglia and their successors, however, have to be confronted with economical issues [74]. In the early stages of reorganization processes hospital treatment was considered to be the most expensive model of mental health care provision. Extended period of hospital treatment, high direct costs of large facilities and underestimation of rates covered by national health insurers brought about enormous level of financial burden for governments [74]. Not surprisingly public policy promoting deinstitutionalization was strongly supported by decision-makers in developed countries like Italy, Great Britain and Germany. However, the early estimations of savings, due to reforms in psychiatric care shift towards community, were highly overestimated [20, 21]. The assessment of potential savings should not have been made solely on the basis of costs of medication, hospitalizations or clinic visits after discharge and outpatients. Unlike other branches of medicine, the costs of mental health proved to be far more indirect than direct. Feasible estimations of economic burden of mental disorders should take into account costs of

- weaker working power,
- reduced educational attainment,
- social support for individuals and their families, as well as
- secondary costs such as expenses on incarceration or consequences of homelessness.

Indirect costs of schizophrenia only, closely related to reduced productivity due to absence at work, early retirement or premature death, account for 50 % of the overall disease-related costs [22, 23]. Additionally, high prevalence of somatic illnesses in patients suffering from serious mental disorders, which lead to frequent acute admissions to emergency wards such as cardiovascular crises or pulmonary diseases and early morbidity (Years of Potential Life Lost - YPLL – between 13 to 32 years), rise indirect costs of mental disorders borne by societies [24, 25]. Hence, on one hand health care systems are lacking epidemiologically reasonable number of psychiatric hospital beds and/or community settings and, on the other, resources spent on mental health care, though increasing, are still insufficient. Special attention should be paid to risk factors and subpopulations marginalized or incapable to demand provision of services available for other social classes. As proved in research projects across the world, access to services is limited for certain groups of patients or persons at risk of mental disorders. Identification of those risk factors associated with higher prevalence of mental disorders through literature review is one main issue of this chapter.

Socioeconomic Status and Prevalence of Mental Disorders

The relationship between socioeconomic status and prevalence of mental disorders has been widely discussed. Research focused on psychotic as well as non-psychotic disorders [26, 27, 28, 29]. Literature distinguishes two main hypotheses regarding social gradient in mental health: the selection hypothesis and social causation hypothesis. According to the first one, mental disorders or specific personality attributes are regarded as a cause of lower socioeconomic status. The second hypothesis implies that low socioeconomic status might itself be a risk factor of mental disorders. Both explanations complement each other to some extent, since personality problems often leading to social life complications are, in many cases, caused by psychological and social deprivation also in childhood. However, important differences - mostly in time-horizons - included in both definitions are expressed in course of mental disturbances the nature of which hypotheses are trying to explain. The selection hypothesis is more likely to be relevant for psychotic disorders i.e. schizophrenia, whereas social causation hypothesis seems to be more relevant for depression (but not for affective bipolar disorder which shares important genetic markers with schizophrenia), other non-psychotic disorders and psychological distress [23, 30]. The mechanisms linking low socioeconomic status and mental disorders are not clear. A number of studies conducted in countries at a different developmental level identified factors influencing or – to some extent – explaining social gradient in mental health. Special attention was drawn to factors regarding material status, since deprivation of goods like ownership of a house, as proven, determined a burden for mental conditions. Other variables linked to psychiatric health are based on psychosocial hypotheses describing factors like perceived job demands and financial hardships, scarce social support and negative life events as important mediators between socioeconomic status and mental health [31, 32, 33]. Authors suggested that lack of control over own life might constitute essential factor influencing occurrence of mental disturbances amongst representatives of lower socioeconomic classes. An inefficient pattern of coping with social and occupational life leads to psychological burden which may influence both somatic and mental health [34]. It has to be mentioned at this point that "sense of control" and similar factors reflecting personality traits cannot independently explain social inequalities in mental health provision. Burdening an individual with the responsibility for achieved socioeconomic position would be a tempting excuse and at the same time a comfortable escape from political challenges. The aim should be to create good lives for citizens and to improve the economy of society [76].

Policy

Mental health policy in general comprises several aspects necessary in structured planning: promotion, prevention, treatment, rehabilitation and advocacy. Data gathered by the WHO showed that only 62.1 % of countries participating in the survey (N=190) had mental health policies (70.6 % of European countries). Authors have found significant association between formal acts and variables such as: substance abuse policy (χ^2 41.8, $p<0.01$), a national mental health programme ($\chi^2=31.6$, $p<0.01$), disability benefits ($\chi^2=12.1$), primary care training facilities in mental health ($\chi^2=22.9$, $p<0.01$), community care facilities in mental health ($\chi^2=7.80$, $p<0.01$) and presence of NGO activities in mental health ($\chi^2=11.2$, $p<0.01$)

[3]. Results explicitly determinate directions of development i.e. necessity to lay legal foundations for service development or at least elaborate drafts of action plans. Even though reduction of inequalities in healthcare is a priority of policy worldwide, general goals cannot be achieved unless particular subpopulations at risk are identified. The World Health Organization's target to reduce the health gap among socioeconomic groups in the European countries by 25 % by 2020 will be only an illusory wish until particular governments are not focused on marginalized social classes [35]. This challenging money- and time-consuming process is additionally hampered by a wide range of identified social determinants e.g. low SES, poverty, unemployment, homelessness or overcrowded housing, lower level of education, etc. which influence on the present stage of social gradient is not clear [36].

Rights of persons with mental disorders have been widely discussed years before antypsychiatry movements initiated deinstitutionalization process worldwide. Inequality in the right to work, to marry, to have a family, to participate in the communities, in an access to education, to health services and in some cases even in the right to live independently were among the most commonly cited issues [37]. Patients' disability was blamed for their disadvantageous social situations and incapacity to participate in public life and profit from goods supplied by the market. Nowadays, the responsibility is assigned to the environmental factors and is not any more attributed to the individuals' impairments. Such shift of liability requires not only legislative tools, which are already prepared in most countries, but predominantly a change of citizens and decision-makers' view of the problem, since discrimination itself rises the level of disability [38, 39]. Disability hampers the human capital and rises financial burden for the societies, due to the need of support provision for vulnerable subpopulation. Thompson et al. showed that care of patients diagnosed with schizophrenic and bipolar disorders devours almost half (43%) of the spending on mental health services, much of which is allocated to inpatients [40].

Gender Aspects

Sociological interpretation of gender differences in concurrent political environment, at least in developed countries, is an identified problem. Legislative regulations oblige the EU states as well as candidate countries to reduce obstacles in equal access to education, varied areas of occupational life, healthcare and social support system. Furthermore, modern politics promotes gender diversity on significant posts through gender parity acts. While governments aim to level social differences between sexes, epidemiology of mental disorders still acts as a diversifier. One of the important issues is how gender correlates with mental health. Depression is more prevalent among woman and according to some authors its occurrence is related to woman's higher exposure to adverse social circumstances and their reactions to these negative experiences [41]. Moreover, woman are disproportionally affected by the poverty, which itself – as already mentioned – is a risk factor of mental disturbance among others - depression [42]. Decedents have to keep in minds that according to World Bank even though poverty rate have been reduced substantially between 1981 and 2005 simultaneously the number of people at risk of falling into poverty has increased from approximately 17 % up to 32 % [The World Bank, Poverty Reduction & Equity]. Unipolar depressive disorders are the leading causes of burden for females aged 15 years and more. Disability Adjusted Life Years coefficient for unipolar depressive disorders in woman equals 8,4 % (first position on list of ten leading causes of disease burden). Striking is the fact that common metabolic disease – diabetes mellitus is listed on the tenth place with 1,9 %. Depression in males constitutes 4,8 % of Disability Adjusted Life Years, reaching forth position [43].

On the other hand suicide attempts are more frequent amongst men [44]. It is noteworthy that, irrespectively of mainstream actions to minimize differences in social competencies between sexes, still much has to be done. Those differences are even more evident in developing countries, especially due to cultural heritage i.e. profound division of competencies, roles and expectations. Overcoming these differences might take more time than experts initially assumed. Public actions aimed at increasing awareness of social equity between sexes and even legislative tools might not be effective enough, unless health care system is focused on prevention and easier access to services and treatment.

Homeless People

As forms of residence influence mental health the late 1980s studies showed that among the rising number of homeless people 30-50 % suffered form severe mental disorders such as mood disorders (19-30 %) and schizophrenia (11-17 %) [45, 46, 47]. To some extent the large proportion of mentally ill was caused by excessive and rapidly performed process of deinstitutionalization. Certainly, early stage of development of social psychiatry cannot solely explain this negative outcome. While assessing factors that could have influence on homelessness, macroeconomic conditions cannot be neglected. Shortage of

- unskilled employment,
- rising costs of housing and
- insufficient social support system

were among additional unfavorable conditions [48]. On the other hand, general sociodemographic predictors of homelessness like male sex, being single, young, poor, less educated and a member of a an ethnic minority resemble risk factors of severe and the most stigmatizing mental disorders like schizophrenia. One should, therefore, consider how these social conditions influence disadvantageous social outcome? Additionally, the same factors may be associated with involvement in criminal justice [49]. Newer results vary dependently on methodology and years in which a particular research was performed. Studies assessing usage of sheltered housing in New York and Philadelphia in the 1990s showed that while admissions during one year follow up in general population were approximately 1 %, the number of the mentally disabled form Medicaid population in Philadelphia who took advantage of such services equaled 3.6 % [50, 51]. Important is the fact that

- poor subpopulations were shown to be more prone to stay in homeless shelters than individuals suffering from severe mental disorder.
- What is more, several research have proved that neither mental disorder nor dual diagnosis constitute direct risk factors of homelessness, the concept of the causative mental disorder has been replaced [52, 53, 54, 55].

Probably specific social position of persons with severe mental disorders should be taken into account while explaining these observations. Development of psychiatric health care – in wealthier countries mostly social psychiatry – has widened the range of services that included varied opportunities of housing and easier access to social support. This might explain decreasing proportions of psychiatric patients among homeless people.

Genetic Aspects of Mental Disorders

Common knowledge in modern psychiatry points to the several factors inevitably connected with occurrence of mental disorders. A lot of interest is nowadays attracted to heredity. Enormous number of studies regards mental illnesses as consequences of certain defects in genome. Specific candidate genes potentially related to concrete diagnoses are being searched. Polygenic heredity of mental illnesses has been confirmed decades ago. Research teams across the whole scientific world continuously test successive gene polymorphisms or examine newly extracted proteins or peptides. Up to now interest has been put to genome regions encoding specified products but only linkages were found – even if conformed in other populations – constitute only components of genetic lesions present in individuals suffering from mental disorders. Undoubtedly, there is still a lot of work to be done in this field. Apart from inherited proneness to mental disorders, a largely debated issue is to what extend a psychiatric disorder occur due to environmental leverage. Current research projects recognize the need to clarify genetic predisposition as well as putative environmental factors in parallel [56, 57]. Diverse factors modifying personal histories of individuals suffering from mental diseases need to be taken into account during psychiatric diagnostic procedures, as the overwhelming majority of schizophrenia cases do not have genetic family burden. Even if these social factors cannot be considered as direct cause of illness, they may certainly modify its course. Such influence on prognosis in case of persistent disorders is of much importance both from medical and economical point of view. Biological medical interventions, according to current observations, are predominantly focused on alleviating psychiatric symptoms severity, prevention of relapses of mental disturbance or improvement in disorder prognosis. Such interventions even though giving quite prompt and tangible results constitute only a part of "healing process". Definition of this term should include not only improvement in mental and – equally important – somatic health, but need to depict social living conditions.

Conclusion

Both medical and social variables together embrace individuals' personal history and only after may be referred to WHO's definition of health i.e. subjective well-being and reduction of disabilities of people with mental disorders. Publication of the results of the *Global Burden of Disease Study* pointed out the significance of mental disturbances in societal aspects [58]. Sartorius reported that mortality due to cardiovascular diseases among psychiatric patients suffering from severe illnesses was higher than due to suicidal attempts in this subpopulation [59]. Disadvantageously, somatic disorders prevalence is not going hand in hand with access to medical services for mentally disturbed persons[60]. Such situations are more common in countries in which mental health system is being rebuilt form stage one (according to historical description proposed by Thornicroft) towards newer models of service delivery i.e. from large separated mental facilities to social psychiatry model [1]. Inequalities of service provision in general are reinforced by economic and systemic obstacles. Such obvious conclusion seems to be only a “technical factor” of social gradient. Furthermore, it may explain inequalities predominantly on the level of between countries, or more precisely between these countries’ economy and governance. As medical actions are focused on an individual while considering social disparities one should take into account patient’s personal level of satisfaction and quality of life.

Costs

The costs of health care are considered one of the challenges in U.S. public policy[61]. In 2006, health care costs reached 16% of the nation’s gross domestic product, on a path to reach 20% by 2016 [62]. While mental disorders contribute to these costs at an estimated 6.2% [63].

Direct world’s costs of schizophrenia only are estimated as 0,5 % to 3,5 % of general national costs of health [64, 65].

Additionally, indirect costs connected with limitation of productiveness due to absence at work or loosing employment, early retirement or premature death, constitute approximately 50 % of overall costs of disorder [66, 67]. Such data are mostly estimated totals, because methods of assessments are far from excellent. Human capital method is based on the assumption that reduction of work effectiveness, temporary or permanent absence at work or working incapacity decrease potential productiveness of a individual in his or her lifetime [68].

In the case of permanent incapacity of working indirect costs estimation include person’s potential earnings till the end of expected employment i.e. retirement. Apart from its transparent manner it has serious limitations, mostly due to the fact that it does not reflect labor market reality. Assumption that the vacancy would not be occupied by another employee hampers its reliability. Friction costs method, however, implies that the vacancy would be occupied by a worker after predefined time interval, which reflects labor market’s conditions, unemployment rate, qualifications required and local economic considerations of a region or country [69, 70]. The differences in estimations of indirect costs of schizophrenia in Germany according to both methods were presented in 1998. According to the human capital method estimation the total equaled 15,5 billion DM (German Mark: DM 1.95583 = €1 in January 1999, according to European Central Bank) whereas the same estimation on the basis of friction costs method gave the total of 10,2 million DM [69, 70]. Moreover between-countries comparison performed by Heider et al. in 2009 showed that direct costs and resource consumption vary significantly depending on the service provision model. The most significant differences in cost estimates were shown for day-clinic use, ranging from 1466 USD-PPP (United States Dollar Purchasing Power Parities) in France to 106 USD-PPP in the UK [71]. It might be explained by the fact that since 1991 the number of beds in hospitals has decreased and the number of day-clinic beds has increased in France [72]. Important variation of hospital inpatient costs was observed: 2333 USD-PPP in the UK to 1399 USD-PPP in France, with Germany falling between. Simultaneously cost for medical outpatient treatment varied from 173 USD-PPP in France to 49 USD-PPP in Germany. Again differences in outgoings on mental health care were explained by model of service provision and differences in rates of overheads [71].

Wide range of economic factors taken into account in assessment of costs of illnesses requires simplified methods, therefore system changes based solely on financial predictors seems to be *a priori* biased.

THE FUTURE OF THE HEALTH CARE SYSTEM-DEMANDS

A Question Rises – Is the Modeling of Health Care System Possible at All?

Multiplicities of factors belonging to theoretically separate branches of scientific fields like sociology, medicine, economy are still regarded too independently. Such kind of methodological reductionism, artificial division of facts reflects common tool of scientific work. The main issue is to arrange "the puzzles" again in order to obtain an expected picture – the real picture. The task may hardly be completed without interdisciplinary approach. The clock is ticking and researchers have to realize that even if they succeed, the outcome still has to be presented to decision-makers and their electorate. Pararell actions should be undertaken to change public view of psychiatry and mentally disturbed patients. Thornicroft et all. in his review showed that amongst possible interventions taken to counteract discrimination and stigma the most effective are: direct contact with persons suffering from a mental disorder (interpersonal level) and informing of the population (social level) [73]. Following this proposal might be a temporary and indispensable action leading to overcoming of inequalities in society. Decision-makers have to match the needs of people moving from institutions, and must take the long view [75]. Even though cost estimations of different approaches in mental service provision (i.e. institutional vs. social psychiatry) show wide variations the essential variable is human well being, quality of life and equity of access to social resources. Similarly as in the case of other branches of medicine the goal might be achieved by improvement in care delivery through innovations in management systems, coordination of actions on political and – what is equally important – business level.

Innovative and flexible strategies in staff training, procurement of founds from diverse sources (pharmaceutical companies, foundations, insurance companies, etc.) and access to beneficiary are important. Certainly private sector only supplements health care system but - especially in the case of developing countries - it might work as benchmark for changes on national level.

REFERENCES

[1] Patel V; Araya R; de Lima M; Ludermir A; Todd C. Women, poverty and common mental disorders in four restructuring societies. *Soc Sci Med.* 1999, 49: 1461-1471.

[2] Saraceno B; Barbui C. Poverty and Mental Illness. *Can J Psychiatry* 1997, 42: 285-290.

[3] Mental Health Atlas 2005, Geneva, WHO, 2005 *http://www.who.int/mental_health/evidence/atlas/global_results.pdf*

[4] Thornicroft G, Tansella M, eds. *The mental health matrix: a manual to improve services.* Cambridge, England, Cambridge University Press, 1999.
[5] Bachrach LL. Deinstitutionalization: promises, problems, and prospects. In: Knudsen HC, Thornicroft G, eds. *Mental Health Service Evaluation*, Cambridge, England, Cambridge University Press, 1996.
[6] Talbott JA. The fate of the public psychiatric system. *Hosp Community Psychiatry* 1985; 36: 46-50.
[7] Searight HR; Handal PJ. The paradox of psychiatric deinstitutionalization: Historical perspective and policy implications. *J Health Hum Resour Admin* 1988, 11(2): 249-266.
[8] Hopper K, Baxter E, Cox S. Not making it crazy: the young homeless patients in New York City. In: Pepper B, Ryglewicz H, eds. *New Directions for Mental Health Services*, no 14, San Francisco, USA, Jossey-Bass 1982; 33-42.
[9] Lamb RH. Lessons learned from deinstitutionalization in the USA. *Br J Psychiatry* 1993, 162: 587-592.
[10] Rossi PH; Wright JD; Fisher GA; et al. The urban homeless: estimating composition and size. *Science* 1987, 235: 1336–1341.
[11] Gelberg L; Linn LS; Leake BD. Mental health, alcohol and drug use, and criminal history among homeless adults. *Am J Psych* 1988, 145: 191–196.
[12] Bachrach LL. What we know about homelessness among mentally ill persons: an analytical review and commentary. *Hosp Community Psychiatr* 1992, 43: 453–464.
[13] Eynan R; Langley J; Tolomiczenko G; et al. The association between homelessness and suicidal ideation and behaviors: results of a cross-sectional survey. *Suicide and Life-Threatening Behavior* 2002, 32: 418–427.
[14] Michaels D; Zoloth S; Alcabes A; et al. Homelessness and indicators of mental illness among inmates in New York City's correctional system. *Hosp Community Psychiatr* 1992, 43: 150–155.
[15] Zapf PA; Roesch R; Hart SD. An examination of the relationship of homelessness to mental disorder, criminal behavior, and health care in a pretrial jail population. *Can J Psychiatr* 1996, 41: 435–440.
[16] Martell DA; Rosner R; Harmon RB. Baserate estimates of criminal behavior by homeless mentally ill persons in New York City. *Psychiatr Serv* 1995, 46: 596–601.
[17] Solomon P; Draine J. Using clinical and criminal involvement factors to explain homelessness among clients of a psychiatric probation and parole service. *Psychiatr Q* 1999, 70: 75–87.
[18] Belcher JR. Are jails replacing the mental health system for the homeless mentally ill? *Community Ment Health J* 1988, 24: 185–195.
[19] Lamb HR; Weinberger LE. Persons with severe mental illness in jails and prisons: a review. Psychiatr Serv 1998, 49: 483–492.
[20] Brenner HD. Stand der Diskussion zur Kosten-Effektivitatsfrage in der Gemeindepsychiatrie und Klinikpsychiatrie. *Schweiz Arch Neurol Psychiatr* 1995, 146(1): 24-32.
[21] Piotrowski P; Kiejna A. Czy system oddzialow dziennych moze byc szansa redukcji kosztow leczenia psychiatrycznego? *Psychiatr Pol 2005*, 39(6): 1067-75.
[22] Tarricone R; Gerzeli S; Montanelli R; et al. Direct and indirect costs of schizophrenia in community psychiatric services in Italy. *The GISESIS study. Health Pol 2000*, 51: 1-18.

[23] Guest JF; Cookson RF. Costs of schizophrenia to UK society. An incidence based cost-of-illness model for the first five years following diagnosis. *Pharmacoeconomics* 1999, 15: 597- 610.

[24] Colton CW; Manderscheid RW. Congruencies in increased mortality rates, years of potential life lost and causes of death among public mental health clients in eight states. *Prev Chronic Dis 2006* VOL3 NO2: 1-14.

[25] Insel TR. Assessing the Economic Costs of Serious Mental Illness. *Am J Psychiatr* 2008, 165: 663-665.

[26] Hunt S; McEwen J; McKenna SP. Social inequalities and perceived health. *Eff Health Care* 1979, 2(4): 151-160.

[27] Kessler RC; McGonagle KA; Zhao S; *et al.* Lifetime and 12-months prevalence of DSM-III-R psychiatric disorders in the United States. *Arch Gen Psychiatry* 1994, 51: 8-19.

[28] Muntaner C; Eaton WW; Miech R; O'Campo P. Socioeconomic position and major mental disorders. *Epidem Rev* 2004, 26: 53-62.

[29] Fryers T; Melzer D; Jenkins R; Brugha T. The distribution of common mental disorders: social inequalities in Europe. *Cl PractEpidem Ment Health* 2005, 1: 14.

[30] Van Snellenberg JX; de Candia T. Meta-analytic evidence for familial coaggregation of schizophrenia and bipolar disorder. *Arch Gen Psychiatry* 2009, 66(7): 748-755.

[31] Hudson CG. Socioeconomic status and mental illness: tests of the social causation and selection hypotheses. *Am J Orthopsychiat* 2005, 75:3-18.

[32] [Stansfeld SA; Head J; Marmot MG. Explaining social class differences in depression and well-being. *Soc Psyciatry Psychiatr Epidemiol* 1998, 33: 1-9.

[33] Dalgard OS. Social inequalities in mental Heath in Nowary: possible explanatory factors. *International Journal of Equity in Health* 2008, 7: 27

[34] Marmot MG. Status syndrome. A challenge to medicine. *JAMA* 2006, 295: 1304-1307.

[35] World Health Organization Health 21. *The Healthor All Policy Framework for the WHO Region, Series 4.* Copenhagen,WHO Regional Office for Europe, 1999.

[36] Araya R; Lewis G; Rojas G; Fritsch R. Education and income: which is more important for mental health? *J Epidemiol Community Health.* 2003, 57(7): 501–505.

[37] Officer A; Groce NE. Key concepts in disability. Lancet 2009, 374: 1795-1796.

[38] Link BG; Yang LH; Phelan JC; Collins PY. Measuring mental illness stigma. *Schizophr Bull* 2004, 30: 511-541.

[39] Thornicroft G. Shunned: *Discrimination against People with Mental Illness.* England, Oxford: Oxford University Press, 2006.

[40] Thompson JW; Belcher JR; DeForge BR; Meyers P, Henderson MJ: Trends in the inpatient care of persons with schizophrenia. *Schizophr Bull* 1995; 21: 75-85.

[41] Piccinelli M; Wilkinson G. Gender differences in depression: critical review. *Br J Psychiatry 2000,* 177: 486–492.

[42] Patel V. Poverty, gender and mental Heath promotion in a globar society. *Promotion & Education 2005*, Supp. 2: 26-29.

[43] World Health Organization. World Health Report 2003: *Shaping the Future.* Geneva, World Health Organization, 2003.

[44] Hawton K. Sex and suicide: gender differences in suicidal behaviour. *Br J Psychiatry 2000*, 177: 484–485.

[45] Koegel P; Burnam MA; Farr RK. The prevalence of specific psychiatric disorders among homeless individuals in the inner city of Los Angeles. *Arch Gen Psychiatr* 1988, 45: 1085–1091.

[46] Breakey WR; Fischer PJ; Kramer M, et al. Health and mental health problems of homeless men and women in Baltimore. *JAMA* 1989, 262:1352–1357.

[47] Susser E; Struening EL; Conover S. Psychiatric problems in homeless men. *Arch Gen Psychiatr* 1989, 46: 845–850.

[48] McQuistion HL; Finnerty M; Hirschowitz J; Susser ES. Challenges for psychiatry in serving homeless people with psychiatric disorders. *Psych Serv* 2003, 54(5): 669-676.

[49] Draine J; Salzer MS; Culhane DP; Hadley TR. Role of social disadvantage in crime, joblessness, and homelessness among persons with serious mental illness. *Psych Serv* 2002; 5(53): 565-573

[50] Culhane DP; Metraux SM. One-year rates of public shelter utilization in New York City (1990, 1995) and Philadelphia (1995). *Popul Res Pol Rev* 1999, 18: 219–236.

[51] Culhane DP; Averyt J; Hadley TR. The rate of public shelter admission among Medicaid-reimbursed users of behavioral health services. *Psychiatr Serv* 1997, 48: 390–392.

[52] Shinn M; Weitzman BC; Stojanovic D; et al. Predictors of homelessness among families in New York City: from shelter request to housing stability. *Am J Publ Health* 1998, 88: 1651–1657.

[53] Bassuk EL; Buckner JC; Weinreb LF; et al. Homelessness in female-headed families: childhood and adult risk and protective factors. *Am J Publ Health* 1997, 87: 241–248.

[54] Sosin MR. Homeless and vulnerable meal program users: a comparison study. *Social Problems* 1992, 39: 170–188.

[55] Toro PA; Bellavia CW; Daeschler CV; et al. Distinguishing homelessness from poverty: a comparative study. *J Consult Clin Psychol* 1995, 63: 280–289.

[56] Wermter AK; Laucht M; Schimmelmann BG et al. From nature versus nurture, via nature and nurture, to gene x environment interaction in mental disorders. *Eur Child Adolesc Psychiatry* 2010, 19(3): 199-210.

[57] Tsuang MT; Bar JL; Stone WS; Faraone SV. Gene-environment interactions in mental disorders. *World Psychiatry* 2004, 3(2): 73-83.

[58] Ustun TB. The Global Burden of the Mental Disorders. *Am J Public Health* 1999, 89(9): 1315-1318.

[59] Sartorius N. *Association for The Improvement of Mental Health Programmes. Presented on: 16th AEP Congress*, 5-9 April 2008, Nice, France.

[60] Thornicroft G. The relationship between anticipated and experienced discrimination. *Presented on: 8th International ENMESH Conference*, 23-25 May 2008, Cracow, Poland.

[61] Catlin A; Cowan C; Hartman M; Heffler S. National Health Expenditure Accounts Team: National health spending in 2006: a year of change for prescription drugs. *Health Aff* (Millwood) 2008; 27: 14–29.

[62] Poisal JA; Truffer C; Smith S; Sisko A; Cowan C; Keehan S; Dickensheets B. Health spending projections through 2016: modest changes obscure Part D's impact. *Health Aff* (Millwood) 2007; 26: w242–w253.

[63] Mark TL; Levit KR; Coffey RM; McKusick DR; Harwood HJ; King EC; Bouchery E; Genuardi JS; Vandivort-Warren R; Buck JA; Ryan K. National Expenditures for Mental Health Services and Substance Abuse Treatment, 1993–2003: SAMHSA Publication SMA 07-4227. Rockville, Md, *Substance Abuse and Mental Health Services Administration*, 2007.

[64] Knapp M; Mangalore R; Simon J. The global costs of schizophrenia. *Schizophr Bull* 2004; 30: 279-293.

[65] Rupp A; Keith SJ. The costs of schizophrenia: Assessing the burden. *Psychiatr Clin North Am* 1993; 16: 413-423.

[66] Tarricone R; Gerzeli S; Montanelli R, et al. Direct and indirect costs of schizophrenia in community psychiatric services in Italy. *The GISESIS study. Health Pol 2000*; 51: 1-18.

[67] Guest JF; Cookson RF. Costs of schizophrenia to UK society. An incidence based cost-of-illness model for the first five years following diagnosis. *PharmacoEconomics* 1999; 15: 597: 610.

[68] Mushkin S. et al. Cost of disease and illness in the United States in the year 2000. *Pub Health Rep* 1978; 93: 493.

[69] Roick C; Kilian R; Angermeyer MC. Indirect costs of schizophrenia. An investigation of the elements and calculation methods for illness related resources-loss. W: Merker N, Göpfert P, Kirch W, Regensburg S (eds) *Public Health Research and Practice: Report of the Public Health Research Association Saxony* 2000-2001. Germany, Roderer Verlag 2001, s. 191-210.

[70] Kilian R; Becker T. Impact of antipsychotic medication on the cost of schizophrenia. *Expert Rev Pharmacoeconomics Outcomes Res* 2005; 5(1): 39-57.

[71] Heider D; Bernert S; et al. Direct medical mental health care costs of schizophrenia in France, Germany and the United Kingdom - findings from the European Schizophrenia Cohort (EuroSC). *Eur Psychiatr* 2009; 24: 216-224.

[72] Verdoux H. The current state of adult mental health care in France. *Eur Arch Psychiatry Clin Neurosci* 2007; 257: 64-70.

[73] Thornicroft G; Brohan E; Kassam A; Lewis-Holmes E. Reducing stigma and discrimination: candidate interventions. *Int J Ment Health Syst* 2008; 2(1): 3.

[74] Piotrowski, P. (2008). Cost-*effectiveness analysis of mental health care in Poland,* PhD Thesis, Wroclaw Medical University. Wroclaw, Poland. Founding: Polish Ministry of Science and Higher Education, grant No. MNiSW N404 068 31/3099.

[75] Knapp, M., Beecham, J,, McDaid, D., Matosevic, T., Smith, M. The economic consequences of deinstitutionalisation of mental health services: lessons from a systematic review of European experience. *Health Soc Care Community* 2010; Dec 10 [Epub ahead of print].

[76] Vallgårda, S. Public health policies: a Scandinavian model? *Scand J Public Health* 2007; 35(2): 205-11.

In: Social Determinants and Mental Health
Editor: Sabine Bährer-Kohler

ISBN: 978-1-61324-353-4

Chapter 14

NUTRITION AND MENTAL HEALTH

Joanna Wyka
Wroclaw University of Environmental and Life Science, Faculty of Food Sciences
Department of Agricultural Technology and Storage, Wroclaw, Poland

ABSTRACT

Nutrition is the intake of food, considered in relation to the body's dietary needs. Nutritional patterns affect significantly man's body at each age. The elderly – with their eating habits and diseases they have overcome – often require specific dietary intervention. A proper and well-balanced diet is an important element of lifestyle that may become a factor facilitating the so-called healthy, successful ageing and delay the development of non-infectious, chronic metabolic diseases that are in majority of cases diagnosed in elder people. Neurodegenerative diseases have been classified amongst chronic diseases yet with still controversial etiology. Nevertheless, it is speculated that some nutritional factors, including the appropriate intake of B-group vitamins, antioxidative vitamins and polyunsaturated fatty acids, are likely to play a significant role in their prevention and therapy. A diet rich in vegetables and fruits, whole-meal bread, milk and dairy products as well as containing fish, plant oils and nuts provides all indispensable nutrients. The appropriate merging of these food products into dishes – widely described in literature as the Mediterranean diet – facilitates leading a long life in health.

Keywords: neurodegenerative diseases, Alzheimer disease (AD), nutritional factors, elderly

1. INTRODUCTION

One factor relating to mental health is nutrition. An adequate, well balanced diet combined with physical and mental activity – is called a cornerstone of good health (WHO, 2010). Jacka et al. document, that a traditional dietary pattern characterized by vegetables, fruit, meat, fish, and whole grains was associated with lower odds for major depression or dysthymia and for anxiety disorders. Nevertheless Jacka et al. and other researchers have demonstrated an association between habitual diet quality and high-prevalence mental disorders, although reverse causality and confounding cannot be ruled out as explanations (Lakhan and Vieira, 2008; Jacka et al., 2010). Concerning fish consumption Hibbeln (1998) postlated that the correlation between apparent fish consumption and lower annual prevalence of major depression does not show that fish consumption can cause differences in the prevalence of major depression or that eating fish or fish oils are useful in treatment. Various cultural, economic, social, and other factors can confound this simple correlational relation. But nutrition is a modifiable risk factor with direct implication on the prevalence of other diseases like cardiovascular ones, which are related in the field of cognitive decline and AD. Without any doubt, the proper nutrition in the older age serves the protective function against chronic diseases, whereas nutrients provided in appropriate quantities support the body in adaptation processes being impaired with age. Extensively described in literature improper eating habits of the elderly are often becoming an additional stress factor and contribute to the advancement of pathological changes. The necessity of balancing increasing nutritional needs of the elderly (among others for antioxidative vitamins, B_{12} and D) and reducing the energy value of a food ration, pose a number of difficulties in the proper planning of food rations, facilitate the occurrence of health disturbances induced by the ill-balanced diet, and indirectly affect the quality and span of life of the elderly (Cannella et al., 2009).

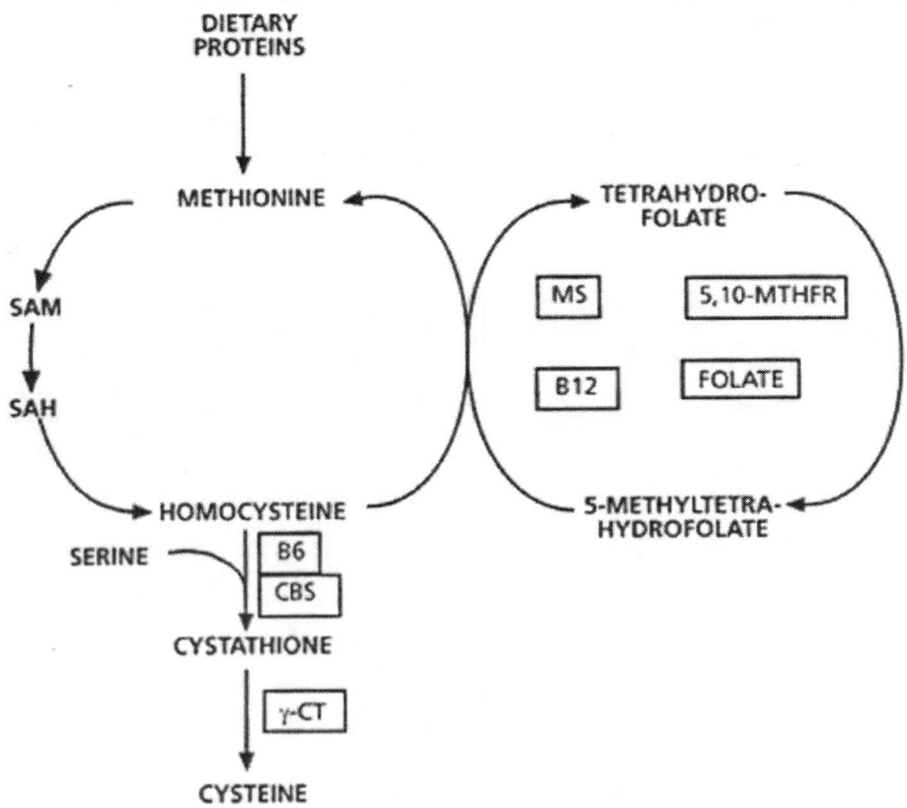

Figure 1. Homocysteine metabolism. Key: CBS – cystathione-β-synthase; γ-CT – γ-cystathionase; MS – methionine synthase; 5,10-MTHFR – 5,10-methylene-tetrahydrofolate reductase; SAM – S-adenosyl-methionine; SAH – S-adenosyl-homocysteine.

2. B-GROUP VITAMINS

B6 and B12 vitamins as well as folic acid play a significant role in metabolism of homocysteine amino acid. It is an intermediate compound between exogenous methionine and endogenous cysteine. In these processes that involve first demethylation followed by transsulfuration a significant function is ascribed to an enzyme called cystathionine β-synthase (CBS), whose coenzyme is the active form of B6 vitamin – pyridoxal phosphate (Fig.1). Cystathione synthesized with these enzymes is then hydrolyzed to cysteine, which in turn is oxidized to sulfate excreted with urine. The second metabolic pathway of homocysteine is re-methylation to non-toxic methionine, with folic acid being a donor of the methyl group and vitamin B12 (cobalamin) being the cofactor of methionine synthase (MS). The concentration of homocysteine in blood serum of a healthy man should range from 5 to 5-15 μmol/L, and its elevated concentration indicates a lower level of MS which may result, besides deficiency of B12 vitamins and/or folic acid, from congenital disorders of homocysteine metabolism linked with polymorphism of genes encoding methylenetetrahydrofolate reductase (5,10-MTHFR), methionine synthase (MS) and cystathionine β-synthase (CBS) (Seshadri et al. 2002; Fudala et al. 2008). Investigations on these dependencies have begun at the 60-ties of the XXth century. However, already at the early 1990-ies, when homocysteine was recognized an independent risk factor of cardiovascular diseases, researches have started addressing its effect on the functioning of the cardiovascular system, development of neural tube defects, but also on the manifestation of psychic disturbances and these of cognitive functions (Harjai 1999; Virtanen et al. 2005). Damage of vessels induced by the increased concentration of homocysteine may directly affect the development of Alzheimer disease and the rate of β-amyloid deposit aggregation in brain or extent of its removal from cerebral tissues to blood circulation. Ischaemia induced by stenosis of brain micro-vessels may additionally stimulate amyloidogenesis and increase the risk of incidence of Alzheimer's dementia (Pluta et al. 1996). One of significant research works confirming a dependency between hyperhomocysteinemia and AD was the Framingham Study, in which the elderly (> 70±7 years, n=1947) were determined for serum level of homocysteine over a twenty-year period (Bostom et al. 1999). It has demonstrated that homocysteine concentration above 14 μmol/L was significantly linked with a twofold higher risk of AD development, and its increase by every 5 μmol/L was elevating that risk by 40%. The elderly with intermittently increasing level of homocysteine since the beginning of the study appeared to be the most susceptible to the development of AD. This risk could have been predicted even 8 years before the appearance of the first disease symptoms. In turn, no significant correlation has been demonstrated between the level of B6, B12 vitamins and folic acid in blood serum and the risk of development of AD-based dementia (Bostom et al. 1999). In another survey, Wang et al. (2001) have determined concentrations of folic acid and vitamin B12 in 370 subjects (>70 years) without senile dementia at the beginning of the study. The low level of these parameters was correlated with an increased risk of AD development, whilst folic acid level below 10 pmol/L and vitamin B12 level below 150 pmol/L were found to double the risk of dementia. In turn, the British survey OPTIMA (Oxford Project To Investigate Memory and Aging) demonstrated a high level of homocysteine and a low concentration of vitamin B12 and folic acid in patients with AD, irrespective of sex, age, social status and the habit of tobacco smoking. A control study conducted 3 years later showed a more rapid progression of the disease in the group of the subjects with a higher initial level of homocysteine (Köseoglu and Karaman, 2007). Corrada et al. (2005) evaluated eating habits of 579 (> 60 years) participants of the Baltimore Longitudinal Study of Aging. Over 9 years of this study, AD was diagnosed in 57 patients. In addition, it proved a significant correlation between high intake of folates (remarkably higher than RDA) and reduced risk of AD development. Such a correlation was, however, not demonstrated for intakes of vitamin C and B12 and carotenoids. In contrast, Reynolds et al. (2002) did not observe any significant correlation between deficiency of folates and vitamin B12 and the development of neurological changes.

A number of surveys have shown a low supply of folates as well as vitamins B6 and B12 in food rations of the elderly, irrespective of age, sex, education and place of living (Pirlich 2001; Haveman-Nies et al. 2001; Marshall et al. 2001; Volkert et al. 2004; Wyka et al. 2010; Wyka et al., 2011). Physiologically-suppressed secretion of hydrochloric acid and digestive enzymes in the stomach and pancreas observed in the older population results in reduced absorption of vitamin B12 and – with trophic changes of stomach mucosa – it impairs the binding of that vitamin with the intrinsic factor (IF) and its absorption (Saunier and Dore, 2002). In turn, folates are characterized by a considerable susceptibility to temperature. Technological processing of food products being a source of folates in diet (green vegetables: broccoli, spinach, Brussels sprouts) causes even 70% losses of that vitamin in food rations.

3. Antioxidative Vitamins

Recent studies have documented the significant role of the inflammatory process and oxidative stress in pathomechanism of a number of chronic, non-infectious metabolic diseases, including i.a.: atherosclerosis, diabetes, neoplasms as well as AD. Free radicals generated ceaselessly, most of all in mitochondria, are highly reactive species that attack primarily cell components. Damage of proteins leads to the loss of the activity of cellular enzymes, membrane transporters and regulatory proteins. In turn, damage to nitric bases constituting DNA may initiate a cascade of reactions leading to uncontrolled proliferation of cells and neoplasm. Peroxidation of membraneous lipids causes the loss of their protective and transport function, whereas oxidation of polyunsaturated fatty acids (PUFAs) additionally contributes to the synthesis of reactive products which destroy, e.g., DNA structure. The generation of free radicals may also be affected by environmental factors, including: tobacco smoking and drinking alcohol as well as diet poor in compounds with oxidoreductive properties.

Under conditions of systemic homeostasis free radicals are inactivated by:

- endogenous antioxidants – (enzymatic: superoxide dismutase, glutathione peroxidase, catalase; and non-enzymatic: polyamides, albumin, Q coenzyme, transferrin, glutathione, and others)
- exogenous antioxidants – vitamins: C, A, E, carotenoids, xanthophylls, polyphenols.

An imbalance between continuous production of reactive oxygen species and their neutralization in enzymatic and non-enzymatic reactions and as a result of the activity of exogenous antioxidants is referred to as oxidative stress. Antioxidative vitamins play the strategic role in the removal of oxidative stress from the body, and their improper intake with foods (fruits, vegetables) may affect, among other things, quicker ageing of the body and development of inflammatory processes. At especially high risk of these processes is the nervous tissue due to high consumption of oxygen and increased mitochondrial density. An additional cause of this risk may be a low concentration of albumin in the cerebrospinal fluid and a high concentration of PUFAs in membranes of nervous cells that are readily subject to peroxidation. Amongst the antioxidative vitamins, the major role in prevention of these processes is ascribed to vitamin E, for it prevents the chain reaction of oxidation of lipids constituting cellular membranes and also oxidation of the LDL – cholesterol fraction responsible for the development of the inflammatory process in atherosclerosis. Schmit et al. (1998) have demonstrated a correlation between vitamin E concentration in blood serum and cognitive functions in a population of 1769 subjects at the age over 60, participants of the Austrian Stroke Prevention Study. Furthermore, Perkins et al. (1999) have found a dependency between vitamin E concentration in blood serum and disorders of cognitive functions amongst 4809 participants of the NHNES study (Health and Nutrition Examination Survey). In contrast, a survey by Perrig et al. (1997) did not confirm a correlation between vitamin E intake and cognitive functions in 442 subjects over 65 years of age, yet such a correlation was noted for vitamin C and carotenoids. In turn, Otrega et al. (2002) have examined 110 respondents at the age of 65-91 years to evaluate their dietary habits over a 5-day period and to determine vitamin E concentration in their blood serum. The subjects with vitamin E intake lower than 50% of RDA and its low concentration in blood serum were observed to make more mistakes in intellectual exercises. Morris et al. (2002) evaluated the intake of vitamin E in 815 healthy individuals over 65 years of age. In the course of the 3.9-year study it has been demonstrated that increased intake of vitamin E from food products was linked with a reduced risk of AD development. Especially protective character of this dependency was observed in the patients without the APOE 4 gene. It is worth emphasizing that the intake of vitamin C, beta-carotene and vitamin E from dietary supplements had no impact on the minimized risk of AD development. Furthermore, participants of the Rotterdam Study (n=5395, >55 years) were assayed for the intake of antioxidative vitamins. Over 6 years of assays, the study revealed 197 cases of dementia, including 146 patients with diagnosed AD. In addition, a high intake of vitamin C and E was demonstrated to be linked with a reduced risk of AD, irrespective of the educational status of the subjects and of whether they possessed the APOE 4 gene (Engelhart et al. 2002). In turn, a research conducted under the Washington Heights-Inwood Columbia Ageing Project amongst 980 older persons showed 242 cases of dementia and no correlation between intakes of carotenoids, vitamins C and C, as well as between diet supplementation with these vitamins or its lack and the risk of AD development (Luchsinger et al. 2003).

Worthy of notice is also the fact that a low intake of vitamins is reported in many populations, however in the elderly it is implicated to affect an especially high risk of health loss. A number of authors point to the health-promoting role of diet supplementation with particular vitamins, but also underline its side effects (Fletcher and Faireld, 2002). Kontush and Schekatolina (2004) have attempted to evaluate the effect of diet supplementation with vitamins on the development of AD based on results of a survey conducted in a total population of 15,948 elderly patients. In the end, 4 out of 6 prospective studies have demonstrated the protective role of using dietary supplements containing both vitamin E and

C in AD development. In contrast, no significant correlation was shown for diet supplementation with single vitamins. Reduced incidence of AD as affected by diet supplementation with vitamins C and E was also reported by Zandi et al. (2004) amongst 4740 elderly patients over 65 years of age. In turn, a review by Boothby et al. (2005) on taking dietary supplements with vitamins E and C has shown that both single vitamins and their complexes were reducing the incidence of AD. Nevertheless, based on data from ample research works these authors do not recommend diet supplementation with these preparations in the prevention of primary and secondary symptoms of AD. Finally, uncontrolled and excessive intake of vitamins in the form of dietary supplements may be the causative agent of increased total mortality amongst both healthy individuals and patients at different age (Bjelakovic et al., 2007).

4. Polyunsaturated Fatty Acids (PUFAs)

From the human health perspective, the most important PUFAs include these with more than two double bonds that belong to the omega-6 family also referred to as *n*-6 family (linolic acid 18:2) and to omega-3/*n*-3 family (α-linolenic 18:3). They are precursors of long-chain polyunsaturated fatty acids (LC-PUFA) and should be consumed every day because in the human body there are no enzymatic systems (Δ^{12}-desaturase and Δ^{15}-desaturase) inserting the double bonds into *n*-6 and *n*-3 positions of the carbon chain. Transformations of PUFAs proceed in endoplasmic reticulum of cells where upon elongation and desaturation processes they are transformed into long-chain metabolites: linolic acid into arachidonic acid (ARA 20:4 n-6), and α-linolenic acid into eicosapentaenoic acid (EPA 20:5 n-3) and docosahexaenoic acid (DHA 22:6 n-3) (Fig.2). In turn, the LC-PUFAs are precursors of the synthesis of active cellular compounds, including: prostaglandins, prostacyclins, tromboxanes, leukotrienes, and additionally are components of cellular membranes, especially in such organs are brain and eye retina (Abbadi et al. 2004). Prostanoids synthesized in excess from arachidonic acid evoke, among other things, increased permeability of blood vessels, local increase in bloodstream and increased aggregation of platelets, as well as affect the intensity and duration of inflammatory processes. Eicosanoids synthesized from eicosapentaenoic acid display the anti-inflammatory effect as well as reduce concentration of very low density triglycerides, VLDL cholesterol and BVLDL apolipoprotein (Apo- B) in blood serum. It should be emphasized that the polyunsaturated fatty acids of the omega-3 and omega-6 family compete for the same enzymes, hence their appropriate intake with food is of great significance.

In man's diet a source of linolic acid are oils from: sunflower (>70%), soybean and maize (>60%), and grape seeds (ca. 80%). The PUFAs of the *n*-3 family, including most of all EPA and DHA, are synthesized in phytoplankton which is ingested by marine fish. They are accumulated in fish liver and muscles (sardines 0.98-1.70 g/3 oz, pink salmon 0.68-1.48 g/3 oz, mackerel 0.34-1.57 g/3 oz, herring 1.7-1.8 g/3oz) (Kris-Etherton et al. 2002). In turn, considerable quantities of α-linolenic acid are provided by linseed oils (55-60%) and walnuts (6%). The proper ratio of omega-6 to omega-3 fatty acids in a diet should reach 4-5:1. Owing to a high intake of plant oils and a low intake of marine fish, their supply is disturbed with their ratio in diets typical of Western Europe and North America countries accounting for 15-30:1.

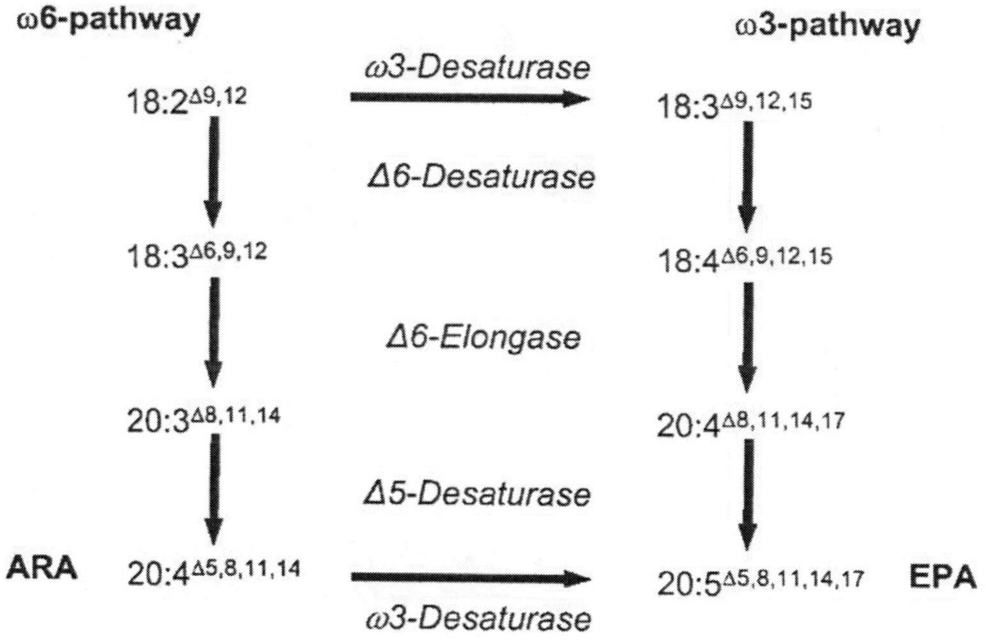

Figure 2. Biosynthesis of LC PUFA from linoleic (18:2) and α-linolenic (18:3) acid.

Population surveys have shown that a high intake of LC-PUFA n-3 originating from fish oils and from marine fish was linked with reduced risk of ischaemic heart disease, myocardial infarction and cerebral stroke and that it may potentially be implicated in reducing the risk of AD development through vascular mechanisms (Bucher et al., 2002; Hu et al., 2002; Mozaffarian et al., 2005). Investigations conducted with old mice have demonstrated that a reduced content of PUFA in brain tissues was eliciting disorders in the functioning of nervous system cell membranes, which resulted in amnesia, a loss of the capability to learn and vision disorders. These symptoms were, however, regressing after mice diet supplementation with fish oils and also directly with DHA (Yehuda et al. 2002). A relationship between a low serum level of DHA and AD incidence in humans has been demonstrated by Conquer et al. (2000). A PAQUID (Personnes Agées QUID) survey conducted with a group of 1416 elderly Frenchmen (>68 years) was aimed at evaluating the effect of the frequency of fish and meat intake on the risk of dementia. Over the 7-year study, a statistically lower risk of diagnosing dementia, including AD, was demonstrated amongst the respondents who were consuming fish and sea fruits at least once a week. Authors of this survey emphasized that symptoms of dementia in the respondents were noted 3 years before diagnosis and that the risk of its incidence could have been affected by improper dietary habits (Bamberger-Gateau et al. 2002). The intake of fish was also assessed amongst 815 healthy individuals at the age of 65-94 years participating in the Chicago Health and Aging Project. In the course of the 2.3-year study, AD was diagnosed in 131 participants. The survey demonstrated that amongst patients who were consuming fish at least once a week or often the risk of AD development decreased to 60% compared to these who were consuming fish rarely or never (Morris et al. 2003). Furthermore, a study by Luchsinger et al. (2002) conducted with 980 healthy individuals at the age of ca. 75 years have shown that over 4 years of the study the annual AD incidence accounted for 6 cases per 100 patients and was attributed to excess intake of dietary energy and fats. This correlation was proved stronger in patients with diagnosed genetically (apolipoprotein E4) higher susceptibility to accumulation of β-amyloid in the brain.

In a number of countries, the intake of fish as a source of LC- PUFA amongst the elderly is insufficient. There are still too few research on the use of EPA+DHA supplements in the prophylaxis of degenerative diseases in men at the advanced age. It seems, however, that recently updated recommendations (Tab. 1) for their intake meet prophylactic objectives of not only cardio-vascular diseases (Kris-Etherton and Hill 2008).

Table 1. Global recommendations for LC – PUFA n-3 and fish

Australia and New Zealand National Health and Medical Research Council (2006)	men and women >19 y 610 mg/day >70y 430mg/day DHA/EPA/DPA
European Society for Cardiology (De Backer et al. 2003)	oily fish and n-3 fatty acids have particular protective properties for primary CV prevention
International Society for the Study of Fatty Acids and Lipids (2004)	a minimum combined intake of 500mg/day EPA and DHA is recommended for CV health
National Heart Foundation of Australia (2004)	at least two portions of fish (preferably oily fish) meals per week
United Kingdom Scientific Advisory Committee on Nutrition (2004)	consume at least two portions of fish per week, of which one should be oily, and provide 450 mg per day EPA+DHA
World Health Organization (2003)	regular fish consumption (one to two servings per week: each serving should provide the equivalent of 200 to 500 mg EPA+DHA)
American Heart Association (Lichtenstein et al.2006)	1 g/day of EPA+DHA
Polish RDA (Jarosz et al. 2008)	2 g α-linolenic acid and 200 mg EPA+DHA

CONCLUSION

Improvement of living standards, nutrition and medical care facilitates the systematic elongation of men life span and contributes to an increase in the percentage of the elderly in the global population. The mode of nutrition and possibilities of covering alimentation demands of older people are – to a significant extent – restricted by their health status. However, most of the elderly are observed to be affected by the highest incidence of chronic, non-infectious metabolic diseases, including psychic disorders. Of significance is also the fact that consequences of pathological processes are coupled with involutional physiological changes proceeding with age, and considerably impair the functioning of all bodily organs and tissues. The observed in the elderly improper nutritional patterns and dietary habits acquired in the childhood and adolescence and reinforced in the adulthood as well as the need to avoid selected food products for different reasons, result in many health implications, deficiencies of nutrients and malnutrition in particular. The improper nutritional status being a consequence of inadequate intake of nutrients with foods, their poor absorption and utilization, as well as effects of extrinsic pathological factors are undoubtedly the basis for, among others, cardiovascular diseases and neoplasms. Although the impact of nutritional factors on cognitive functions of man has not been explicitly recognized yet, it seems that propagation of a balanced diet from the childhood is likely to delay by a couple of years the development of diseases with confirmed nutritional etiology, and indirectly also these linked with impairment of the cognitive functions.

Eating is one of the few joys in man's life, especially in life of an elder person. It may also serve a function of the so-called "protective factor", but also become an additional negative stressor. Therefore, principles of appropriate selection of food products that would provide adequate quantities of all nutrients indispensable for health, especially B-group vitamins, antioxidative vitamins and polyunsaturated fatty acids, should be widely propagated. These recommendations were formulated and presented in the form of a health pyramid addressed to the elderly and well as their caregivers (Fig.3.). Diet providing both food products contained in the health pyramid for the elderly and the number of due rations of particular groups of food products enables the assumed reduction of energy intake and assures high nutritional density. The pyramid promotes fruits and vegetables as sources of antioxidants and minerals, as well as bread and whole-meal cereals enriched with vitamins. Wholesome protein is provided by appropriate rations of poultry, fish, legume grains and eggs. In addition, the pyramid recommends 8 glasses of fluids a day, diet supplementation with vitamin D and B12, and calcium, as well as physical activity necessary for maintaining health and desired life quality. It seems that, apart from physical activity, the elderly should also undertake everyday intellectual activities, e.g. reading with comprehension, memorizing poems or doing crosswords.

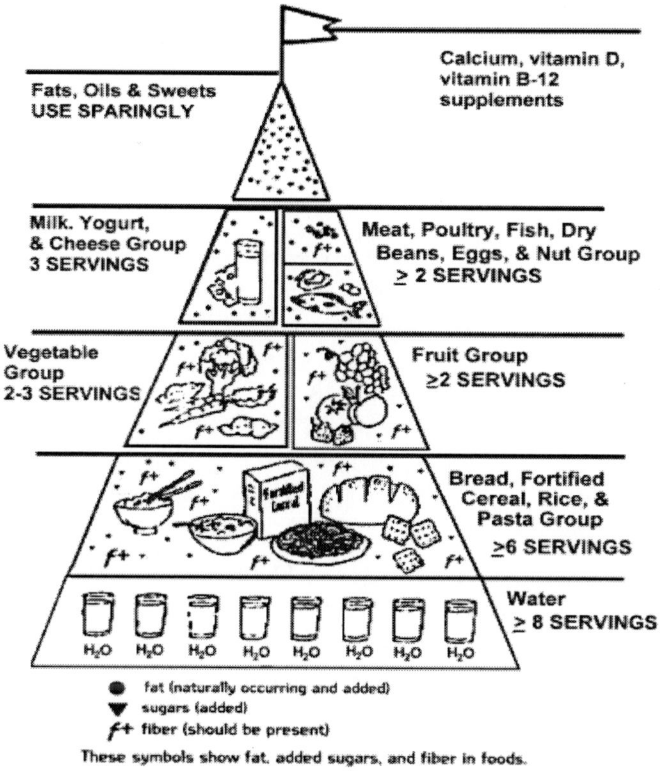

Figure 3. (Continued).

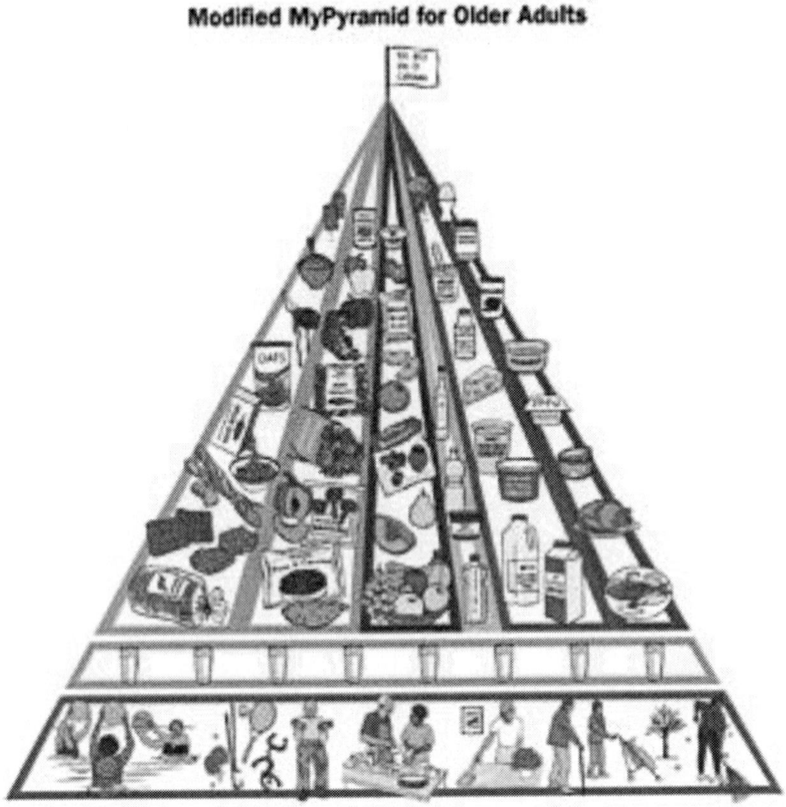

Figure 3. Healthy eating pyramid for persons over 70 years of age (Russell et al. 1999; Lichtenstain et al. 2008).

REFERENCES

Abbadi A., Domergue F., Bauer J., Napier J.A. et al. (2004) Biosynthesis of Very-Long – Chain Polyunsaturated Fatty Acids in Transgenic Oliseeds: Constraints on Their Accumulation. *The Plant Cell* 16, 2734-2748

Barberger-Gateau P., Letenneur L., Deschamps V. et al. (2002). Fish, meat and risk of dementia: cohort study. *BMJ* 325, 932-933

Bjelakovic G., Nikolova D., Gluud L.L. et al. (2007) Mortality in randomized trials of antioxidant supplements for primary and secondary prevention. *JAMA* 297, 842-857

Boothby L.A., Doering P.L (2005) Vitamin C and vitamin E for Alzheimer's disease. nn. *Pharmacother*. 39(12), 2073-2079

Bostom A.G., Rosenberg I.H., Silbershatz H et al. (1999) Nonfasting plasma total homocysteine levels and stroke incidence in elderly persons: the Framingham *Study. Ann Intern. Med.* 131, 352-355

Bucher H.C et al (2002) Polyunsaturated fatty acids in coronary heart disease: meta – nalysis of randomized controlled trials. *Am. J. Med.* 112,298-304

Cannella C., Savina C., Donini L.M (2009) Nutrition, longevity and behavior. *Arch. Gerontol. Geriatr*. Suppl.1, 19-27.

Corrada M.M., Kawas C.H., Hallfrisch J., Muller D, Brookmeyer R. (2005) reduced risk of alzheimer's disease with high folate intake: The Baltimore Longitudinal Study of Aging. *Alzheimer's & Dementia* 1, 11-18

Engelhart M.J., Geerlings M.I., Ruitenberg A., Van Swieten et al.(2002) Dietary intake of antioxidants and risk of Alzheimer disease. *JAMA* 287,3223-3229

Fletcher R.H., Fairfield K.M (2002) Vitamins for chronic disease prevention in adults. *JAMA* 287(23), 3127-3129

Fudala M., Brola W., Przybylski W., Czernicki J (2008) Is research in homocysteine and cyanocobalamine levels likely to become the key to diagnosing and treating Alzheimer diseases? *Med. Stud.* 10, 53-58.

Harjai K.J. (1999) Potential New Cardiovascular Risk Factors: Left Ventricular Hypertrophy, Homocysteine, Lipoprotein (a), Triglycerides, Oxidative Stress, and Fibrinogen. *Ann. Intern. Med.* 131, 376-386

Haveman-Nies A., Tucker K.L., de Groot L. et al. (2001) Evaluation of dietary quality in relationship to nutritional and lifestyle factors in elderly of the US Framingham Heart Study and the European SENECA study. E. *J. Clin. Nutr.* 55, 870-880

Hibbeln, J.R., (1998). Fish consumption and major depression. *The Lancet* 351, 1110-1213

Hu F.B.et al. (2002) Fish and omega -3 fatty acid intake and risk of coronary heart disease in woman. *JAMA* 287,1815-1821

Jacka F.H., Pasco J.A., Mykletun A et al. (2010) *Association of western and traditional diets with depression and anxiety in women.* 167, 244-247

Jarosz M., Bułhak-Jachymczyk B.(2008) Normy żywienia człowieka. *Podstawy prewencji otyłości i chorób niezakaźnych*. PZWL, Warsaw

Kontush A., Schekatolina S (2004). Vitamin E in neurodegenerative disorders. *Ann. New York Acad. Sci.* 1031, 249-262

Köseoglu E., Karaman Y. (2007). Relations between homocysteine, folate and vitamin B12 in vascular dementia and in Alzheimer disease. *Clin. Biochem*. 40, 859-863

Kris-Etherton P.M., Harris W.S., Appel L.J. (2002) Fish Consumption, Fish Oil, Omega-3 fatty Acids, and Cardiovascular disease. *Circulation* 106, 2747-2757

Kris-Etherton P.M., Hill A.M (2008) N-3 fatty acids: food or supplements? *JADA* 108 (7), 1125-1130

Lakhan S. E., Vieira K.F. (2008) Nutritonal therapies for mental disorders. *Nutr. J.* 7, 2

Lichtenstein A.H., Appel L.J., Brands M., et al. (2006) Diet and lifestyle recommendations revision 2006. A scientific statement from American Heart Association. *Nutrition* Committee. Circulation, 114, 1-15

Lichtenstein A.H., Rasmussen H., Yu W.W et al (2008) Modified MyPyramid for older adults. *J. Nutr.* 138, 5-11

Luchsinger J.A., Tang M-X., Shea S., Mayeux R.(2002). Caloric intake and the risk of Alzheimer Disease. *Arch. Neurol.* 59, 1258-1263

Luchsinger J.A., Tang M-X., Shea S., Mayeux R (2003) Antioxidant vitamin intake and risk of Alzheimer disease. *Arch. Neurol.* 60, 203-208

Marshall T., Stumbo P. J., Warren J. J., Xie X-J. (2001) Inadequate nutrient intakes are common and are associated with low diet variety in rural, community-dwelling elderly. *J. Nutr.* 131,2192-2196

Morris M.C., Evans D.A., Bienias J.L et al. (2002) Dietary intake of antioxidant nutrients and the risk of incident Alzheimer diseases in a Biracial Community Study. *JAMA* 287, 3230-3237

Morris M.C., Evans D.A., Bienias J.L. et al. (2003) Consumption of fish and n-3 fatty acids and risk of incident Alzheimer disease. *Arch. Neurol.* 60, 940-946

Mozaffarian D et al. (2005) Fish consumption and stroke risk in elderly individuals: The Cardiovascular Health Study. *Arch. Intern. Med.* 165, 200-206

Otrega R.M., Requejo A.M., Lopez-Sobaler A.M., Andres P., et al.(2002) Cognitive Function in Elderly People is influenced by vitamin E status. *J. Nutr.* 132,2065-2068

Perkins A.J., Hendrie H.C., Callahan C.M., et al (1999) Association of antioxidants with memory in a multiethnic elderly sample using the Third National Health and Nutrition Examination Survey. *Am. J. Epidemiol.* 150, 37-44

Perrig W.J., Perrig P., Stahelin H.B.(1997) The relation between antioxidants and memory performance in the old and very old. *J. Am. Geriatr Soc.* 45,718-724

Pirlich M.(2001) Nutrition in the elderly. *Best Practie &Res.Clin. Gastroenter.* 15(6), 869-884

Pluta R., Barcikowska M., Januszewski S et al. (1996) Evidence of blood brain barrier permeability/leakage from circulating human Alzheimer's beta-amyloid(1-42)-peptide. *Neuroreport* 7, 1261-1265

Russell R.M., Rasmussen H., Lichtenstein A.H (1999) Modified food guide pyramid for people over seventy years of age. *J. Nutr.* 129, 751-753

Saunier K., Dore J (2002) Gastrointestinal tract and the elderly: functional foods, gut microflora and healthy aging. *Digest. Liver dis.* 34, 19-24

Schmidt R., Hayn M., Reinhard B et al.(1998) Plasma antioxidants and cognitive performance in middle-aged and older adults: results of the Austrian Stroke Prevention Study. *J. Am. Geriatr. Soc.* 46, 1407-1410

Seshadri S., Beiser A., Selhub J., Jacques P.F et al. (2002) Plasma homocysteine as a risk factor for dementia and Alzheimer's disease. *N. Engl. J. Med.* 346 (7), 476-483.

Virtanen J.K., Voutilainen S., Alfthan G., Korhonen M.J., Rissanen T.H., et al. (2002) Homocysteine as a risk factor for CVD mortality in men with other CVD risk factors:
The Kuopio Ischaemic Heart Disease Risk factor (KIHD) *Study. J. Intern. Med.* 257(3), 255-262

Volkert D., Kreuel K., Heseker H., Stehle P. (2004) Energy and nutrient intake of young-old, old-old and very-old elderly in Germany. *Euro.. J. Clin. Nutr.* 58, 1190-1200

Wang H.X., Wahlin A., Basun H. et al. (2001) Vitamin B12 and foliate in relation to the development of Alzheimer 's disease. *Neurology* 56 (9), 1188-1194

World Health Organization (2003). Diet, nutrition and the prevention of chronic diseases. *Report of Joint WHO/FAO Expert Consultation* , no.916, Geneva.

World Health Organization (2010). Setting priorities for global mental health research.

Wyka J., Biernat J., Kiedik D. (2010). Nutritional determination of the health status in polish elderly people from an urban environment. *Journal of Nutrition, Health and Aging*, 14 (1), 67-71

Wyka J., Biernat J., Mikołajczak J., Piotrowska E. (2011). Assessment of dietary intake and nutritional status (MNA) in Polish free-living elderly people from rural environments. *Arch. Gerontol. Geriatr.* (accepted to print)

Yehuda S., Rabinovitz S., Carasso R.L., Mostofsky D.I. (2002). The role of polyunsaturated fatty acids in restoring the aging neuronal membrane. *Nerurobiol. Aging*. 23,843-853

Zandi P.P., Anthony J.C., Khachaturian A.S., Stone S.V. et al (2004) Reduced risk of Alzheimer disease in users of antioxidant vitamin supplements. *Arch. Neurol*. 61, 82-88

In: Social Determinants and Mental Health
Editor: Sabine Bährer-Kohler
ISBN: 978-1-61324-353-4

Chapter 15

Rural Communities and Mental Health

[1]Sarah M. Buila, Terry L. Shirley[2] and Elaine T. Jurkowski[3]
[1]Southern Illinois University College of Education and Human Services, School of Social Work, Carbondale, US
[2]Missouri State University, Community Counseling Center, Southeast Cape Girardeau, US
[3]Southern Illinois University College of Education and Human Services School of Social Work, Carbondale, US

Introduction

According to the United Nations (2008), 49.4 percent (3,411,951,000) of the world's population live in rural areas. These individuals present unique challenges and strengths for maintaining mental health. This chapter explores the nature of what it means to live in a rural community and how the rural context influences mental health across the lifespan. Social factors unique to rural dwellers include: resource deprivation, agrarian societies, employment and education disparities as compared to urban dwellers. From the vantage point of social determinants of health: economics, the physical and social environments, and lifestyle all play roles in the mental health of individuals living in rural communities. This chapter attempts to capture what is unique in the lifestyles and living conditions of rural dwellers compared to those living in urban and metropolitan areas and how these social determinants influence mental health. Special attention is given to the needs of the elderly and the incidence of suicide amongst rural inhabitants. Of all the disparities between rural and urban dwelling factors, the most disturbing is the higher rate of completed suicide. The intervention approach based on behavioral/mental health literacy is explored as well as the strengths that come from the rural environment. The consequences of untreated mental health conditions are of great concern to mental health service providers, researchers, and policy makers. Governments should consider incentives for increasing services and the location of mental health professionals in rural areas. Other implications for improving mental health outcomes in rural communities are discussed.

Defining Rural

The definition of rural or rural communities lacks consensus worldwide (Dolea, Stormant, Shaw, Zum, & Braichat, 2009). Most often "rural" is defined as "not urban." (USDA, 2008; Dax,1996). Most definitions consider population density, availability of economic resources and distance from an urban area (Dolea, et al, 2009). An early definition of rural, adopted by the European Conference on Rural Hygiene (1931) referred to rural as "an area or a district where agriculture is the chief or even the sole industry, and where all other industries are of small importance and, in the main, dependent on agriculture" (Quoted in Bridgman, 1955. p.12). While this definition may be accurate, in a developing context, primary focus on the agrarian may unintentionally limit the scope of what constitutes rural. For example, in most developing countries, farming is the industry that dominates the rural economy but this is no longer true in the United States (McGrahahan, 2003). Some explain this as a trend of farm consolidation and improved technology resulting in a wider gap between small farm earnings and commercial operation earnings. Small farms in the United States depend more on off farm incomes. Thus, rural economies in the United States depend more on machinery manufacturing, recreation, telemarketing, prisons, and health services (Ghelfi & McGranahan, 2004). In a recent study in Australia by Frager and colleagues (2010), attention is brought to the wide variation of occupations held by rural dwellers and the high proportion of retired persons. Hoyt and colleagues (Hoyt, Conger, Valde, & Weihs, 1997) challenge the point that persons living in contemporary rural areas are homogenous. For the purpose of this chapter rural is defined as non-urban, primarily but not solely, agriculturally based.

Living in a rural area can often mean living away from resources such as health and mental health facilities (Morton, 2003; Bodor, 2009). It can mean long distances and transportation problems limit access to care. Living in rural areas can also mean differences in employment and income, education quality and availability; differences which also impact poverty rates. These variables interact and compound one another. While some aspects of living in a rural setting may have health and mental health protective influence, others intersect to have detrimental effects on one's mental health. Variables impacting mental health are explored, including: social factors, behavior and lifestyle related variables followed by employment, economics, and education related variables.

Social Factors, Behavior, and Lifestyle

Rural dwellers encounter many barriers to seeking mental healthcare; for example less anonymity, misconceptions about mental illness, and higher stigma associated with mental illness. Hoyt and colleagues (1997) conducted interviews with rural dwellers from a range of rural environments with populations under 2,500 to those over 50,000. Farm and non-farm households were included in the sample of 1,735. They found that persons in rural places expressed higher levels of stigma. Persons with higher levels of depressive symptoms were more likely to hold a stigmatized view of services. Older respondents and women who had used mental health services had lower levels of stigma. Social support was associated with a greater likelihood of seeking mental health services. Stigma toward mental health service use was significantly associated with the willingness to seek such services (Hoyt et al, 1997). Ramirez-Ferrero (2005) has also identified multiple barriers to help-seeking for mental health issues. He conducted an ethnographic study of farming communities in the mid-western United States. Like Hoyt et al, Ramierz-Ferrero (2005) found widespread stigma associated with mental illness. This stigma, he suggests, may be related to lack of information. For example, many subjects associate mental illness with the most severe and disabling conditions such as schizophrenia and are not aware of services for persons experiencing depression, anxiety, or stress. An exploratory study by Fuller, Edwards, Proctor, and Moss (2000) which utilized key informants helps to articulate the issue of defining mental illness versus mental distress. Informants spoke of mental health problems as circumstantial problems in everyday living rather than disease or illness. Other barriers include the fear of losing one's freedom, lack of health insurance, and the characterization of social service professionals as outsiders (Ramirez-Ferrero, 2005).

What Ramirez-Ferrero (2005) identifies as barriers to help-seeking, especially for male farmers, can be described as self-stigma as well as public stigma. Based on his study, a need for services of any kind is considered an expression of weakness and dependency. The choice to seek help is culturally conditioned and conceptions of masculinity are at the core. The farmer withdraws and as a consequence has little social support when he needs it the most. Ramirez-Ferrero (2005) points out that farmers' use of health services was tied to the agricultural seasons and that the definition of health or illness was not necessarily based upon symptoms but rather functioning. Other studies have identified this emphasis on role performance, the ability to work productively, as the indicator of what constitutes health to rural dwellers (Weinert & Long, 1987; Elliot-Schmidt & Strong, 1997). Hoyt et al (1997) point out that "agrarian values," specifically "self-reliance and rugged individualism are not conducive to seeking formal care" (p. 452).

In an Australian sample, purposely selected from small rural towns and adjacent farming environs, Judd, Jackson, Komiti, Murry, Fraser, Grieve, and Gomez (2006), looked at the attitudes of stoicism, self-efficacy, perceived stigma and attitudes towards seeking professional psychological help. While this study did not find perceived stigma or attitudes towards seeking professional help for psychological problems to influence lifetime help-seeking, it did find higher levels of stoicism and self-efficacy associated with the lower likelihood of seeking help for mental health problems. The study by Fuller et al, (2000) echoed findings that stigma and a "culture of self-reliance" impact help-seeking behaviors of rural dwellers.

Some persons living in rural settings may belong to marginalized groups that face barriers to services despite the setting, only to have those barriers exaggerated by proximity issues and a scarcity of resources in the rural setting. For example, First Nations indigenous peoples in Canada (Bodor, 2009) and immigrants or migrating farm workers in the United States (Martinez-Brawley, 2009). Harvey (2009) suggests that even the unique needs of rural women go unnoticed and unaddressed because of how mental health is conceptualized and how these women are stereotyped as stoic and self-reliant.

EMPLOYMENT, ECONOMICS, AND EDUCATION

Employment, education, and economics are closely related. Employment and education cannot be separated from poverty, nor poverty from mental health. Those with less education suffer higher rates of poverty (Jensen, McLaughlin, & Slack, 2003). Those who are poor have less opportunity for education or skills development. It has been consistently replicated that there is a negative relationship between socioeconomic status and mental illness (Hudson, 2005) and poverty has been shown to be associated with higher rates of childhood psychiatric disorders (Mcleod & Shananhan, 1996; Department of Health, 1999; Costello, Keeler, & Argold, 2000).

The World Bank (2007) estimates that three-quarters of the developing world's poor live in rural areas when assessed by international poverty lines. In the United States, the poverty rate has been higher in rural counties every year from 1959-2009 (USDA, 2010). Economics and political power are entangled, perpetuating poverty for disadvantaged rural poor. Rural dwellers have less ability to compete with others in a global economy as unskilled workers. Rural dwellers in the United States have historically lagged behind in education attainment and the disparities become more pronounced when examined by race and ethnicity (Beaulieu, Israel, & Wimberley, 2003). Related to poverty, unemployment increases the rate of psychiatric disorders and substance abuse (Murali & Oyebode, 2004).

In the United States, the types of employment available have changed. Traditional rural industries, farming, mining, and timber have all declined since the 1920's and the major industrial shift has been from agriculture to support services (McGranahan, 2003). Note that the decline of these industries has been simultaneous with increases in poverty due to low paying jobs utilizing low-skilled workers. This shift has also affected the rural male work force. For example, increased jobs in the apparel industry, which more typically hires women equates to differences in who is employed and for what wage (McGranahan, 2003).

Efforts to combat poverty with "welfare to work" welfare reform in the United States impacted rural poor differently than their urban counterparts because of greater differences between the welfare recipient's skill or education level mismatched to the jobs available, as well as child care and transportation difficulties (Zimmerman & Hirschl, 2003). In less developed parts of the world, there is less attention to addressing the problems of poverty. Poverty impacts disadvantaged groups disproportionately worldwide. These groups include women, children, ethnic minorities, and indigenous people (International Fund for Agricultural Development, 2011). Social and political inequalities perpetuate the poverty cycle. For example, discrimination impedes employment, education, and financial services. Social expectations for women to marry young coupled with poverty interfere with education, which then impedes work opportunities. Children in poor households are needed to work in order to contribute to family household income. Tragically, there is a negative correlation between child labor and achievement of education (Allais & Hagemann, 2008). Without education, a child's opportunities for more gainful employment are compromised later in life. Child labor is a problem worldwide with the most children aged 5-14 working in Asia but the highest percentage in Africa. Of the total child labor force, 70.4 percent are working in agriculture (World Bank, 1999).

Related to education disparities is the practice of industries of taking advantage of unskilled (inexpensive) labor in rural areas (McGranahan & Ghelfie, 1998). These industries tend to provide the lowest pay, and require long hours under poor working conditions. These conditions in turn impact the mental health of individuals and families. Frager and her colleagues (2010) examined how employment and occupation make a difference in distress among rural residents of New South Whales, Australia. Among their sample of 2639 residents, they found the greatest distress remained with those permanently unable to work (57%) and those unemployed (69%). These groups of people suffer considerable stress because there are limited mental health care and health promotion resources within rural areas those there are may be linked to employment.

Rural Elderly

According to the U. S. Census, International Population Report, virtually every nation is experiencing growth in their number of older persons with developing countries increasing more rapidly (Kinsella & He, 2009). Individuals aged 65 and older comprise a higher percentage of the population in rural areas as compared to urban centers in the United States (Clifford et al., 1985; Glasgow, 1988; Glasgow, 2000). This is true also in many developing countries. In a study that looked at differences in the share of persons 65 and over versus total population, living in rural areas of 39 countries, 27countries had higher percentages of all elderly living in rural areas (Kinsella & Velkoff, 2001). This disproportionate concentration of older people in rural areas is related to the out-migration of younger people from some rural regions (Glasgow, 2000; Kinsella & He, 2009). Many older people living in rural areas often have no adult children living nearby. This lack of face-to-face contact with their children, who in many cases are the primary candidates as family caregivers, affects the overall intergenerational relationships of families in many rural areas.

The small population size and low population densities characteristic of rural areas limit the development of social relationships. Rural dispersion and distance limit opportunities for social interaction (Hofferth & Iceland, 1998). Social and economic well-being suggests relatively greater need for care-giving among rural older people. Because of this, older persons who live alone in rural areas are at greater risk of not having their care-giving needs met.

Compared to older adults living in urban areas, those living in the rural setting are at increased risk for social factors such as widowhood, lower income, and lower educational levels. (Coward, Netzer & Peek, 1996). Historically, per capita incomes have been lower and poverty rates have been higher among rural older adults (Glasgow & Brown, 1998). These factors have important implications for social support systems, economic and overall well-being. It is estimated that 80% of rural in home-care of older persons is provided by informal support systems (Stoller, 1996). This informal support consists mostly of family members, but may also include, church networks, friends, and neighbors (Kivett, Stevenson, & Zwane, 2000). Some authors speculate as to whether rural elders' under use of formal services is a matter of inaccessibility of services or rather it is a matter of rural values (Kivett, Stevenson, & Zwane, 2000). For example, do strong informal networks or a lack of formal services in rural areas contribute to the high level of informal support use? (Stoller, 1996). Either way, there may be undesired consequences for older adults in rural communities. They may go without care or face placement in a long term care facility. "Deficiencies in community-based home care in rural areas possibly have lead to the premature institutionalization of the very old" (Kivett, Stevenson & Zwane, 2000, p. 60). This is an issue in industrialized countries due to the lack of available workforce and social support to provide care for elders (Jurkowski, 2008).

Rural Suicide

Of all the disparities between rural and urban dwelling factors, the most disturbing is the higher rate of completed suicide. This tragedy exists despite national context. For example, in Australia rural suicide rates were 2.7 times higher than urban rates (Sankaranarayanan, Carter, & Lewin, 2010) and suicide rates in Australian rural communities has steadily increased from 1985-2005 (Judd, Cooper, Fraser, & Davis, 2006). Suicide rates are ½ to 3 times greater in rural areas of the United States (Yenerall, 2009). Gallager and Sheehy (1994) note higher rates of suicide and greater increases in suicide rates for rural dwellers as opposed to urban in the United Kingdom, Sweden, and Denmark. Epidemiology reports show higher rates of suicide in rural areas than urban areas for China, India, the Republic of Korea and Sri Lanka (Hendin et al, 2008). Kurosu (1991) found higher rates of suicide in sparsely populated areas of Japan.

The phenomenon of suicide in rural areas can be understood by considering contributing factors. As noted above, persons living in rural environments have less access to mental health services coupled with higher stigma associated with mental health conditions. While most suicides are the result of multiple factors, untreated depression is of primary concern. About 90 percent of persons who have completed suicide had some kind of psychiatric disorder (Cavanagh, Carson, Sharpe, & Lawrie, 2003). In addition to mental illness, poverty, unemployment, older age, alcohol misuse, availability of means for suicide, and social isolation all contribute to higher risk for suicide (Hawton & van Heeringen, 2009).

Availability of means is different for different localities. In developing countries, chemical pesticides are more commonly used for self-harm where as in developed countries, self-poisoning involves medications. Depending on firearm availability for some countries, the most lethal method used is a gun. Relevant to rural farmers, chemical pesticides, including insecticides, fungicides and soil fumigants, have been associated with symptoms of clinical depression (Stallones & Beseler, 2002). For one class of insecticides, organophosphates, either regular cumulative exposure or a poisoning incident was significantly associated with diagnosed depression (Beseler, et al, 2008). Fatal pesticide poisoning is estimated to account for one third of completed suicides worldwide (Gunnell, Eddleston, Phillips, & Konradsen, 2007). This is a particular problem in rural agricultural areas where access to pesticides is poorly controlled, most significantly those areas within developing countries (London, Flisher, Wesseling, Mergler & Kromhout, 2005; Gunnell & Eddleston, 2003; Dinham & Malik, 2003). London and colleagues (2005) make a compelling argument based on extensive literature review, that organophosphates (pesticides) not only pose a risk as an agent of suicide but act "in a biological/toxicological sense as a cause of suicide" because of the association with depression (p.315).

Access to means might lead a person from suicidal thoughts to suicidal acts (Hawton & Heeringen, 2009). The lethality of the means results in more completed suicides as opposed to failed attempts. Firearms present one of the most lethal means and suicide using a firearm is more frequent in countries where household ownership is more common (Ajdacic-Gross, et al, 2006). More people own guns in the United States then any other country (United Nations, 2010). Not surprisingly, in United States the most common method of suicide is the use of a firearm (Brent & Bridge, 2003) and it is rural households in the United States that are more likely to own a gun (Connor, 2005; Lott, 2010). Comparatively, the most common methods of suicide in European countries are by hanging and poisoning (Brock & Griffith, 2003; Varnik, 2009).

MENTAL HEALTH LITERACY

Understanding how the lack of knowledge and awareness about mental health is related to myths about self-reliance is crucial as this impacts receptivity to interventions. The behavioral health literacy approach, also called "mental health literacy" is defined by Jorm and colleagues as "knowledge and beliefs about mental disorders which aid their recognition, management or prevention" (Jorm et al, 1997, p.182). Stansbury et al (2010) utilized this conceptual framework of mental health literacy in their exploratory study. The participants, who identified as African American pastors in predominantly rural churches, answered interview questions based on vignette related to geriatric African American Alzheimer's disease and mental health literacy (Stansbury et al. 2010). According to vignette results, all nine clergy members stated that they would refer congregants with Alzheimer's Disease (AD) to resources such as "visitation," "support groups," and "respite care" as a valuable church involvement, while the other five preferred to refer congregants with AD to their church's "internal health care ministry" or "nursing ministry" (Stansbury et al. 2010). This study provides a rural location and demographic specific effort towards understanding mental health literacy needs.

Kermode and colleagues (2009) conducted another such study. According to this study, "Attitudes to people with mental disorders: a mental health literacy survey in a rural area of Maharashtra, India," the role health literacy plays in limiting the stigma associated with mental disorders is complex and varies culture to culture. Kermode et al utilized a vignette-based questionnaire in order to determine community views about those with mental disorders, particularly depression and psychosis. The researchers hoped to use the findings to develop a mental health-training program for village health workers (VHWs). The study involved 129 female and 111 male randomly selected community members and 60 female VHWs. There were no male VHWs available for the study. The sample was chosen purposefully from 10 communities within rural Maharashtra (Kermode et al, 2009). They found that despite being accepting, the community still harbored negative and incorrect beliefs about persons with mental disorders. The majority of the test subjects felt that mental health issues such as those in the vignettes were not "real medical illness." Kermode et al (2009) concluded that providing mental health training that is contextually and culturally relevant to village health workers would be more effective than "promoting bio-medical explanations for mental disorders" (p.1087). This approach would enable the VHWs to communicate and model positive attitudes towards persons with mental disorders.

Behavioral/Mental health literacy includes education about suicide prevention, understanding risks, warning signs and options to intervene. A primary and effective effort towards the prevention of suicide is to limit access to the means (Daigle, 2005; Mann et al, 2005). Persons who act on impulse, even those less suicidal would not complete suicide without the means. There is some support for the assumption that periods of high suicide risk are short (Florentine & Crane, 2010). Not having immediate access to lethal means may delay an attempt and can provide a window of time where intervention can occur. The implications indicated here are for policy makers and practitioners. Gunnell & Eddleston (2003) have listed strategies for addressing the issue of pesticide poisoning. These include: reduce the availability of toxic pesticides by restricting use to less dangerous chemicals and prohibiting sales of those lethal to humans, licensing users and requiring locked storage, reduce use in agricultural practice, appoint village elder, teacher or police to hold storage, public education, require label warnings and providing access to immediate remedies such as antidotes or charcoal.

The Strengths of a Rural Community

There are strengths related to living in a rural environment. Gorman et al (2007) conducted an exploratory study in order to identify stressors associated with living in a rural environment and to identify factors that enhance resilience to mental illness. The subjects, all men from Queensland, had identified themselves as having been through a period of extreme emotional difficulty, depression, and suicidal thoughts for some. Although the sample was small (n=10), this particular population is difficult to recruit, hence this study gives a rare glimpse of potential risk and protective factors which can be used for further research. The study identified positive thinking, self-awareness, self-control, the meaning of life and appreciation of life and hope as factors related to the individual and their inner strength that helped with coping with adversity (Gorman et al, 2007). In addition, the study identified support and strategies which helped the men cope. These were: seeking help and treatment, talking to others, making life changes, support from friends and family, being needed and taking a break from everyday drudgery (Gorman et al, 2007).

Wainer identified "determinants of positive mental health in rural contexts" by talking with rural doctors (referenced in Wainer and Chesters, 2000). Here too, are clues to the resilience of rural dwellers and insights for further study. The indicators that rural individuals and communities "do well" are: sense of belonging, closer community ties, possibility of self-determination, connection with the earth and the seasons, and an ability to deal confidently with conflicts that arise between individuals and society (Wainer, and Chesters, 2000). While practitioners explore strengths unique to rural dwellers, it should be evident there exists great diversity within the rural landscape. As Philo, Parr and Burns remind us "to take seriously… the sheer variability in the rural…" (2003, p.278). To reiterate, Hoyt and colleagues (1997), this is not a homogenous group. Practitioners and researchers alike need to investigate the "local circumstances" and adapt accordingly (Pugh, 2009).

IMPLICATIONS

Implications for improving mental health outcomes for rural communities include those for practitioners, for policy makers, and for researchers. Practitioners' most immediate task in is to address the lack of knowledge about mental health in rural areas through public education which targets stigma. The media such as the local newspaper and radio or television stations can be useful venues for public education interventions. Practitioners can also use a behavioral health literacy approach, which can be targeted towards individuals and communities. Policy makers need to recognize the practice differences and disparities in resources of rural communities. Tertiary care centers with educational and prevention resources can be critical to supplement the lack of mental health care providers. Mobile services may also be a feasible option for serving rural communities. Finally, researchers can contribute to the practice evidence for intervention in rural communities.

Policies that address poverty, education, and overall health and well-being are implicated in order to improve the mental health of persons living in rural areas. Governments should consider incentives for increasing services and the location of mental health professionals in rural areas. Then attention must be given to the impact of services provided as the response of rural populations may differ from those from urban settings. Finally, policy makers should consider policies that limit access to the most lethal means for suicide.

To better inform practitioners and policy makers there are areas indicated for further research. Researchers can contribute to the paucity of resources for intervention and lack of evidence generated from rural communities in a number of ways. Comparative research between urban and rural settings could help to build a scientific basis for our practice knowledge base. Comparative research could also showcase the unique features and outcomes that rural settings create in terms of mental health outcomes. This includes the investigation of behavioral/mental health literacy as exemplified by Stansbury et al, and Kermonde et al. above. Education needs must give specific attention to region and culturally relevant information in order to better inform behavioral/mental health literacy efforts. There needs to be continued surveillance in rural areas for mental health conditions and suicide attempts, the changing age, race, gender and cultural demographics, and the location of mental health providers to better inform decisions about resource allocation. Key to understanding the mental health needs of rural dwellers is understanding how they define mental health, their beliefs about mental disorders, the strengths inherent in their environment, and the mental health resource context specific to various regions.

REFERENCES

Ajdacic-Gross, V., Hepp, U., Gadola, E., Bopp, M., Lauber, C., Schnyder, U., et al. (2006). Changing Times: A longitudinal analysis of international firearm suicide data. *American Journal of Public Health, 96*(10), 1-4.

Allais, F. B. & Hagemann, F. (2008). Child labour and education: Evidence from SIMPOC surveys. Working Paper, International Programme on the Elimination of Child Labour (IPEC). Geneva: International Labour Office.

Beaulieu, L.J., Israel, G.D. & Wimberley, R.C. (2003). Promoting educational achievement: A partnership of families, schools and communities. In Brown, D. L., & Swanson, L. E. (Eds.), *Challenges for rural America in the twenty-first century*. (pp. 273-289). University Park, Pennsylvania: The Pennsylvania University Press.

Beleler, C L., Stallones, L., Hoppin, J. A., Alavanja, M. C., Blair, A., Keefe, T., & Kamel, K. (2008). Depression and pesticide exposures among private pesticide applicators enrolled in the agricultural health study. *Environmental Health Perspectives, 116*(12), 1713-1719.

Bodor, R. (2009). The future of social work and mental health in rural Northern Canada. *Rural Society, 19*(4), 289-292.

Brent, D. A. & Bridge, J. (2003). Firearms availability and suicide: Evidence, interventions, and future directions. *American Behavioral Scientist, 46*(9), 1192-1210.

Bridgeman, R. F. (1955). The rural hospital: Its structure and organization. Geneva: World Health OrganizationMonograph available from *http://who.libdoc.who.int/monograph/WHO_MONO_21 _ (part1).pdf. Retrieved 2* January, 2011.

Brock, A. & Griffith, C. (2003). Trends in suicide by method in England and Whales: 1971-2001. *Health Statistics Quarterly,* Winter 2003, 20, 7-18. Available from www.statistcs.gov.uk/products/p6725.asp

Cavanagh, J., T., O., Carson, A., J., Sharpe, M., & Lawrie, S. M. Psychological autopsy studies of suicide: A systematic review. *Psychological Medicine, 33*(3), 395-405.

Clifford, W. B., Heaton, T. B., Voss, P. R., & Fugitt, G. V. (1985). The rural elderly in demographic perspective. In R. T. Coward & G.R Lee (Eds.), The elderly in rural society: Every forth elder (pp. 25-55). New York: Springer.

Connor, S. (2005). The association between presence of children in the home and firearm-ownership and storage practices. *Pediatrics, 115*(1). 38-43.

Costello, E. J., Keeler, G. P., & Argold, A. (2000). Poverty, race/ethnicity, and psychiatric disorder: A study of rural children. *American Journal of Public Health, 91*(9), 1494-8.

Coward, R. T., Netzer, J. K. & Peek, C. W. (1996). Obstacles to creating high-quality long term care services to rural elders. In G. D. Rowles, J. C. Beaulieu, & W.W. Myers (Eds.), Long term care for the rural elderly (pp. 10-34). New York: Springer.

Daigle, M. (2005). Suicide prevention through means restriction: Assessing the risk of substation: A critical review and synthesis. *Accident Analysis and Prevention, 37*(4), 625-632.

Dax, T. (1996). Defining rural areas: International comparisons and the OECD indicators. *Rural Society, 6*(3), 3-18.

Dinham, B. & Malik, S. (2003). Pesticides and human rights. *International Journal of Occupational and Environmental Health, 9*(1). 40-52.

Department of Health, (1999). Saving lives: Our healthier nation. London: Stationary Office, available at http://www.archive.officialdocument.co.uk/document. Retrieved 2 January 2011.

Dolea, C., Stormant, L., Shaw, D., Zum, P. & Braichat, J. M. (2009). Increasing access to health workers in remote and rural areas through improved retention. Geneva: World Health Organization, available at *http://www.who.int/hrh/migration/backgroundpaper.pdf. Retrieved 2 January 2011).*

Elliot-Schmidt, R. & Strong, J. (1997). The concept of well-being in a rural setting: Understanding health and illness. *Australian Journal of Health and Illness, 5*(2), 59-63.

Florentine, J. B. & Crane, C. (2010). Suicide prevention by limiting access to methods: A review of theory and practice. *Social Science & Medicine, 70*(10), 1626-1632.

Fragar, L., Stain, H., Perkins, D., Kelly, B., Fuller, J., Coleman, C., Lewin, T. J., & Wilson, J. M. (2010). Distress among rural residents: Does employment and occupation make a difference? *Australian Journal of Rural Health, 18*(1), 25-31.

Fuller, J., Edwards, J., Proctor, N. & Moss, J. (2000). How definition of mental health problems can influence help seeking in rural and remote communities. *Australian Journal of Rural Health, 8*(3). 148-153.

Gallager, A. G. & Sheehy, N. (2006). Suicide in rural communities. *Journal of Community and Applied Social Psychology, 56*(4), 145-155.

Ghelfi, L. & McGanahan, D. (2004). One in five rural counties depend on farming. *Amber Waves*, 11. USDA Economic Research Services . Retrieved from *www.ers.usda.gov/publications/forces/rural.pdf.*February 1, 2011.

Glasgow, N. (1988). The nonmetro elderly: Economics and demographics status (RDRR-70). Washington, D. C.: United States Department of Agriculture.

Glasgow, N. (2000). Rural/Urban patterns of aging and caregiving in the United States. *Journal of Family Issues, 21*(5), 611-631.

Glasgow, N. & Brown, D. (1998). Older, rural and poor. In R. T. Coward and J. A. Krout (Eds.), *Aging in Rural Settings*, (pp. 187-207). New York: Springer Publishing Company.

Gorman, D., Buikstra, E., Hegney, D., Pearce, S., Rogers-Clark, C., Weir, J. & McCullagh, B. (2007). Rural men and mental health: Their experiences and how they managed. *International Journal of Mental Health Nursing, 16*(5), 298-306.

Gunnell, D. & Eddleston, M. (2003). Suicide by intentional ingestion of pesticides: A continuing tragedy In developing countries. *International Journal of Epidemiology, 32*(6), 902-909.

Gunnell, D., Eddleston, M., Phillips, M. R. Konradsen, F. (2007). The global distribution of fatal pesticide self-poisoning: Systematic review. *Brittish Medical Council Journal, http://www. Biomedcetnral.com/1471-2458/7/357, 7(357).*

Harvey, D. (2009). Conceptualising the mental health of rural women: A social work and health promotion perspective. *Rural Society, 19*(4), 353-362.

Hawton, K., & Heeringen, K. van (2009). Suicide. *Lancet, 373*(9672) 1372-1381.

Hendin, H., Vijayuakumar, L, Bertolate, J., Wang, Phillips, M. & Pirhis, J. (2008). Epidemiology of Suicide in Asia. In Herdin, H., Phillips, M,. Vijayuakumar, L., Pirkis, J., Wang, H., Yip, P., Wasserman, K., Bertolate, J., & Fleischmann, A., (Eds.), *World Health Organization, Department of Mental Health and Substance Abuse* (pp.7-18). Geneva, Switzerland: WHO Documentation Services.

Hofferth, S. & Iceland, J. (1998). Social capital in rural and urban communities. *Rural Sociology, 63*(4), 574-575.

Hoyt, D. R., Conger, R. D., Valde, J., G. & Weihs, K. (1997). Psychological distress and help seeking in rural America. *American Journal of Community Psychology, 25*(4), 449-470.

Hudson, C. G. (2005). Socioeconomic status and mental illness: Tests of the social causation and selection hypotheses. *Journal of Orthopsychiatry, 75*(1), 3-18.

International Fund for Agricultural Development (2011). *Rural poverty report 2011.* Available from http://www. Ifad.org/rpr2011/index.html. Retrieved 11 January 2011.

Jensen, L., McLaughlin, D. K. & Slack, T. (2003). Rural poverty: The persisting challenge. In Brown, D. & L., Swanson, L. E. (Eds.), *Challenges for rural America in the twenty-first century.* (pp. 118-131).University Park, Pennsylvania: The Pennsylvania University Press.

Jorm, A. F., Korten, A., E., Jacomb, P. A. Christensen, B. R., Rodgers, B. & Pollitt, P. (1997). "Mental health literacy": a survey of the public's ability to recognize mental disorders and their beliefs about effectiveness of treatment. *Medical Journal of Australia, 166*(4), 182-186.

Judd, F. Cooper, A. M., Fraser, C. & Davis, J. (2006). Rural suicide-people or place effect? *Australian and New Zealand Journal of Psychiatry, 40*(3), 208-216.

Judd, F., Jackson, H., Komiti, A., Murray, G., Fraser, C., Grieve, A. & Gomez, R. (2006). Help-seeking by rural residents for mental health problems: the importance of agrarian values. *Australian and New Zealand Journal of Psychiatry, 40*(9), 769-776.

Jurkowski, E. (2008). *Policy and program planning for older adults: Realities and visions.* New York, New York: Springer Publications.

Kermode, M., Bowen, K., Arole, S., Pathare, S., & Jorm, A. F. (2009). Attitudes to people with mental disorders: A mental health literacy survey in rural area of Maharashtra, India. *Social Psychiatry and Psychiatric Epidemiology, 44*(12) 1087-96.

Kinsella, K. & He, W. (2009). U. S. *Census Bureau, International Populations Reports,* P95/09-1 An aging world: 2008. Washington, D. C.: U. S. Government Printing Office.

Kinsella, K., & Velkoff, V. A. (2001). U. S. Census Bureau, P95/01-1 An aging world: 2001. Washington, D. C.: U. S. Government Printing Office.

Kivett, V. R., Stevenson, M. L. & Zwane, C. H. (2000). Very-old rural adults: Functional status and social support. *The Journal of Applied Gerontology, 19*(1). 58-77.

Kurosu, S. (1991). Suicide in rural areas: The case of Japan 1960-1980. *Rural Sociology, 56*(4), 603-618.

London, L., Flisher, A. J., Wesseling, C., Mergler, D. & Kromhout, H. (2005). Suicide and exposure to Organophosphate insecticides: Cause or effect? *American Journal of Industrial Medicine, 47*(4), 308-312.

Lott, J. R. (2010). *More guns, less crime: Understanding crime and gun-control laws.* Third Edition. Chicago: University of Chicago Press.

Mann, J.J., Apter, A., Bertolote, J. Beautrais, A., Currier, D., Haas, A. et al. (2005). Suicide prevention strategies: A systematic review. *Journal of the American Medical Association, 294*(16). 2064-2074.

Martinez-Brawley, E. (2009). 'The world is flat': is U. S. rural social work flattening too? *Rural Society, 19*(4), 286-288.

McGranahan, D. A. (2003). How people make a living in rural America. In Brown, D. L., & Swanson, L. E. (eds.), *Challenges for rural America in the twenty-first century.*(pp.135-151). University Park, Pennsylvania: The Pennsylvania University Press.

McGranahan, D. A. & Ghelfie, L. M. (1998). Current trends in the supply and demand for education in rural and urban areas. In Gibbs, R. M., Swaim, P. L. & Teixeria, R., (Eds.), *Rural education and training in the new economy: The myth of the rural skills gap,* (pp. 131-171).Ames, Iowa: Iowa State University Press.

McLoed, J. D. & Shananhan, M. J. (1996). Trajectories of poverty and children's mental health. *Journal of Health and Social Behavior, 37*(3), 207-220.

Morton, L. W. (2003). Rural health policy. In Brown, D. L., & Swanson, L. E. (eds.), *Challenges for rural America in the twenty-first century* (pp. 290- 302). University Park, Pennsylvania: The Pennsylvania University Press.

Murali, V. & Oyebode, F. (2004). Poverty, social inequality and mental health. *Advances in Psychiatric Treatment, 10*(3), 216-224.

Philo, C., Parr, H., & Burns, N. (2003). Rural madness: A geographical reading and critique of the rural mental health literature. *Journal of Rural Studies, 19*(3), 259-281.

Pugh, R. (2009). Social work and rural mental health in the UK. *Rural Society, 19*(4), 283-285.

Ramirez-Ferrero, E.(2005). *Troubled fields: Men, emotions, and the crisis in American farming*. New York: Columbia University Press.

Sankaranarayanan, A., Carter, G., & Lewin, T. (2010). Rural-Urban differences in suicide rates for current patients of a public health services in Australia. *Suicide and Life Threatening Behavior, 40*(4), 376-382.

Stallones, L. & Beseler, C. L. (2002). Pesticide poisoning and depressive symptoms among farm residents. *Annuals of Epidemiology, 12*(6), 389-394.

Stansbury, K. L., Harley, D. A., & Brown-Hughes, T. (2010). African-American urban clergy's literacy of Alzheimer's disease. *Social Work in Mental Health, 8*(3), 254-266.

Stoller, E. P. (1996). The role of the family in rural long-term care. In G. D. Rowles, J. C. Beaulieu, &W.W. Myers (Eds.). Long term care for the rural elderly (pp. 35-63). New York: Springer.

United Nations. (2008). World *urbanization prospects: The 2007 revision population database*. Available from http://esa.un.org/unup/. Retrieved November 10, 2010

United Nations (2010). *United Nations Office on Drugs and Crime. Firearms*. Available from www.unodc.org/documents/data-and-analysis/tocta/6.Firearms.pdf Retrieved January 12, 2011.

United States Department of Agriculture, National Agricultural Library (2010). *Rural income, poverty, and welfare: Poverty geography.* Retrieved November 14, 2010 from http://www.nal.usda.gov/ric/ficpubs/what_is_rural.shtml

United States Department of Agriculture, National Agricultural Library (2008). *What is rural?* Retrieved November 14, 2010 from *http://www.nal.usda.gov/ric/ficpubs/what_is_rural.shtml*

Varnik, A., Kolves, K., Allik, J., Arensman, E., Aromaa, E., van Audenhove, C., et al. (2009). Gender issues in suicide rates, trends and methods among youths aged 15-24 in 15 European countries. *Journal of Affective Disorders, 113*(3), 216-226.

Wainer, J. & Chesters, J. (2000). Rural mental health: Neither romanticism nor despair. *Australian Journal of Rural Health, 8*(3), 141-147.

Weinert, C. & Long, K. A. (1987). Understanding the health care needs of rural families. *Family Relations, 36*(4), 450-455.

World Bank (2007). *New evidence on the urbanization of global poverty*, by M. Ravaillion, S. Chen & P.Sangraula. Policy research working paper 4199, April. Washington, DC: Retrieved December 14, 2010 from http://www.wds.worldbank.org/external/default/WDSContentServer/WDSP/IB/2007/08/27/000158349_20070827111606/Rendered/PDF/wps41990lupdate1.pdf

World Bank (1999). Facts and figures on child labour. International Labour Office. Retrieved from info.worldbank.org/etools/docs/library/237384/toolkitfr/pdf/facts.pdf

Yenerall, J. D. , 2004-08-14 "Surge in Suicide Rates in Rural Areas: A Sociological Analysis" *Paper presented at the annual meeting of the American Sociological Association, Hilton San Francisco & Renaissance Parc 55 Hotel, San Francisco, CA,*

Online <.PDF>. 2009-05-26. Retrieved November 15, 2010. from http://www.allacademic.com/meta/p109584_index.html

Zimmerman, J. N. & Hirschl, T. A. (2003). Welfare reform in rural areas: A voyage through uncharted waters. In Brown, D. L., & Swanson, L. E. (Eds.), *Challenges for rural America in the twenty-first century* (pp. 363-374). University Park, Pennsylvania: The Pennsylvania University Press.

In: Social Determinants and Mental Health
Editor: Sabine Bährer-Kohler

ISBN: 978-1-61324-353-4

Chapter 16

LIFESPAN PERSPECTIVE – CHILD MENTAL HEALTH*: SOCIOECONOMIC INEQUALITIES AND FAMILY RESOURCES

***Simone Gonçalves de Assis*[1], *Raquel de Vasconcellos Carvalhaes de Oliveira*[2], *Joviana Quintes Avanci*[1] and *Renata Pires Pesce*[1]**

[1]Latin American Centre for Studies on Violence and Health (CLAVES), Oswaldo Cruz Foundation, Brazil

[2] Laboratory of Clinical Epidemiology Research Institute Evandro Chagas/ Oswaldo Cruz Foundation FIOCRUZ/ Health Ministry, Rio de Janeiro, Brazil

ABSTRACT

The objective of this chapter is to analyze in which way socioeconomic inequalities and family resources affect children's mental health. The research investigates children's development in São Gonçalo (Rio de Janeiro/Brazil) and their families over three years (2005, 2006 and 2008), in a period of solid and paced social and economic development. Those responsible for the children responded to a multidimensional questionnaire. Valid information was gathered on 278 children in the three years of follow-up on: social demographic variables, family resources and total behavior problems. Exploratory analysis and *logistic mixture model* were performed and the results indicate that there is a reduction of members within the nuclear family, improvement in the family income, and reduction of total behavior problems. The resulting model indicates that the absence of maternal employment increases 61.7 times the likelihood of children behavioral problems; it also acts by reducing the probability of behavior problems in children of jobless mothers. Social and economic investments in the first years of life are essential, but these actions must still be provided throughout the course of development, involving the intimate realm of the family towards the broader socioeconomic context shaped by the governments, international agencies and civil society. The maintenance of continuous public policies of redistribution of income and more access to mental health services for

* The research had the support of the National Council of Scientific and Technological Development (CNPq) and the Carlos Chagas Filho Research Support Foundation of the State of Rio de Janeiro (Faperj), Brazil.

children are key considerations that enable children to have guaranteed rights to live in healthy families and cohesive communities.

INTRODUCTION

Social, political, economic and cultural conditions are factors that affect the ways in which people are born, grow, live, work and age, including the health system. These impact the health condition, the people's expectation and quality of life and are mostly responsible for health inequities [WHO, 2007]. Income and social status, social networking, educational level, insertion in the workplace, health practices, childhood development, gender and culture are examples of social determinants of health [PHAC, 2009].

Children are especially dependent on socioeconomic inequalities, since: they are in their physical, emotional and cognitive development; they live in a period of high vulnerability, with total dependency on the environment that is offered; suffer the consequences of poverty that may impact until adulthood [Siegrist & Marmot, 2006]. The initial period of life is particularly sensitive, depending on the brain and biological development to directly relate to the quality of received stimulation, of support and nurture of the social environment in which the child lives, learns and grows [Richter, 2004].

Socioeconomic gradient is related to the occurrence of problems in the childhood development and disorders in their physical and mental health, such as obesity, depression, anxiety and participation in crime [WHO, 2005; WHO, 2007; Sloat & Willms, 2002]. Living in poverty during childhood affects adulthood by mechanisms of latency, cumulative effects and pathways, for example, early life social origins influence readiness for school, and then, cognitive, emotional, and behavioral readiness for school subsequently affect school success and social adjustment [Kohen, Hertzman & Brooks-Gunn, 1998].

To the situation of poverty is added family difficulties (death, divorce, diseases, violence), communities (precarious sanitation, transport and social support network) and environmental issues (natural disasters), affecting even more the childhood mental health. The accumulation of traumatic events contributes in increasing the vulnerability of the childhood psychopathology [Garmezy, 1993; Rutter, 1996].

Pathways: From Poverty to Children´S Behavior Problems

Mental health problems affect between 10-20% of children worldwide, placing it among the five leading causes of illness in children over five years of age [Bird, 1996; Murray & Lopez, 1996]. Among these, the most important are the behavior problems, characterized by emotional and behavioral difficulties, whose prevalence varies among countries and methodology. National research with Canadian children reports a prevalence of 19.1%; in Brazil, the rates range between 12.7% and 35.2%, with attention, hyperactivity and emotional disorders being the most frequent behavior problems [Assis, Avanci & Oliveira, 2009; Cury & Golfeto, 2003; Fleitlich-Bilyk & Goodman, 2004].

The childhood cognitive and emotional development is influenced by environmental levels closely inter-related and non-hierarchical: family, neighborhood and the broader societal level [WHO, 2005]. The family is an important micro system in which the child interacts and learns a pattern of roles, of activities and of relationships that are associated with certain behaviors and social expectations, inserted in larger systems that influence each other, such as work, social support network and community [Bronfenbrenner, 1996].

The gradient effect of family resources are the most powerful explanation for differences in children's well-being within societies, and these resources profoundly affect all other aspects of the family environment [Siddiqi, Kawachi, Berkman, Subramanian, & Hertzman, 2007]. Family functioning, parenting styles, parents' commitment to parenting and social support are fundamental for working in the most immediate level of the child's interaction, encouraging and managing their contact with the external environment [Sloat & Willms, 2002; Richter, 2004].

Parents living in poverty are vulnerable to mental health problems, due to demands and daily frustration [Patel, DeSouza & Rodrigues, 2003]; in this context, important parent-child interactions may be impaired, resulting in fewer opportunities for learning experiences [Willms, 2003]. Siegrist and Marmot [2006] explain that maternal mental health problems resulting from poverty are situational; becoming serious when causing limitations by favoring the permanence of poverty and when becoming a way of life that extends to future generations.

Poverty in a Brazilian City

Despite the crisis that hit the worldwide economy in recent years, social and economic conditions in Brazil have evolved gradually, with successive decrease in income inequality between 2001 and 2010. The proportion of people living in poverty decreased from 35.3% in 1993 to 18.1% in 2007, equivalent to approximately 34 million people with income below US$80 month [Neri, 2010].

The economic growth of the last decade has enabled a significant number of Brazilians living in poverty to achieve a greater access to goods and public services, depending on the increase of job opportunities and education policies, health and income transfers, which stimulated the development of social protection network. Concomitantly, the growth of the availability of credit increased the proportion of people with bank accounts, in addition to the elevated commitment of the Brazilian State in increasing access to basic services such as sewage, garbage, water and electricity [Torres, Bichir & Carpin, 2006].

Profound changes have also taken place in the age composition and the pattern of illness and death of the Brazilian population. In less than 50 years, Brazil went from a mortality profile typical of a young population to a pattern of complex and costly typical of older ages. Also, coexisting infectious and parasitic diseases, non contagious diseases and specially accidents and violence have been on the rise since the 1980s.

This changing context directly affects the profile of the Brazilian families. By the end of the 2000 decade, there are more women in the labor market, fewer people per household (3.3 persons), specially through the reduction of fertility in the country, currently averaging 1.9 children per woman. Another aspect to be considered is that the number of families characterized as "single mother with children" is nearly a third of the total. Thus, poor mothers who do not work, often have no income; if they work, they cannot take care of their children. They also live with low monthly income [IBGE, 2010].

Despite the changes affecting the Brazilian society, living conditions and family health still depend on the socioeconomic status they belong to, the region of the country, city and neighborhood in which they live, the degree of social inclusion and the opportunity to enjoy the possibility of access to public services [Cohen, Janicki-Deverts, Chen & Matthews, 2010].

The city of São Gonçalo, studied in this chapter, is situated in the metropolitan region of the State of Rio de Janeiro. It has an approximate population of one million and a high concentration of low-income families, limited availability of water supply and sanitation, low coverage of public services, relevant pattern of urban violence and social exclusion [IBGE, 2010].

This chapter has outlined childhood development of children of São Gonçalo and their families over three years, trying to understand how socioeconomic inequalities and family resources affect children's mental health.

METHOD

This chapter presents data from a longitudinal study (2005, 2006 and 2008) following schoolchildren of public elementary schools in São Gonçalo (Rio de Janeiro/Brazil). Five hundred children were initially selected to participate in the study through multi-stage cluster sampling: schools, classes and students. Valid information was gathered on 278 children in the three years of follow-up for all the variables investigated in this chapter, corresponding to 834 observations. Over the years a total of 53 participants who left the study were of a similar profile to those that remained in groupings related to sex, age and family income.

Those responsible for the children (mostly mothers) responded to a multidimensional questionnaire.

Socioeconomic and demographic variables: a) sex; b) age; c) child's skin color (white or non-white); d) family structure (mother and father; mother and stepfather or father and stepmother; with only one parent; without father and mother); e) maternal employment (formal, informal, jobless); f) monthly household income per capita (in US$), composed by the ratio of the sum of all amounts received by family members, including welfare programs, divided by the number of the family members. Thereafter, the income was classified as up to US$ 2.00/day or more than US$2.00/day.

Family resources: a) maternal psychological distress [Self Reported Questionnaire; Harding, 1980]. Alpha of Cronbach=0.84; b) General Functioning Scale of the McMaster Family Assessment Device [Epstein, Baldwin & Bishop, 1983]. Low values of one standard deviation below average correspond to a precarious family functioning. Alpha of Cronbach=0.81; c) support from close friends/family with whom the caregiver is comfortable to talk; d) external support for the caregiver [church, community, health services, etc].

Total problems: used *Child Behavioral Checklist* which measures total behavioral problems (T score higher or equal to 60) of children, which includes internalizing, externalizing, thought, attention and social problems [Achenbach & Rescorla, 2001].

Statistical analysis was performed through the description of frequencies, median of age and monthly per capita income over time. The variables were gathered in different moments over time (Table 1).

Subsequently an exploratory analysis describes the effects of variables on behavior problems in the first year of the study and the logistic mixture model includes fixed and random effects and incorporates repeated measures in all years of follow-up. For this, random factors were considered, where the *intercept* and *slope* representing the time of data collection with different effects for children, depending on repeated measures being used within 3 years for each child. For the final model, successive analysis stages are presented to show the inclusion of socioeconomic and demographic variables (Model A); successive inclusion of variables that measures family resources in all significant variables of Model A, obtaining the final explicative model of the behavior problems (Model B). In all stages sex and age were included, in order to adjust the other effects.

The method of estimation of the model was the Laplace Method. The inclusion of variables was determined by the likelihood ratio test between nested models. Finally the fit of the model was verified by comparing the values of the *Akaike criterion* (AIC); lower values indicate better fitting models.

The magnitude of the effects of the variables on the occurrence of behavior problems was measured by the description of the OR; p-values<0.05 indicate significant values in statistical tests.

Ethical approval was obtained from Oswaldo Cruz Foundation Ethics Committee. Written informed consent was obtained from the caretaker, the school principal and the local education government.

RESULTS

Description of the Social and Family Context and Behavior Problems

Children's socioeconomic and demographic profile (Table 1) shows that there are more children in the 9 years old range, male and non-white. Regarding family structure, there is a reduction of members within the nuclear family and an increase of family members throughout new marriages of parents in three years of follow-up. It is also worth mentioning that in 2008, 23% of children lived with only one of their parents, almost exclusively with their mothers. The growth of the number of mothers in the work force is also evident, strengthening the economic and social inclusion of their families. It also confirms that one in three mothers remain jobless, with no contribution to the family income. The increase in the family income during the period studied can be seen by the larger number of families having two dollars per capita daily in order to survive.

Referring to the family resources (Table 1), we found that 13.7% of households showed a precarious family functioning, characterized by the distrust, lack of communication, misunderstandings, rejection of others and difficulty in making family decisions. The presence of psychological distress was observed in 36.3% of mothers with symptoms of anxiety, depression and somatic complaints. The lack of support from someone close to share feelings and difficulties were reported by about 21.9%-31.9% of the caretakers. Social isolation is much larger (though declining) in relation to the support of persons in service or institutions, reaching 55.4% of the caretakers in 2008.

In Table 1 it is observed that there is a further reduction of total behavioral problems of children throughout the years, reaching 14.4% of children in 2008.

Figure 1 shows the evolution of the monthly income provided by the families, with 50% in family income between 2005 and 2008, reaching US$ 103.55 per capita in 2008.

Table 1. Description of children and families characteristics over the years. São Gonçalo/Brazil

Variables	Categories	2005		2006		2008	
		N	%	N	%	N	%
SOCIOECONOMIC AND DEMOGRAPHIC PROFILE							
Sex of children[1]	Male	148	53.2%	-	-	-	-
	Female	130	46.8%	-	-	-	-
Child's skin color[1]	White	97	34.9%	-	-	-	-
	Non-white	181	65.1%	-	-	-	-
Family structure	Father and Mother	167	60.1%	161	57.9%	149	53.6%
	With step-parent	40	14.4%	51	18.3%	53	19.1%
	Only one of the parents	62	22.3%	58	20.9%	66	23.7%
	Without father or mother	9	3.2%	8	2.9%	10	3.6%
Type of work of the mother	Formal	65	23.4%	70	25.2%	95	34.2%
	Informal	71	25.5%	83	29.9%	82	29.5%
	Jobless	142	51.1%	125	45.0%	101	36.3%
Per capita family income	Less than US$2/day	122	43.9%	116	41.7%	56	20.1%
	More than US$2/day	156	56.1%	162	58.3%	222	79.9%
FAMILY RESOURCES							
General Family Functioning[1]	Poor	38	13.7%	-	-	-	-
	Regular/Good	240	86.3%	-	-	-	-
Maternal Psychological suffering[1]	No	-	-	177	63.7%	-	-
	Yes	-	-	101	36.3%	-	-
Support of close friends/family	Yes	217	78.1%	191	68.7%	213	76.6%
	No	61	21.9%	87	31.9%	65	23.4%
External Support	Yes	99	35.6%	119	42.8%	124	44.6%
	No	179	64.4%	159	57.2%	154	55.4%
BEHAVIOR PROBLEMS							
Total Problems	Normal	225	80.9%	228	82.0%	238	85.6%
	Borderline+ Clinical	53	19.1%	50	18.0%	40	14.4%

1Evaluated in one wave of the Longitudinal Study [fixed]

Note: age of the child in 2005 = median of 9 years [interquartile range = 8-10 years; variation of 6-14 years].

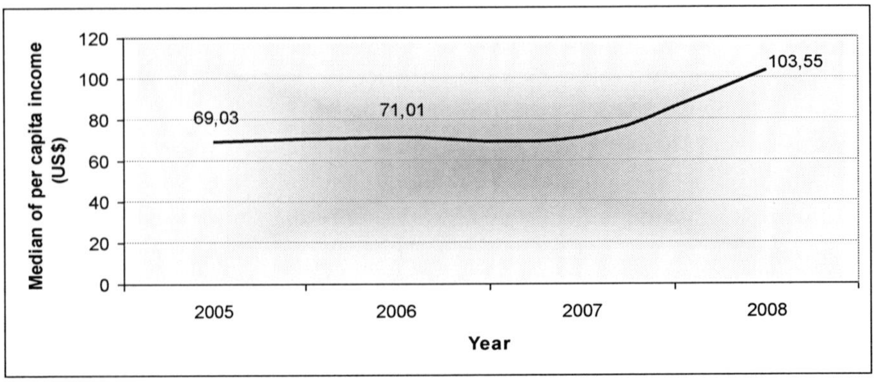

Figure 1. Monthly household income per capita [US$], 2005-2008.

Effects of Social and Family Context in the Emergence of Behavior Problems in Children

Table 2 shows the crude effects obtained by the exploratory analysis in 2005 and those adjusted by the logistic mixture regression models.

No variable in the socioeconomic and demographic context was associated to behavior problems in the exploratory analysis. Family resources are more associated with behavior problems: precarious family functioning, psychological distress of the caretaker and the lack of support from close friends/family.

Analyzing–Model A it appears that in the socioeconomic context, maternal work is the only explanatory variable of the outcome. In considering the family resources (Model B), emphasis is placed on the precarious family functioning, which increases 61.7 times the probability of the emergence of behavior problems. It also works by reducing the probability of the outcome between children born of jobless mothers, moving from 17.4 to 11.1.

Table 2. Socioeconomic and demographic profile, family resources and behavior problem

Variables	Categories	Exploratory		Model A		Model B	
		OR[1]	p-value	OR	p-value	OR	p-value
SOCIOECONOMIC AND DEMOGRAPHIC PROFILE							
Sex	Male	1.92	0.038	2.62	0.719	3.04	0.478
Skin Color	Non-White	1.45	0.263	1.48	0.895	-	-
Age	-	1.27	0.117	1.39	0.777	1.52	0.531
Family Structure	With step-parent	1.88	0.119	1.30	0.875	-	-
	With only one of the parents	1.19	0.647	1.48	0.815	-	-
	No father and mother	1.42	0.652	4.25	0.622	-	-
Type of work of mother	Informal	1.12	0.810	12.59	0.088	5.43	0.108
	Jobless	1.53	0.280	17.44	0.042	11.14	0.014
Monthly income per capita	Less than US$2	1.07	0.820	3.24	0.144	-	-
FAMILY RESOURCES							
Family Functioning	No	4.55	<0.001	-	-	61.65	0.014
Psychological Distress	Yes	3.11	<0.001	-	-	7.74	0.191
Family Support	No	2.71	0.002	-	-	-	-
External Support	No	0.89	0.720	-	-	-	-
Variance[2]	Intercept [individual]	-		125.01		46.84	
	Slope per year of follow-up	-		14.25		5.51	

[1]OR crude in the first observation of each child [OR simple].

[2]Variance of random effects in *log-odds* of behavioral problems.

Note: Coefficients that are statistically significant [p<0.05] appear in boldface.

Model B shows a better adjustment than Model A, assessed by: smaller variance of intercept; less random effect for each year of follow-up; the likelihood ratio test ($p<0.05$) and; lower AIC value (Model A=578.8 and Model B=565.9). These results indicate that the variables of family resources explain the improvement between socioeconomic/demographic variables and behavioral problems in children. The inclusion of psychological distress adjusts the regression model (likelihood ratio: $p<0.05$), although it shows no statistical significance (Model B).

CONCLUSION

Children studied in this chapter live in a context of social exclusion, presenting characteristics that facilitate the study of the impact of poverty on children's mental health. The findings relating indicators of low socioeconomic condition to behavioral problems in children have been reported in several countries, indicating the complexity and dynamics involved when children's development is followed over the years [Najman *et al.*, 2004; Huston, 1991; Anselmi *et al.*, 2008].

Maternal work stood out for being sensitive to show social and economic differences related to the emergence of behavioral problems in children studied. It is emphasized that the socioeconomic indicators measure differentiated and interconnected facets of social and economic integration, as an example of frequent association between family income and maternal work.

Within a period of three years, there had been significant changes in family structures as well as increased income and greater access to public policies for income generation and employment [Neri, 2010; Assis. Avanci & Oliveira, 2009]. In addition, poverty situation in the studied families remains more severe than that observed in the Brazilian population: 20.1% of households receive less than US$ 2 per capita per day, compared to the 12.7% observed in the Brazilian population [UNDP, 2009].

As established in this chapter, Racine and Boyle [2002] found out that precarious family functioning enables the emergence of behavioral problems in Canadian children, mediating the effect of poverty experienced by families. Lack of maternal employment and consequent lack of economic and material resources enables the emergence of emotional difficulties that affect the ability to deal with their children and favor the creation of an unsuitable environment. Moreover, the lack of employment can generate personal dissatisfaction and feeling of helplessness, causing problems in parents and children [Huston, 1991].

To understand the impact of social and economic context on children's health and on their living conditions is an important step for prevention and intervention. Investments in the first years of life, the critical phase for emotional, cognitive, and social development of human being is essential. Also, actions must be provided throughout the course of development, involving the intimate realm of the family towards the broader socioeconomic context shaped by governments, international agencies, and civil society [Siegrist & Marmot, 2006; WHO, 2007].

It is necessary to integrate sustainable programs and services directed to child development, focusing on mental health actions and protection policies to ameliorate the effects of growing up in poverty. Survey of the World Health Organization shows that the shortage of resources to promote childhood mental health in the world involves: human and economic aspects, weakness in customer service, lack of professional training programs and absence of specific mental health policies for this age group. In Brazil, as well as in many other countries there are no significant experiences in the inclusion of the childhood mental health services in the services [WHO, 2001; BMA, 2006].

Children´s protection policies are essential and include services directed to children, such as daycares, preschools, home and community-based child development centers. It can also act indirectly through the support provided for caretakers, which includes parenting programs, home support or home visiting, and other family support programs (WHO, 2005).

Little progress will be achieved for children and their families if there is no guarantee of continuous public policies of inçome redistribution which is a crucial problem in countries with high inequality, such as Brazil. The fundamental element for children is to have their rights guaranteed to live in healthy families and cohesive communities. This will only happen if the Brazilian Federal Constitution and the modern children's protection laws have been met faithfully. To this end, it is necessary to invest funding and knowledge to expand and strengthen the institutions and professionals responsible for the well-being of children, adolescents and their families.

REFERENCES

Achenbach, T. M. & Rescola, L. A. (2001). *Manual for the ASEBA School-age forms & profiles.* Burlington, VT: University of Vermont, Research Center for Children, Youth & Families.

Anselmi, L., Fernando, C. B., Maycoln, L. M., Teodoro, C. A. Piccinini, A. M. B., Menezes, C. L. & Araujo, L. A. R. (2008). Continuity of behavioral and emotional problems from pre-school years to pre-adolescence in a developing country. *Journal of Child Psychology and Psychiatry, 49(5)*, 499-507.

Assis, S. G., Avanci, J. Q. & Oliveira, R. V. C. (2009). Desigualdades socioeconômicas e saúde mental infantil. *Rev Saúde Pública, 43(1)*, 92-100.

Bird, H. R. (1996). Epidemiology of childhood disorders in a cross-cultural context. *J. Child Psychol Psychiatry, 37(1)*, 35-49: 1469-7610.

BRITISH MEDICAL ASSOCIATION. (2006). *Child and adolescent mental health*: a guide for health care professionals. England: British Medical Association.

Bronfenbrenner, U. (1996). Ecological systems theory. In R.Vasta (Ed.), *Six theories of child development* (pp. 187-249). Londres: Jessica Kingsley Publishers.

Cohen S., Janicki-Deverts, D., Chen E., & Matthews, K. A. (2010) Childhood socioeconomic status and adult health. *Annals of the New York Academy of Science, 1186*, 37-55.

Cury, C. R., & Golfeto, J. H. (2003). Strengths and Difficulties Questionnaire (SDQ): A study of children in Ribeirão Preto. Revista Brasileira de Psiquiatria, *25(3)*, 139-145.

Epstein, N. B., Baldwin, L. M., & Bishop, D. S (1983). The McMaster Family Assessment Device. *Journal of Marital and Family Therapy, 9,* 171–180.

Fleitlich-Bilyk, B., & Goodman, R. Prevalence of Child and Adolescent Psychiatric Disorders in Southeast Brazil (2004). *Journal of the American Academy of Child & Adolescent Psychiatry, 43(6)*, 727-734.

Garmezy, N. (1993). Children in Poverty: resilience despite risk. *Psychiatry, 56,* 127-136.

Harding, T. W. (1980). Mental Disorder in Primary Health Care: A Study of Their Frequency and Diagnosis in Four Developing Countries. *Psychological Medicine*, *10*, 231-241.

Huston, A. C. (org.). (1991). *Children in Poverty*. Cambridge: Cambridge University Press.

INSTITUTO BRASILEIRO DE GEOGRAFIA E ESTATÍSTICA (BR) (2010). *Suplemento Acesso a Transferências de Renda de Programas Sociais - Pesquisa Nacional por Amostra de Domicílios.* Retrieved on April 26, 2010, from http://www.sidra.ibge.gov.br/pnad/

Kohen, D. E., Hertzman, H., & Brooks-Gunn, J. (1998). *Neighbourhood influences on children's school readiness*. In Applied Research Branch, Human Resources Development Canada Working Paper No (W-98-15E).

Murray, C. J. L., & Lopez, A. D. (1996). *The global burden of disease*. Geneva: World Health Organization.

Najman, J. M., Aird, R., Bor, W., O'Callaghan, M., Williams, G. M., & Shuttlewood, G. J. (2004). The generational transmission of socioeconomic inequalities in child cognitive development and emotional health. *Soc Sci Med., 58(6)*,1147-58.

Neri, M. C. (2010). *Poverty and the new middle class in the decade of equality*. Retrieved on November 03, 2010, from *http://www3.fgv.br/ibrecps/retcm/index_eng.htm*

Patel, V., De Souza, N., & Rodrigues, M. (2003). Post-natal depression and infant growth and development in low income countries: a cohort study from Goa, India. *Archives of Disease in Childhood, 88*, 34–37.

PUBLIC HEALTH AGENCY OF CANADA (PHAC) (2009). *What determines health?* Retrieved March 17, 2009, from http://www.phacaspc.gc.ca/ph-sp/determinants/index-eng.php

Racine, Y., & Boyle, M. H. (2002). Family Functioning and children's behavior problems. P. 199-209. In: Willms J. D. (Eds). *Vulnerable children*. (pp.199-209).

Richter, L. (2004). *The importance of caregiver-child interactions for the survival and healthy development of young children: a review.* Geneva: World Health Organization.

Rutter, M. (1996) Stress research: Accomplishments and tasks ahead. In: Haggerty, R.; Sherrod, L.R.; Garmezy, N., & Rutter, M. *Stress, risk, and resilience in children and adolescents. Processes, Mechanisms, and Interventions*. Cambridge, UK: Cambridge University Press.

Siddiqi, A., Kawachi, I., Berkman, L., Subramanian, S.V. & Hertzman, C. (2007). Variation of socioeconomic gradients in children's development across advanced capitalist societies: analysis of 25 OECD nations. *International Journal of Health Services*, *37 (1)*, 63 –87.

Siegrist, J., & Marmot, M. (2006). *Social inequalities in health*. New York: Oxford University Press.

Sloat, E., & Willms, J. D. (2002) A gradient approach to the study of childhood vulnerability. In: Willms J.D. (editor). *Vulnerable children*. (pp.23-44). Canada: The University of Alberta Press.

Torres, H.G, Bichir, R. M., & Carpin, T. P. (2006). Uma pobreza diferente? Mudanças no padrão de consumo da população de baixa renda. *Novos Estudos, 74*, 17-22.

United Nations Development Programme. *Human Development Report (2009). Overcoming barriers: Human mobility and development.* Retrieved January 11, 2010, from *http://hdr.undp.org/en/media/HDR_2009_EN_Complete.pdf*.

Williams, J. D. (2003). *Ten hypotheses about socioeconomic gradients and community differences in children's developmental outcomes.* In Applied Research Branch, Strategic Policy, Human Resources Development.

WORLD HEALTH ORGANIZATION (WHO) (2001). *The Mental Health Report 2001: mental health: new understanding new hope*. Geneva: World Health Organization.

WORLD HEALTH ORGANIZATION (WHO) (2005). *Knowledge network for early child development Analytic and Strategic Review Paper: International Perspectives on Early Child Development.* Geneva: World Health Organization.

WORLD HEALTH ORGANIZATION (WHO) (2007). *Final Report for the World Health Organization's Commission on the Social Determinants of Health.* Geneva: World Health Organization.

In: Social Determinants and Mental Health
Editor: Sabine Bährer-Kohler
ISBN: 978-1-61324-353-4

Chapter 17

LIFESPAN PERSPECTIVE – BETWEEN RISK AND PROTECTION: SOCIAL INFLUENCES ON ADOLESCENTS' MENTAL HEALTH

Bernd Dollinger[1] and Henning Schmidt-Semisch[2]
[1]University of Siegen, Faculty of Pedagogy and Psychology, Siegen, Germany
[2]University of Bremen, Department of Human and Health Science, Bremen, Germany

ABSTRACT

Dimensions of social integration and their connection with individual well-being have been broadly discussed in the literature. A variety of theoretical and empirical studies examine the relationship of societal and social factors and their bearing on positive and more often negative consequences on mental health. It appears evident that poverty, unemployment, discrimination, etc. represent problematic and wearing circumstances of socialization that may lead to psychic turbulences. But looking behind the surface of plausibility of current empirical research studies, it becomes evident that 'social influences' do not represent a homogenous set of factors, which can be isolated and scrutinized easily. Apart from the well known fact that 'mental health' is difficult to define, there are specific challenges for research on social influences that this paper will discuss.

INTRODUCTION

In the following discussion, we highlight four problems which should be considered when social influences on adolescents' mental health are studied.

First, theories which are trying to sort possible social influences and their relevance to individual well-being are not seeded in the same level (Franke 2006). Theoretical assumptions range from macrosocial conditions (e.g., unemployment, social inequality, race discrimination, social change) to microsocial specifications which refer to nearby influences on individuals (e.g., family ties, relationships). It is worth mentioning that between these two dimensions there exists a mesosocial level of organizational and intermediate aspects (e.g., peer involvement, school related characteristics, neighborhood influences) raising the question how the different perspectives can be integrated (Alexander et al. 1987). Even though there are prominent integrative conceptions such as Coleman's "methodological individualism" (Coleman 1986), Giddens' "theory of structuration" (Giddens 1984) or Bourdieu's "habitus" and "field theory" (Bourdieu 1984), which all attempted to overcome the gap between macro and micro theories, no consensus has been achieved. Empirical studies are reliant on theoretical background knowledge, so the enduring controversies may cause problems in the interpretation of statistical findings. For instance, it is problematic to determine causality: does poverty cause mental challenges, or do mental challenges cause poverty? Or is poverty only relevant if it is accompanied by an individual's poor coping skills which themselves can be traced back to a variety of individual and social factors? To decide about these questions it is necessary to be theoretically informed on possible connections of a variety of independent and dependent factors.

Second, the confusion relating to social factors' impact on individual well-being is intensified by the fact that single factors can hardly be isolated. Generally speaking, poverty does not occur only as poverty, but is associated with unemployment, family problems, educational disadvantage, etc. Social factors which are relevant for mental health interact, build up and unfurl over a long period of time and consequently have a devastating impact due to a complex interaction of a variety of factors (Lantz et al. 1998).

Third, it has to be taken into account that relevant variables cannot be dichotomized as occurring or not-occurring but have to be measured in degrees of intensity or severity. To cite poverty again as an example, it is evident that a short period of indigence may have a fundamentally different impact on adolescents than a chronic inability to maintain one's livelihood although both phenomena can be categorized as 'poverty'. In order to conduct an empirical study, decisions have to be made whether a potential factor with a specific intensity is identified as a relevant variable or not. According to this fact, there is a normative and cultural bias in every empirical study dealing with social influences on mental health because a merely 'objective' methodology is unrealistic (Ravens-Sieberer et al. 2008, 155).

Fourth, it has to be kept in mind that individuals do not respond uniformly to external influences. Cognitive stress theories identify stress not as a function of a stressor's objective qualities but as a result of complex cognitive appraisals in which potential stressors are individually evaluated and related with options to handle them on the basis of personal and/or social resources (Lazarus/Folkman 1984). Thus, stress and an impairment of an individual's well-being are dependent on subjective appraisals and individual coping styles and traits (Lazarus 1998). Evaluating adolescents' mental health, it is important to pay attention not only to an adolescent's way to appraise and cope with external influences but also to scrutinize the mediating impact of possibly supportive or harmful effects of family life, school related influences, and involvement in peer contexts.

These problems illuminate the difficulties arising from the need to examine social influences on mental health. Despite a variety of sophisticated empirical studies (e.g. Lampert et al. 2006; Ravens-Sieberer 2008), there is still more theoretical and empirical research to be done. It is not sufficient to rely on plausibility but empirical evidence is needed to evaluate the relevance of specific factors to specific subgroups. In the following, we present pieces of empirically tested evidence which have been assembled to date and which are robust enough to be seen as convincing influences.

EMPIRICAL EVIDENCE

A first and highly influential aspect on mental health is a person's socio-economic status. In a research review, Mielck (2005, 42) states that despite varying definitions of psychic morbidities in different studies they concur in the result that mental health is declining with a low social status. An underprivileged socio-economic position is accompanied by a relative high likeliness to suffer from a psychic dysfunction. The effect appears to be meaningful for men and women and all age groups.

The "KIDSCREEN study" (Ravens-Sieberer et al. 2008) which collected representative data on children's and adolescents' (aged 8 to 18 years) mental health in twelve European countries provides an effectual account. Prevalence of mental health problems varied significantly between the countries, the highest rates occurred in the UK and Hungary and the lowest rates in Germany and Switzerland. Regarding social factors, a low socio-economic status (measured by a family's car and computer ownership, frequency of family holidays, and an adolescent's own bedroom) was associated with a high risk of suffering from mental health challenges. The same effect was found for poor parental relation, parental mental health problems, and deficient social support. Especially a low level of social support proved to be a very important factor for poor mental health across the countries (ibid., 161).

A strong relevance of the social status was also found in the study "Health Behaviour in School-aged children" (HBSC), coordinated by the World Health Organization (WHO). The study is measuring adolescents' health and health behavior in a recurring survey. At present, there are 43 regions and countries participating in the study (HBSC 2010). The identification of social inequality is undertaken by instruments similar to measures used in the KIDSCREEN study. Additionally, in HBSC information on parents' occupational status and the type of school attended by an adolescent is collected. Findings were also compared with the Gini-index which is a measure of income inequality. It is stated that "countries with lower mental health mean scores ... have higher Gini coefficients, indicating higher income inequality. Only in two countries is higher income equality and lower mental health observed. Most of the countries with higher positive mental health ... have Gini coefficients lower than 32, indicating higher income equality" (WHO 2008, 38). All in all, adolescents living in underprivileged circumstances report a comparatively low health status and show a greater amount of psychosomatic symptoms than adolescents with an average or high status of affluence (Lampert/Richter 2009, 216; see also Bohn et al 2010; Lampert et al. 2006).

These seminal cross national studies leave no doubt that adolescents' mental health is strongly related to socio-economic factors. The findings are robust and theoretically plausible with reference to, e.g., health related stress theories (e.g. Antonovsky 1987). But despite the non-ambiguous character of the results they must be specified because adolescence is not a homogeneous status but a conglomeration of very different lifestyles, attitudes, and social relations. Furthermore, adolescents are living in complex social relations and institutional networks so that the connection of socio-economic influences and adolescents' mental health is not immediate, particularly as poverty and social exclusion can be handled competently and constructively (Steinert/Pilgram 2007). This is not to downplay the relevance of social inequality and its very often detrimental effect on individual well-being and mental health, but it pays tribute to the complex interaction of social inequality and mental health and the difficulty to predefine causalities. If it is taken into account that health is not a state but a complex multidimensional process (e.g., Engel 1977), and if it is taken seriously that social interactions have relevant impact on mental health, than the ascription of deficits can be an integral part of the constitution of mental health problems. Thus, connecting poverty and mental health and ascribing it categorially to social groups can stigmatize and bring about a self-fulfilling prophecy (Merton 1967, 421ff). A variety of studies have not only proved mental illness to be a highly relevant stigma (e.g., Martin et al. 2000), especially if mental illness is ascribed to adolescents (Martin et al. 2007), but also demonstrated that labeling people mentally ill can be harmful, produce social stress, and lead to ongoing mental challenges (e.g., Link et al. 1997; Wright et al. 2000). According to Markowitz (1998, 336), "labeling and stigma indirectly leads to sustained illness", because „in order to avoid rejection, persons who are labeled engage in coping-strategies, such as secrecy, disclosure, or social withdrawal, which may constrict social networks, leading to unemployment and lowered income."

Following this account, adolescents are in a state between risk and protection: They are at risk if they belong to a disadvantaged subgroup of society. If this social situation is perceived by others, young people are not necessarily granted protection from further harm. In contrast, even support can be stigmatizing if it relies upon the categorial ascription of deficits. Consequently, even though social inequality has to be taken seriously as a negative impact on mental health, the connection of inequality and mental health must be interpreted as a complex interactive process which is not determinate but contingent upon a variety of factors. According to empirical findings, there is no imperative that young people living in poverty or a state of social exclusion will suffer from mental health problems. They can successfully handle their precarious environment. But to do so, they need social support, acknowledgment, and resources, e.g. social networks, involvement in peer and friendship groups, social capital (Klocke 2006: 212; Barry/Friedli 2010; Bengel et al. 2009; Hawe/Shiell 2000).

Social interactions and networks are not automatically protective. According to an investigation by Ueno focusing on adolescent depressive symptoms, a wide range of friendships was negatively associated with depressive symptoms, but "the relationship between having more friends and fewer depressive symptoms was largely mediated by a sense of belonging" (Ueno 2005, 484; correspondingly Wight et al. 2006; Heponiemi et al. 2006). This important role of subjectively experienced support and belonging is consistent with findings that bullying at schools can have a fundamental negative impact on adolescents' mental health. E.g., in a large school survey in Germany, a focal point was bullying at schools. 29.6 % of the adolescents in ninth grade reported that they had been a victim of bullying (Baier et al. 2010, 207). Being a victim of bullying was significantly associated with low self-esteem and a poor mental state. The authors indicate that with an increased intensity of bullying the victims' mental health is more and more seriously affected (ibid., 213). Despite the comparatively high mental pressure on these adolescents they remained relatively inconspicuous because they did not engage heavily in alcohol consumption or violent behavior. This indicates the need to distinguish thoroughly between different – e.g., internalizing and externalizing – styles of coping with social strains.

CONCLUSION

Although there is well-founded empirical evidence regarding social influences on adolescents' mental health (e.g. low socio-economic status, parental mental health problems or poor social support), these studies are not encompassing enough.

First, research findings and correlations are based on logic of risk-factors and, correspondingly, can only be interpreted as statistic probabilities: It's possible to make statements about probable consequences if specific or cumulated risk factors occur but these statements are not automatically valid to claim causalities or to forecast individual behavior. Risk-factors define specific categories of persons at risk and identify them. This categorization can initiate processes of stigmatizing and labeling people as mentally ill, irrespective of their actually mental health status. Fitzgibbon (2007; 2010) designates this phenomenon as "actuarial fallacy" meaning that even if a specific group of persons at risk is identified, there is no substantiated possibility to predict that an individual group member will in fact suffer from a mental health problem.

A second problem arises from interventions which are being implemented in order to overcome risk factors. As mentioned above, risk factors of mental health usually emerge over a long period of time; they interact and differ in their impact on specific mental health problems and mental diseases. Thus, it is hardly possible to decide about the distinct effects of specific interventions on mental health; it can only tentatively be assessed if measurements affect a specific kind of behavior in particular cases. Taken the complexity of social interactions and social change into account, it is almost impossible to appraise the definite status of findings. Given the fact that an experimental design – as an ideal standard in evidence based medicine – can not be applied when measuring complex social influences, it is only possible to attain more or less plausible and preliminary explanations.

Third, research findings suggest that highest evidence is given for correlations between mental health and the socio-economic status of a person. Since this statement refers to the relevance of socio-structural determinants in the field of adolescents' mental health problems, it is not satisfactory to intervene solely on the level of individuals or families. This is also true for interventions which are undertaken to empower adolescents or make them more resilient against social strains and stress. As Franke (2006: 175) states, research on resilience seeks to identify which specific adolescents have the ability to adapt to the norms of a society but it is not asked whether these norms are conducive to the mental, social, or physical health of children and adolescents. Much more time and activity should be invested to investigate how social conditions can be made beneficial for individuals' mental health: "As a society, we distribute important goods – such as education, housing, jobs, income, wealth, opportunity, political participation, and a sense of community – very unequally across subgroups that differ by race, ethnicity, gender, or class. These social and economic inequalities then produce health inequalities through complex mechanisms that we are just beginning to understand. We could, if we had the appropriate political understanding and will, limit these inequalities, or at least mitigate their effects through other social politics and practices" (Daniels 2008: 13).

In a society which restricts the access to health for many children and adolescents on a socio-structural level, a focus on risk and resilience factors as well as on corresponding interventions can be reductionistic and ethically questionable.

LITERATURE

Alexander, J.C., Giesen, B., Münch, R. & Smelser, N.J. (1987). *The Micro-macro Link* (2. ed.). Berkeley: University of California Press.

Antonovsky, A. (1987). *Unraveling the mystery of health: How People Manage Stress and Stay Well.* San Francisco: Jossey-Bass.

Baier, D., Pfeiffer, C., Rabold, S., Simonson, J. & Kappes, C. (2010). Kinder und Jugendliche in Deutschland: Gewalterfahrungen, Integration, Medienkonsum. Hannover. *(http://www.kfn.de/versions/kfn/assets/fob109.pdf; download 04.10.2010).*

Barry, M. & Friedli, L. (2010). The influence of social, demographic and physical factors on positive mental health in children, adolescents and older people. In: C.L. Cooper, J.G. U. Field, R. Jenkins & B.J. Sahakian (Eds.), *Mental capital and wellbeing* (pp. 475-484). Oxford: Wiley-Blackwell.

Bengel, J./Meinders-Lücking, F./Rottmann, N. (2009): Schutzfaktoren bei Kindern und Jugendlichen – Stand der Forschung zu psychosozialen Schutzfaktoren für Gesundheit. Forschung und Praxis der Gesundheitsförderung, Bd. 35 hrgg. v. *Bundeszentrale für gesundheitliche Aufklärung: Köln.*

Bohn, V., Rathmann, K. & Richter, M. (2010). Psychosoziale Gesundheit bei Kindern und Jugendlichen in Nordrhein-Westfalen: Die Bedeutung von Alter, Geschlecht und Schultyp. In: *Das Gesundheitswesen*, Vol. 72, 293-300.

Bourdieu, P. (1984). *Distinction: A Social Critique of the Judgement of Taste*. London: Routledge & Kegan Paul.

Coleman, J.S. (1986). Social Theory, Social Research , and a Theory of Action. In: *American Journal of Sociology*, Vol. 91, 1309-1335.

Daniels, N. (2008).Just health. Meeting Health Needs Fairly. Cambridge: University Press

Engel, G.L. (1977). The need for a new medical model. A challenge for biomedicine. In: *Science*, Vol. 196, 129-136.

Fitzgibbon, W. (2007). Risk Analysis and the New Practitioner: Myth or Reality? In: *Punishment and Society*, Vol. 9, 87-97.

Fitzgibbon, W. (2010). Risikoträger oder verletzliche Individuen: Über die präemptive Kriminalisierung von Menschen mit psychischen Problemen. In: B. Paul & H. Schmidt-Semisch (Eds.), *Risiko Gesundheit. Über Risiken und Nebenwirkungen der Gesundheitsgesellschaft* (pp. 227-240). Wiesbaden: VS.

Franke, A. (2006). *Modelle von Gesundheit und Krankheit*. Bern: Huber.

Giddens, A. (1984). *The constitution of Society. Outline of the theory of structuration.* Cambridge: Polity Press.

Hawe, P./Shiell, A. (2000): Social Capital and Health Promotion: a Review. In: *Social Science and Medicine* 51: 871-885.

Health Behaviour in School-aged children (HBSC), (2010). Overview. *(http://www.hbsc.org/overview.html; download 04.10.2010).*

Heponiemi, T. et al. (2006): The longitudinal effects of social support and hostility on depressive tendencies. In: *Social Science & Medicine*, Vol. 63, 1374-1382.

Klocke, A. (2006): Gesundheitsrelevante Verhaltensweisen im Jugendalter. Sozioökonomische, kulturelle und geschlechtsspezifische Einflussfaktoren im internationalen Vergleich. In: Wendt, C./Wolf, C. (Eds.): Soziologie der Gesundheits.

Sonderheft 46/2006 der Kölner Zeitschrift für Soziologie und Sozialpsychologie, *Wiesbaden: VS Verlag*: 198-223.

Lampert, T. & Richter, M. (2009): Gesundheitliche Ungleichheit bei Kindern und Jugendlichen. In: K. Hurrelmann/M. Richter (Eds.): *Gesundheitliche Ungleichheit.* (2. ed., pp. 209-230). Wiesbaden: VS.

Lampert, T./Richter, M. & Klocke, A. (2006): Kinder und Jugendliche: Ungleiche Lebensbedingungen, Ungleiche Gesundheitschancen. In: *Das Gesundheitswesen*, Vol. 68: 94-100.

Lantz, P.M., House, J.S., Lepkowski, J.M., Williams, D.R., Mero, R.P. & Chen, J. (1998). Socioecomic Factors, Health Behaviours, and Mortality. Results From a National Representative Prospective Study of US Adults. In: *JAMA*, Vol. 279, 1703-1708.

Lazarus, R.S. (1998). Coping from the Perspective of Personality. In: *Zeitschrift für Differentielle und Diagnostische Psychologie,* Vol. 19: 213-231.

Lazarus, R.S. & Folkman, S. (1984). *Stress, appraisal, and coping*. New York: Springer.

Link, B.G., Struening, E., Phelan, J.C., Rahav, M. & Nuttbrock, L. (1997). On Stigma and Its Consequences: Evidence from a Longitudinal Study of Men with Dual Diagnoses of Mental Illness and Substance Abuse. In: *Journal of Health and Social Behavior,* Vol. 38, 177-190.

Markowitz, F.E. (1998). The Effects of Stigma on the Psychological Well-Being and Life-Satisfaction of Persons With Mental Illness. In: *Journal of Health and Social Behavior*, Vol. 39, 335-347.

Martin, J.K., Pescosolido, B.A., Olafsdottir, S. & McLeodJane D. (2007). The Construction of Fear: Americans' Preferences for Social Distance from Children and Adolescents with Mental Health Problems. In: *Journal of Health and Social Behavior*, Vol. 48, 50-67.

Martin, J.K., Pescosolido, B.A., Tuch, S.A. (2000). Of Fear and Loathing: The Role of „Disturbing Behavior", Labels, and Causal Attributions in Shaping Public Attitudes Toward Persons with Mental Illness. In: *Journal of Health and Social Behavior*, Vol. 41, 208-223.

Merton, R.K. (1967). Social Theory and Social Structure (2. ed.). New York: Free Press.

Mielck, A. (2005). *Soziale Ungleichheit und Gesundheit*. Bern: Huber.

Ravens-Sieberer, U., Erhart, M., Gosch, A., Wille, N. & The European KIDSCREEN Group (2008). Mental Health of Children and Adolescents in 12 European Countries – Results from the European Kidscreen Study. In: *Clinical Psychology and Psychotherapy*, Vol. 15, 154-163.

Steinert, H. & Pilgram, A. (Eds.) (2007). *Welfare policy from below. Struggles against social exclusion in Europe.* Aldershot: Ashgate.

Ueno, K. (2005). The effects of friendship networks on adolescent depressive symptoms. In: *Social Science Research*, Vol. 34, 484-510.

Wight, R.G., Boticello, A.L., Aneshensel, C.S. (2006). Socioecenomic Context, Social Support, and Adolescent Mental Health: A Multilevel Investigation. In: *Journal of Youth and Adolescence,* Vol. 35, 115-126.

Wright, E.R., Gronfein, W.P. & Oewns, T.J. (2000). Deinstitutionalization, Social Rejection, and the Self-Esteem of Former Mental Patients. In: *Journal of Health and Social Behavior*, Vol. 41, 68-90.

World Health Organization (WHO) (2008). *Social cohesion for mental well-being among adolescents.* Copenhagen: WHO Regional Office for Europe.

In: Social Determinants and Mental Health
Editor: Sabine Bährer-Kohler

ISBN: 978-1-61324-353-4

Chapter 18

Lifespan Perspective: Social Determinants of Health and Promotion of Mental Health in Old Age

Carlos Augusto de Mendonça Lima
Department of Psychiatry and Mental Health, Centro Hospitalar do Alto Ave, E.P.E.
Guimarães, Portugal

Abstract

Social determinants of health are the conditions in which people are born, grow, live, work and age and which are shaped by the distribution of money, power and resources at global, national and local levels (4). These social determinants are associated with mental disorders by contributing to its onset or course. Social determinants of health are influenced by policy choices and are primarily responsible for disparities in health. The goal of this chapter is to describe how the interaction among social determinants, mental health and well-being of older persons were considered on recent selected statements, policies, declarations or other public health documents with the aim to promote a better mental health.

Introduction

Since the World Health Organization (WHO) has defined health as a state of complete physical, mental, and social well-being, not merely the absence of disease (1) and mental health as a state of well-being in which the individual realizes his or her own abilities, can cope with the normal stresses of life, can work productively, and is able to make a contribution to his or her community (2) that the well-being dimension became central in policies and strategies of Health and Mental Health.

Mental well-being is an asset of individuals, communities and populations whose value can change throughout the life course. Someone's mental health is affected by a range of determinants throughout life, such the genetic heritage, personal experiences, and the environment in which the person lives (3).

Social determinants of health are the conditions in which people are born, grow, live, work and age and which are shaped by the distribution of money, power and resources at global, national and local levels (4). These social determinants are associated with mental disorders by contributing to its onset or course. A list of these social determinants should include at least:

- Cultural and spiritual references
- Education and literacy
- Physical environment
- Social status and security
- Financial resources including income security
- Food and housing security and quality
- Health system
- Justice system, including respect of Human Rights
- Employment and working conditions
- Leisure and personal development
- Spiritual development
- Discrimination and stigma
- Inequalities
- Social, political and physical exclusion and marginalization
- Violence, abuse, neglect, abandon

Social determinants may play a role as risk factors for mental health (unemployment, poverty, inequalities, stigma and discrimination, poor housing, poor early years experience, violence, abuse, drug and alcohol abuse, poor general health, caring duties), while others may be protective factors (employment, social protection, resilience, social networks, positive community engagement, positive spiritual life, hope, optimism, good general health, good quality parenting, positive relationships in childhood) (3).

By acting on social determinants of health, it is possible to contribute to a better subjective mental health and well-being of people, to build the capacity of communities to manage adversity, and to reduce the burden and consequences of mental health problems. Disadvantages because of mental health problems damage the social cohesion of communities and societies by decreasing interpersonal trust, social participation and civic engagement (5).

The goal of this chapter is to describe how the interaction between social determinants and mental health and well-being of older persons were considered on recent selected statements, policies, declarations or other public health documents with the aim to promote a better mental health. These documents were grouped in four levels. Those promoting a better health and well-being (i) for all; (ii) for older persons and during the ageing process, (iii) for persons with mental disorders, and (iv) for older persons with mental disorders.

Better Health and Well-Being For All

The Report of the WHO Commission on Social Determinants of Health (CSDH) (4)

The CSDH was set up with the task to collect, collate, and synthesize global evidence on the social determinants of health and their impact on health inequity, and to make recommendations for action to address that inequity (4).

Social justice is a matter of life and death: it affects the way people live, their consequent chance of illness, and their risk of premature death. The development level of a society can be estimated by the quality of its population's health, how fairly health is distributed across all levels of a society, and the degree of protection provided from disadvantage as a result of ill-health.

The health inequities in a social group, the social gradient in health within countries, and the marked health inequities between countries are caused by *the unequal distribution of power, income, goods, and services, globally and nationally, the consequent unfairness in the immediate, visible circumstances of peoples lives – their access to health care, schools, and education, their conditions of work and leisure, their homes, communities, towns, or cities – and their chances of leading a flourishing life.* This unequal distribution of health-damaging experiences is not caused by 'natural' reasons: it is the consequence of a *toxic combination of poor social policies and programmes, unfair economic arrangements, and bad politics* (4).

The Commission's overall recommendations to action on the social determinants of health to promote a better health include:

1. Improve Daily Living Conditions
2. Tackle the Inequitable Distribution of Power, Money, and Resources
3. Measure and Understand the Problem and Assess the Impact of Action

CSDH aspires to reduce the world health inequities in a generation. For this it is necessary to involve a progressive flattening of the health gradient by improving the health of all social groups to a level closer to that of the most advantaged.

Better Health and Well-Being for Older Persons and During the Ageing Process

The United Nations Political Declaration and Madrid International Plan of Action on Ageing 2002 and the Follow-Up to the Second World Assembly on Ageing 2010

The Second World Assembly on Ageing (II WAA) (6) produced two relevant documents: the Political Declaration on Ageing and the Plan of Action on Ageing.

The Article 7 of the Political Declaration (6) describes the consequences of poverty on older persons' life and recognizes the importance of placing ageing in the development agendas, as well as in strategies for the eradication of poverty and in seeking to achieve full participation in the global economy of all developing countries.

It was committed to provide older persons with universal and equal access to health care and services, including physical and mental health services.

This Political Declaration was completed by the United Nations Plan of Action on Ageing (6). At its issues *Health promotion and well-being throughout life* and *Mental health needs of older persons* this plan gives a more specific contribution to promote the mental health in old age. According to them health promotion activities and equal access of older persons to health care and services is the cornerstone of healthy ageing. In order to attain these objectives it is necessary not only specific actions to affect individual health but also improvements in the economic and social situation of older persons.

Besides the significant progress brought by both United Nations Political Declaration and Madrid International Plan of Action on Ageing 2002, the defense of Human Rights of Older Persons is still considered as not good enough. Human Rights, and their protection, are an important basic social determinant of health (8). The Universal Declaration of Human Rights (9) addresses the rights of all human beings, but the rights and needs of certain groups are not adequately covered by it. The United Nations General Assembly decided in 16 November 2010 (7) a Follow-up to the II WAA (World Assembly on Ageing). This decision includes the establishment of a working group for the purpose of strengthening the protection of the human rights of older persons.

Better Health and Well-Being for Persons with Mental Disorders

The WHO World Report 2001 (2)

The World Health Report 2001 (2) describes how the social factors have been associated with the development of mental and behavioral disorders. The nature of modern urbanization may have deleterious consequences for mental health through the influence of increased stressors and adverse life events. Migration frequently causes high rates of unemployment and bad living conditions, exposing migrants to increased risk of mental disorders. Isolation, lack of transport and communications, limited educational and economic opportunities, absence of mental health services are common difficulties in rural areas.

The poor and the deprived have a higher prevalence of mental and behavioural disorders. This higher prevalence may be explainable both by (i) higher causation of disorders among the poor and by (ii) the drift of the mentally ill into poverty. The overall lack of mental health services and the barriers faced by certain socioeconomic groups in accessing care can contribute to this.

Women are in general at greater risk of experiencing mental and behavioural disorders than others in the community because of the burden of the multiple roles they have to play and by the fact they face significant gender discrimination, associated poverty, hunger, malnutrition, overwork and domestic and sexual violence.

Racism is related to the perpetuation of mental problems. People victim of racism are at higher risk of mental problems and people who practice racism are found to develop certain kinds of mental disorders.

The WHO Report on Promoting Mental Health (10)

This report, prepared by the WHO Department of Mental Health and Substance Abuse in collaboration with the Victorian Health Promotion Foundation and the University of Melbourne (10) recognizes that:

- people who are more socially isolated and people who are disadvantaged have poorer health than others;
- more socially cohesive societies are healthier, with lower mortality.

The report criticizes traditional way of understanding the relations between socioeconomic epidemiological data and health. An immediate challenge for society's leaders is to create or refine the social structures and processes we use to evaluate the available evidence and to mobilize resources to promote mental health.

Better Health and Well-Being for Older Persons with Mental Disorders

WHO and WPA Consensus Statements on Psychiatry of the Elderly

Mental disorders in older persons assume some specificities, such their age of onset: persons with late onset mental disorders are more able to keep a better functioning in the activities of daily living because their occupational and social roles have not been interrupted by the disorder earlier in life and their skills may remain, while the early onset increases the risk of becoming poor, remaining unmarried, of separation what can contribute for social isolation later in life (11). Older persons are more reluctant to ask for psychiatric help and they commonly complain of diffuse physical symptoms as expression of their mental suffering.

The following documents tried to take into account these specificities. The social determinants of mental disorders in old age were mentioned at them as follows.

WHO and WPA Consensus Statement on Psychiatry of the Elderly (12)

The authors of this statement (12) recognized that an elderly suffering from mental health problems often has a combination of psychological, physical and social needs. These factors, together with the biological, social and cultural changes associated with ageing may significantly alter the clinical presentation of mental illness in old age. Therapeutic interventions to encourage autonomy should include retraining in daily living skills and improving safety at home. Provision of practical support and information including social and legal rights' advice to patients and their supporters make an important contribution.

WHO and WPA Technical Consensus Statement on Organizing Services in Psychiatry of the Elderly (13)

To prepare for increasing life expectancy calls for significant social innovations at the individual and societal level, which must be founded on a knowledge base drawn from contributions by, and collaboration among, the medical, behavioral, psychological, biological and social sciences (13).

Patients with severe mental illness may need considerable support in maintaining self-care and activities of daily living. The ability of informal carers to meet these needs, and the resultant burdens on carers need to be monitored closely and emerging problems addressed promptly.

The legal rights and financial and other personal interests of such patients must be protected. Some older people with mental disorders may not be able effectively to represent their interests, manage their affairs or agree to what is proposed for them: . This is particularly problematic for patients who are alone and where there is a conflict between individual and family interests (14).

Housing of older persons with mental disorders can become particularly problematic: though care should be provided in patients' homes as long as possible, care in an alternative residential setting may be the only way of meeting patients needs effectively.

The place of the spiritual needs of older people with mental health problems is recognized. Meaningful and appropriate recreational and leisure activities may contribute substantially to quality of life.

WHO and WPA Technical Consensus Statement on Educating in Psychiatry of the Elderly (15)

To educate professionals, caregivers and the lay public in mental health issues in old age is necessary to reduce the burden of mental disorders. A first statement on this topic (15) proposed a general knowledge based curriculum to help the development of educating programmes. It included the special significance in old age of the interdependence of mental, physical and social factors and the prevention and health promotion including recreational and spiritual issues.

Skill-Based Objectives for Specialist Training in Old Age Psychiatry (16)

The precedent statement was completed by a skill-based objectives curriculum, prepared by a group of experts for the European context (16). According to this curriculum, specialists should demonstrate the ability to deliver appropriate, good quality and cost-effective physical, psychological and social interventions in the management of mental illness in older people living in the community, residential or hospital settings. They should demonstrate an understanding of the social, economic and cultural changes associated with the ageing process, taking into account of the cultural, spiritual and ethnic issues in the recognition, assessment, diagnosis and management of mental health problems in the older person.

They should have the ability to run a multi-disciplinary community oriented service for older people with all forms of mental health problems which ensures equity of access to care and be able to work effectively and efficiently in different settings.

Specialists should be able to evaluate stress and burden in carers and their determinants and should demonstrate the ability to organize appropriate support packages.

In this context specialists should demonstrate an understanding of all aspects of elder abuse and the ability to recognize and manage elder abuse in a range of different settings.

WHO and WPA Technical Consensus Statement on Reducing Stigma and Discrimination Against Older People with Mental Disorders (17)

The role of stigma and discrimination of older persons with mental disorders as a social determinant of health was developed in one statement (17). It recognized that stigma against older people occurs in many societies; there is in this case therefore a 'double jeopardy' (because of the old age and because of the mental disorders) and both issues need to be addressed in anti-stigma strategies for this age group.

Actions against stigma should form part of the promotion of good mental health by professional training and public education, and should be a major component of all levels of a health and social care programme.

Stigma against older people with mental disorder is *reinforced* by:

- Cultural factors
- Social and economic instability and crisis
- The actual or perceived absence or inadequacy of preventive strategies and treatments for mental disorders;
- The lack of information systems to educate both professionals and the general public;
- Gender discrimination;
- Any rewards for those who stigmatize.

The negative attitudes against older persons with mental disorders may lead in turn to *discrimination* against individuals, their families and those who care for them in terms of:

- poor quality treatment and care,
- marginalization within care systems,
- 'warehousing' outside the health care system,
- low status of professionals, services providing care,
- staff recruitment, retention problems,
- inadequate funding at national and local levels,
- inequity in reimbursement for treatment,
- negative impact on families,

- victimization, abuse, neglect,
- unnecessary institutionalisation,
- social distancing and exclusion of the sufferers and lack of familiarity with their experiences,
- poor quality of life,
- exclusion from research, and consequent lack of evidence to inform policy and practice,
- adverse economic effects,
- discriminatory legislation,
- unemployment, in societies where older people typically remain in the workforce,
- material and financial inequity,
- government neglect, and lack of legislative protections,
- derogatory language.

Two main goals of a strategy to reduce stigma and discrimination in the context of mental disorders in old age are to:

- ensure that appropriate health and social care systems are in place that can meet the needs of older people with mental disorder and their carers;
- position mental health of older people on the public agenda – mental disorder is as important in old age as in earlier life.

Other Relevant Documents

Two Thematic Conferences were recently organized to implement the European Pact for Mental Health and Well-being.

The first was on the *Promotion of social inclusion and the combat of stigma for better mental health and well-being* co-organised by the European Commission's Directorate for Health and Consumers and Portuguese Ministry of Health with the support of the Belgian Presidency of the EU in November 2010 at Lisbon (18).

According to the final document, good mental health is critical to the success of communities and nations. Promoting social inclusion and protection, promotes the subjective mental health and well-being of people, builds the capacity of communities to manage adversity, and reduces the burden and consequences of mental health problems. Widespread disadvantage damages the social cohesion of communities and societies by decreasing interpersonal trust, social participation and civic engagement. Social protection systems with a reasonable minimum wage and a well-regulated financial system guarantee a socially acceptable minimum income and avoid financial exclusion.

The availability of accessible primary care mental health services is a precondition to the social inclusion of people with mental health problems. Holistic community-based health services should be age and gender appropriate and delivered as part of a community partnership which includes government, civil society and social protection services.

The second thematic conference, on the theme *Promotion of Mental health and Well-being in Older People – making it happen*, was co-organized by the European Commission's

Directorate for Health and Consumers and the Ministry of Health and Social Affaires of Spain, with the support of the Presidency of Spain of the European Union, and realized in Madrid, on June 2010 (19). It was stressed that it is a duty of all to give greater priority to promoting mental health and well-being and to tackle mental health problems.

Five themes were debated:

1. Mental health promotion in old age: a healthy lifestyle, safe living environment and participation in society and community are important protective factors for mental health and well-being. Support from families and peers promote mental health by reducing isolation and loneliness.
2. Prevention of mental disorders and promotion of autonomy: to prevent mental disorders in old age means to address the risk factors and to improve help seeking, quality of services, early detection and intervention.
3. Older people in vulnerable situations: certain older people face higher risk of mental health problems such older women, persons with disabilities, those in situation or at risk of poverty, with chronic illness, suffering abuse and belonging to minorities.
4. Health systems for care and treatment: care systems have to be community and outpatient oriented, to include collaboration between the treatment systems for mental and physical disorders as well between health and the social sectors. Primary care should be used to proactively pursue the goal of improving mental health and well-being in older people.
5. Supporting the informal carers: support the role of informal carers by training them and protecting their well-being.

Conclusion

Social determinants of health are primarily responsible for disparities in health. They are influenced by policies choices which influence the development of public service systems. These systems, in their turn, shape the social determinants of health through the development of programmes, resource allocations and organization of services. The influence of negative social determinants of health often is caused by bad political choices and the consequent unequal distribution of resources.

The establishment of good policies is the first step to produce changes. This chapter shows a considerable number of documents, produced at several different levels, in collaboration among different sectors and disciplines, in an effort to point the direction to change social inequalities which are at the origin of social injustice, suffering, illness and premature death.

The growing mental health needs of an ageing population may require additional policies, in particular for care and treatment, the promotion of healthy lifestyles and supportive environments. But the most important for the implementation of the presented texts are the political will and courage to induce changes.

REFERENCES

[1] World Health Organization (1948). *Constitution of the World Health Organization.* Geneva, World Health Organization.

[2] World Health Organization (2001). *World Health Report 2001. Mental Health: New Understanding, New Hope*. Geneva, World Health Organization.

[3] Stengard, E (2010). Key principles for Mental Health Promotion and Mental Disorder Prevention in Older People: ProMenPol and DataPrev projects. In: European Communities. *Mental Health and Well-Being in Older People – Making it Happen. Conclusions from the Thematic Conference* (pp: 5-6). Luxembourg, European Communities.

[4] Commission on Social Determinants of Health (2008). *Closing the gap in a generation: health equity through action on the social determinants of health. Final Report of the Commission on Social Determinants of Health.* Geneva, World Health Organization.

[5] O'Sullivan, C (2010). Social determinants of Mental Health. In: European Communities. *Background document for the thematic conference: "Promoting Social Inclusion and Combating Stigma for better Mental Health and Well-being"* (pp.: 9-14). Luxembourg, European Communities.

[6] United Nations (2002). *Report of the Second World Assembly on Ageing. Madrid, 8-12 April 2002.* New York: United Nations.

[7] United Nations General Assembly (2010). *Follow-up to the Second World Assembly on Ageing.* New York: United Nations.

[8] World Health Organization (2006). *WHO Resource book on Mental Health, Human Rights and Legislation.* Geneva: World Health Organization.

[9] United Nations (1948). *Universal Declaration of Human Rights.* New York: United Nations.

[10] World Health Organization (2004). *Promoting mental health: concepts, emerging evidence, practice : summary report / a report from the World Health Organization, Department of Mental Health and Substance Abuse in collaboration with the Victorian Health Promotion Foundation (VicHealth) and the University of Melbourne*. Geneva: World Health Organization.

[11] Mechanic, D. & McAlpine, D. D (2002). The influence of social factors on mental health. In: Copeland, J. R. M., Abou-Saleh, M. T. & Blazer, D. G. *Principles and Practice of Geriatric Psychiatry* (2nd edition, pp.: 95-98). Chichester: John Wiley & Sons, Ltd.

[12] World Health Organization & World Psychiatric Association (1996). *Psychiatry of the elderly: a consensus statement.* Geneva: World Health Organization.

[13] World Health Organization & World Psychiatric Association (1997). *Organization of care in Psychiatry of the elderly: a technical consensus statement.* Geneva: World Health Organization.

[14] Katona, C., Chiu, E., Adelman, S., Baloyannis, S., Camus, V., Firmino, H., Gove, D., Graham, N., Ghebrehiwet, T., Içelli, I., Ihl, R., Kalasic, A., Leszek, L., Kim, S., de Mendonça Lima, C. A., Peisah, C., Tataru, N. & Warner, J. (2009). World psychiatric association section of old age psychiatry consensus statement on ethics and capacity in older people with mental disorders. *Int J Geriatr Psychiatry, 24 (12)*: 1319-1324.

[15] World Health Organization & World Psychiatric Association (1998). *Education in Psychiatry of the elderly: a technical consensus statement.* Geneva: World Health Organization.

[16] Gustafson, L., Burns, A., Katona, C., Bertolote, J. M., Camus, V., Copeland, J. R. M., Dufey, A. F., Graham, N., Ihl, R., Kanowski, S., Kühne, N., de Mendonça Lima, C. A., Mateos Alvarez, R., Rutz, W., Tataru, N. L., Tudose, C. (2003). Skill-based objectives for specialist training in old age psychiatry. *Int J Geriatr Psychiatry, 18*: 686-693.

[17] Graham, N., Lindesay, J., Katona, C., Bertolote, J. M., Camus, V., Copeland, J. R. M., de Mendonça Lima, C. A., Gaillard, M., Nargeot, M. C. G., Gray, J., Jacobsson, L., Kingma, M., Kühne, N. O'Loughlin, A., Saraceno, B., Taintor, Z., Wancata, J. (2003). Reducing stigma and discrimination against older people with mental disorders: a technical consensus statement *Int J Geriatr Psychiatry, 18*: 670-678.

[18] European Communities (2010). *Background document for the thematic conference: "Promoting Social Inclusion and Combating Stigma for better Mental Health and Well-being"* (pp.: 9-14). Luxembourg: European Communities.

[19] European Communities (2010). *Mental Health and Well-Being in Older People – Making it Happen. Conclusions from the Thematic Conference* (pp: 5-6). Luxembourg: European Communities.

In: Social Determinants and Mental Health
Editor: Sabine Bährer-Kohler

ISBN: 978-1-61324-353-4

Chapter 19

LIFESPAN PERSPECTIVE – IMPORTANCE OF SOCIAL DETERMINANTS TO THE ELDERLY: THE CASE OF THE SUPER-AGED SOCIETY OF JAPAN

Masatoshi Takeda
Osaka University Graduate School of Medicine, Faculty of Medicine, Department of Integrated Medicine Osaka, Japan
President of International Psychogeriatric Association, US

INTRODUCTION

With the steady expansion of lifespans in the world, society has been aging. Along with economic development, developing countries in Asia and Africa will have to face various problems caused by the aging society, which were not necessarily well managed by developed Western countries. Since human society is quite different in traditional and cultural values, each country is expected to solve the problems caused by the rapid increase in the elderly population.

LIFESPAN AND ECONOMIC DEVELOPMENT

The average lifespan of the human being has steadily expanded owing to the development of science and technology, especially after the industrial revolution in the latter half of the 18th century. Improvements in the living environment, e.g. urban infrastructures and public hygiene as well as the development of antibiotics and medical technology have significantly contributed to the prolongation of the average lifespan in the last two centuries.

The average lifespan in a country correlates with its GDP (Figure 1), with lifespans increasing more in developing countries and less in developed countries. It is interesting to note that the greater the GDP the longer the average lifespan of a country.

It is important to note that economic development prolongs the average but not the maximum lifespan of the human being. Economic development helps more people to live longer but does not increase the maximum lifespan of an individual. So the expansion of the average lifespan with the same maximum lifespan implies that a society will have a larger elderly population. In other words, economic development makes for a society where more people live out their lives.

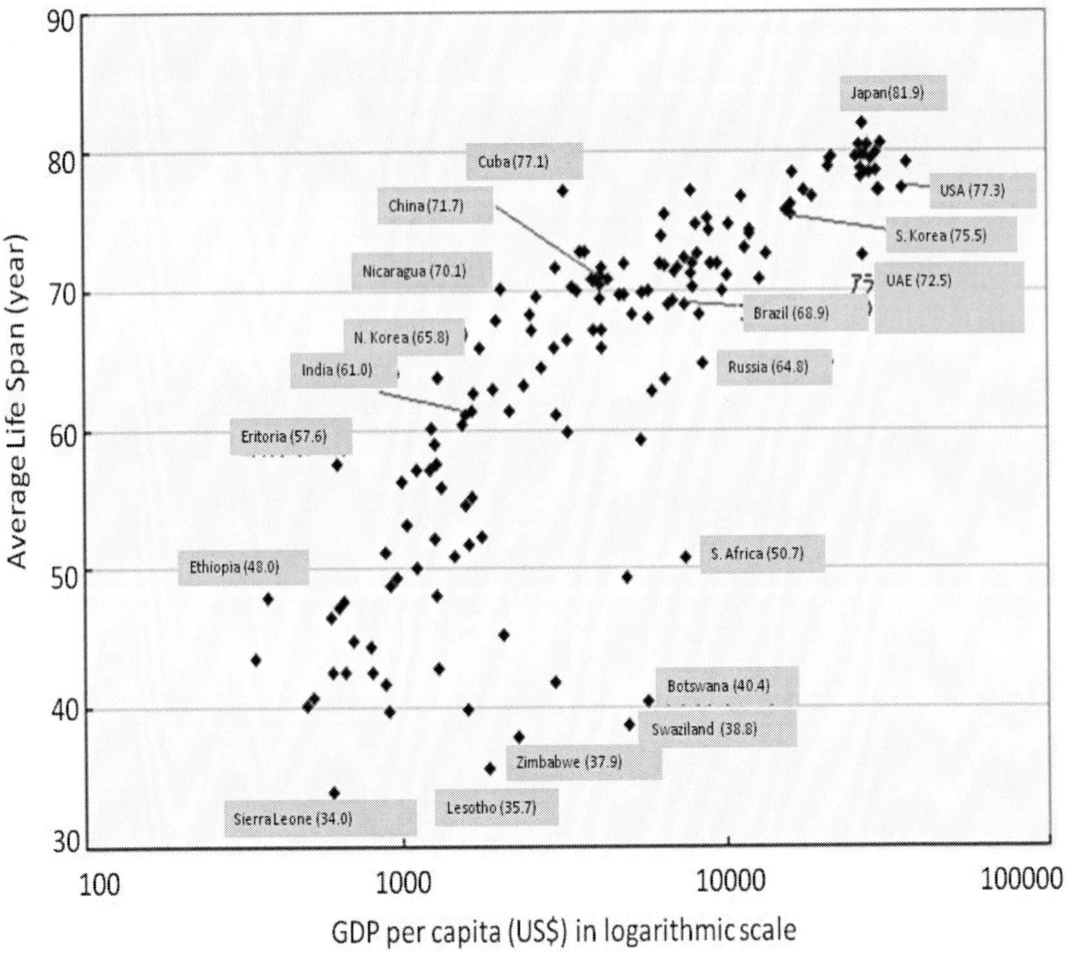

Figure 1. Average lifespan and gross domestic product (GDP) in 149 countries. The average lifespan of 149 countries with populations of one million and over plotted against GDP (gross domestic product) per capita (US$) on a logarithmic scale.

Economic development may have another impact on society. As is shown in Figure 2, birthrates have shrunk significantly in all countries in the world in these 60 years. The reduction of the birthrate is more drastic in Japan and South Korea than in European countries. In South Korea the birthrate was 6.0 in 1958, and it was drastically reduced to 1.08 in 2006. The birthrate of Japan was 3.7 in 1950, and it was down to 1.32 in 2006. The sharp drop of the Japanese birthrate in 1966 can be explained by a traditional superstition based upon the Chinese zodiac calendar, which says that a woman born in the year of Hinoeuma, which happened to be 1966, will be rash-tempered and will not make a good wife. Most Asian countries experienced significant reductions in their birthrate in these years along with economic development of the country. When a society changes from a primitive economy to capitalism and commercialism, women tend to have jobs to earn money, so that fewer children are born. As it is said ironically, capitalism is the best birth-control pill.

In 1950, sixty years ago, there were 131 million elderly in the world, comprising only 5.2% of the total population, a figure which increased to 477 million (7.3%) in 2005 and will increase again to 1,492 million (16.2%). In the 100 years after 1950, the number of elderly people in the developed countries will increase 5.1 times, but in the developing countries it will increase 17.4 times in the same period, which implies that significantly more elderly people will be living there in the near future.

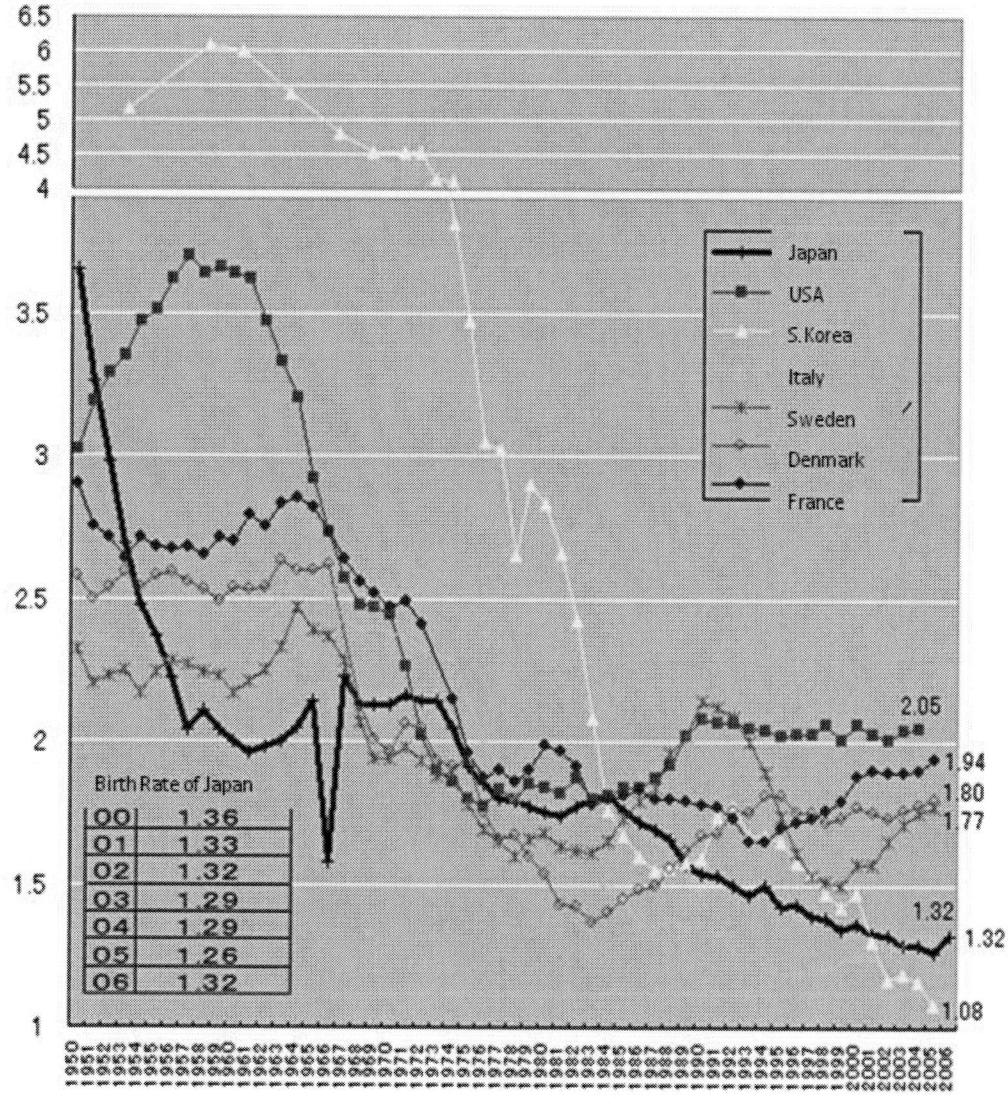

Figure 2. Change in birthrate by country between 1950-2006.

In 2005 there were 185 million elderly people in developed countries, and 292 million in developing countries. The distribution of the elderly people among developing and developed countries changed from near-equivalence in 1950 to 1.6 times more in 2005, and 3.6 times more in 2050. Due to the more rapid increase in the elderly population in the developing countries, the elderly population there will be 1,166 million by 2050, 3.6 times more than in the developed countries (326 million). The problem of aging will become more important in developing than in developed countries in the near future. (Table 1)

Table 1. The elderly population in developed and developing countries in 1950, 2005, and 2050

	1950	2005	2050
(A)Developed country (million)	64	185	326
Ratio of the elderly	7.9%	15.3%	26.1%
(B)Developing country (million)	67	292	1,166
Ratio of the elderly	3.9%	5.5%	14.7%
(C)Elderly Population (A+B) (million)	131	477	1,492
Ratio of the elderly (C/D)	5.2%	7.3%	16.2%
(D)Total Population (million)	2,535	6,515	9,191
life span (male) (year)	45.0	63.9	73.1
life span (female) (year)	47.8	68.3	77.8
birth rate (%)	5.0	2.7	2.0

Developed countries include Europe, North America, Japan, Australia, and New Zealand. Developing countries include Africa, Asia (excluding Japan), Central and South America, Melanesia, Micronesia, and Polynesia. Total populations together with lifespan by sex as well as birthrates are listed for reference.

Source: UN, World Population Prospects: The 2005 Revision.

An Aging Society and Economic Development – The Case of Japan

Japan now enjoys the longest lifespan in the world (79.59 years for men and 86.44 for women in 2011). There are 25 million elderly people, comprising 20% of the total population of Japan. The ratio of the elderly population is now the highest in the world, and it will continue to be significantly higher than in most Western (Figure 3a) and Asian countries (Figure 3b). The third characteristic of the Japanese society is the high ratio of the most aged sector of the population (75 years old and above) among the elderly. The share of this group was 9.0% in the year 2005, and it will rise to 12.5% by 2015. These characteristics are partly due to the rapid aging of the society.

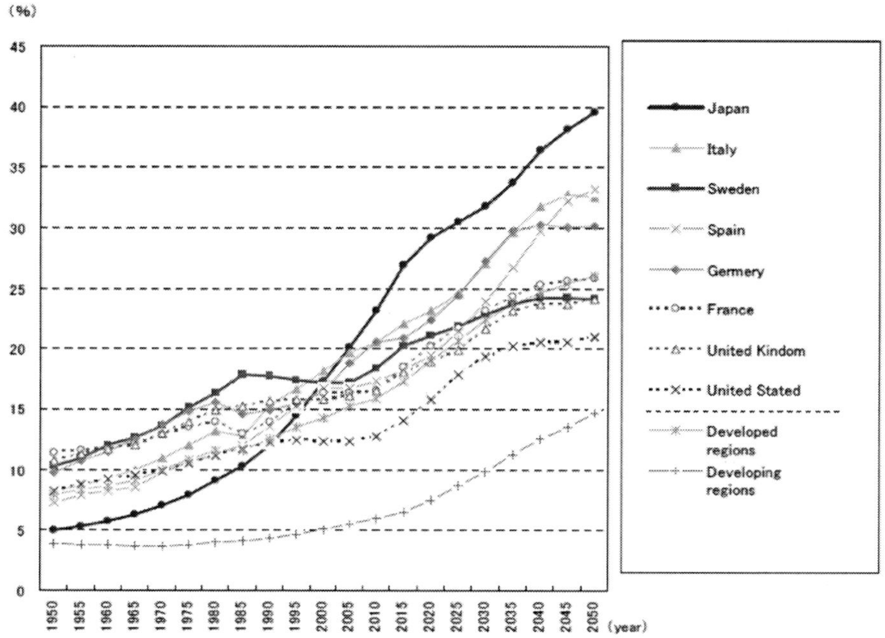

(a)

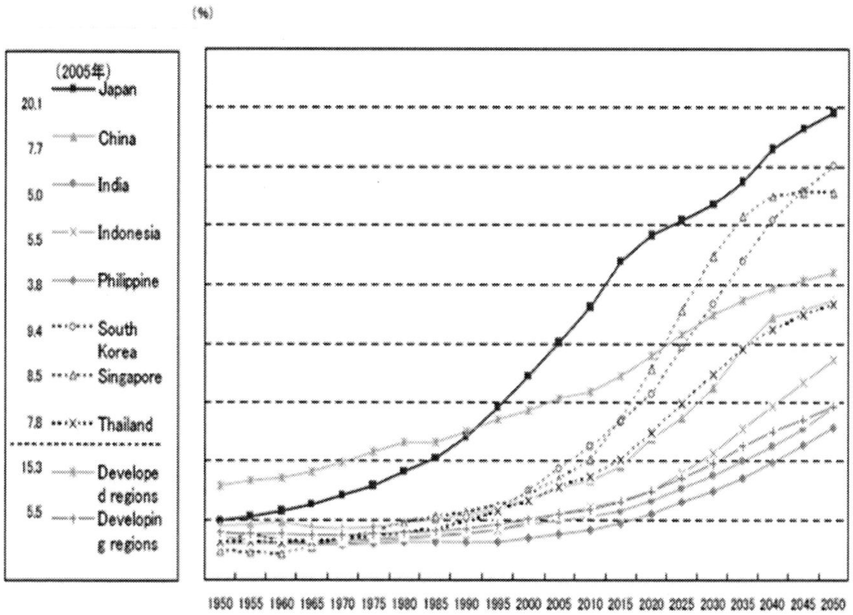

(b)

Figure 3. Ratio of elderly population by country (a) Japan and European countries, (b) Japan and Asian countries. Source: for Japan: National Census of Japan (Ministry of Internal Affairs and Communications) and on the projected population of Japan (National Institute of Population and Social Security Research) on the assumption that birth and death rates are ranked medium (estimated in December 2006). Developed regions include North America, Japan, Europe, Australia and New Zealand. Developing regions include Africa, Asia (other than Japan), Central and South America, Melanesia, Micronesia, and Polynesia.

A society is called "aging" when the elderly population exceeds 7%, "aged" at 14%, and "super-aged" at 20% or more elderly people.

It took only 24 years (1970 to 1994) for Japan to change from an aging (7% elderly people) to an aged society (14% elderly), which is in sharp contrast to most Western countries where the transition takes 40-120 years. It took 40 years (1932 to 1972) in Germany, 47 years in the United Kingdom (1929 to 1976), 61 years in Italy (1927 to 1988), an expected 71 years in the USA (1942 to 2013), and 115 years in France (1864 to 1979) (Table 2). Rapid aging has caused a strain in Japanese society for which academia, industry, public service, and government policy-makers are struggling to find a solution. A similar, even more rapid transition to an aging society is expected in Singapore and South Korea. In most developed countries there will an elderly population of more than 20% after the year 2030.

Table 2. Speed of societal aging

	Year the elderly population reaches 7%	Year the elderly population reaches 14%	Year the elderly population reaches 20%	E Period from 7% to 14% (year)	F Period from 14% to 20% (year)	E+F Period from 7% to 20% (year)
S Korea	**2000**	**2019**	**2026**	19	7	26
Japan	**1970**	**1994**	**2006**	24	12	36
China	**2000**	**2030**	**2039**	30	9	39
Germany	**1932**	**1972**	**2012**	40	40	80
UK	**1929**	**1976**	**2021**	47	45	92
Italy	**1927**	**1988**	**2007**	61	19	80
USA	**1942**	**2013**	**2028**	71	15	86
France	**1864**	**1979**	**2020**	115	41	156

The Unique Cultural Background of the Japanese Society

Japanese culture is a mixture of the Western and the Oriental. Westernization suddenly occurred in 1868 (the Meiji Restoration, which opened the door to the Western culture) and Americanization in 1945 (end of World War 2), causing drastic changes in all aspects of societal values, such as morals, esteem, and respect for the elderly.

The traditional Japanese living style was nurtured by Shinto and Buddhism for more than a thousand years, during which loyalty to the authority and respectfulness to the elderly were highly valued. According to the lifestyle of the people believing in Shinto or Buddhism, living in a large family is very common, and elderly people are treated with respect and dignity due to their experience, wisdom, knowledge, and accumulated common sense.

Japanese people live their lives under an absolute family chief, who pays great respect to the elderly parents.

The majority of Japanese believe in Shinto (107 million) and Buddhism (89 million), while only 3 million are Christians (National Census by the Japanese Ministry of Education, 2010). Even though the philosophical thinking of the Japanese is still heavily influenced by oriental religion and culture, the lifestyle of the Japanese people has significantly changed since the end of World War 2.

Social Determinants of the Lifestyle and Care of the Japanese Elderly

As shown in Figure 4, the living arrangements of the elderly Japanese have changed from living with children to a new style, where couples live alone. In 1980, about 70% of the elderly lived in families with children. However, the number of elderly people living in three-generation families dropped to 44% in 2006, in sharp contrast to the increase in the number of elderly couples living alone.

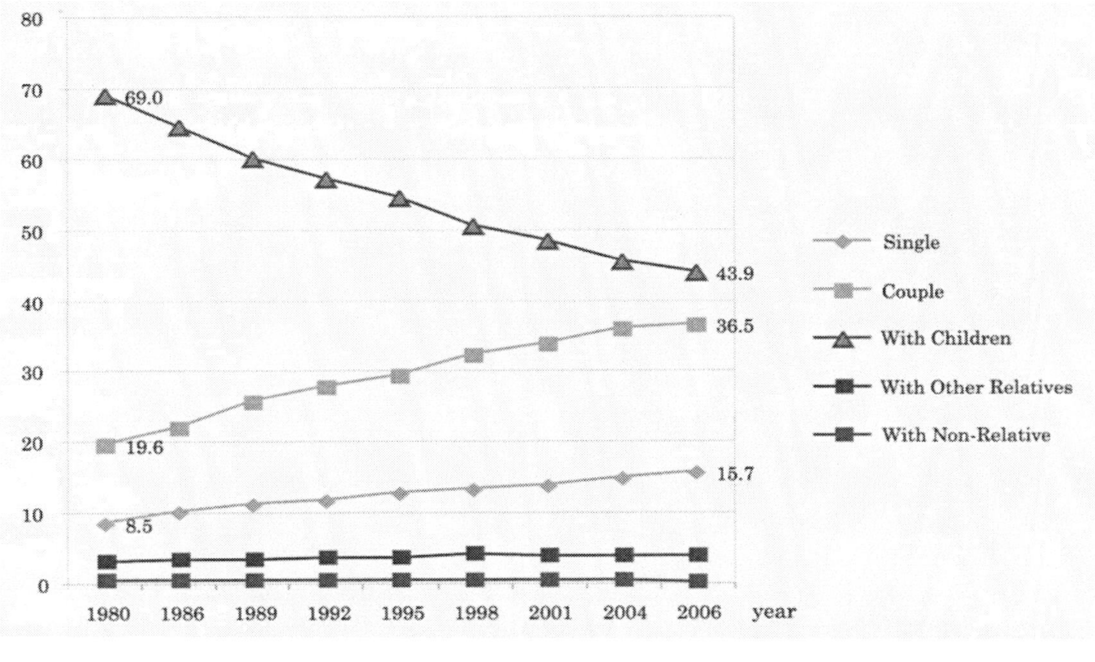

Figure 4. Living arrangements of individuals aged 65 and over (%).

A change in the preferred relations with children may explain the actual change in the living arrangements of the Japanese elderly. As shown in Figure 5, 60% of the elderly people wanted a living situation in which they hoped to always live together with their children and grandchildren in 1960, but this percentage has declined year by year, and in 2005 more than half of the elderly people wanted to live apart from their children, keeping frequent contact for meals and conversation. The preference of the elderly has changed from living in a three-generation family to independent living and keeping up a close relationship with their children. This trend indicates that the elderly prefer a more independent lifestyle in a separate family, with less intimate relationships with their children and grandchildren.

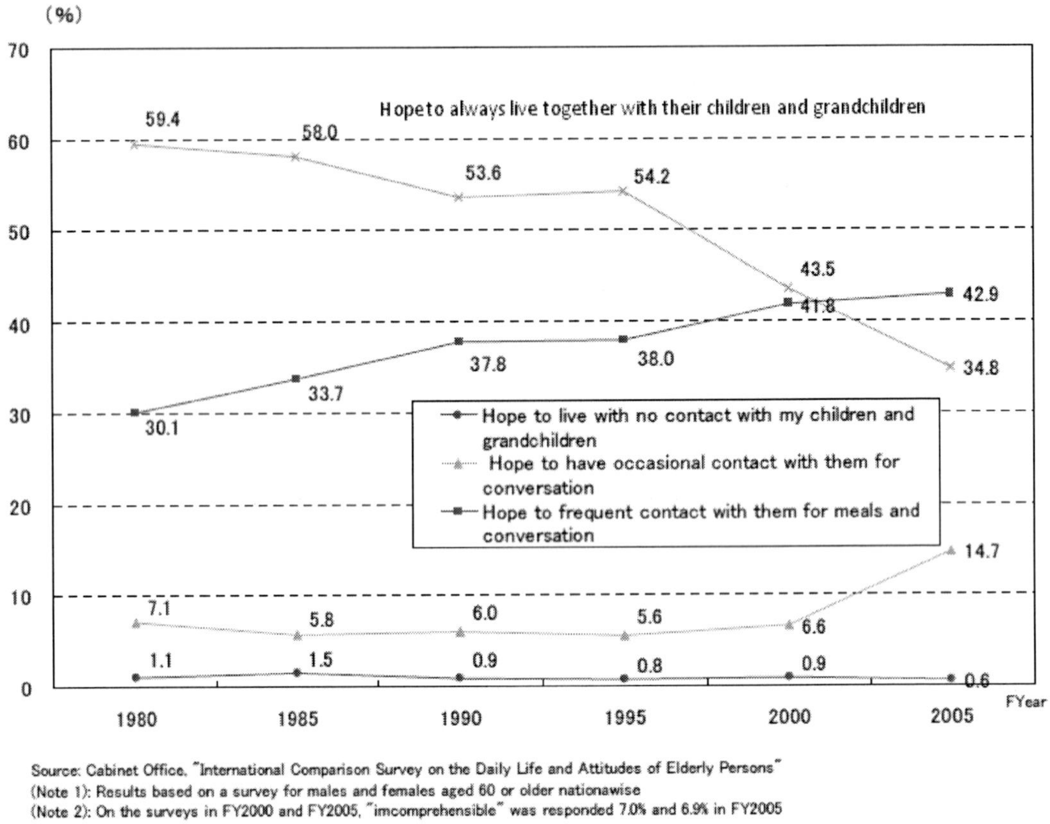

Figure 5. Change of relationships with families of the Japanese elderly.

This change in lifestyle is reflected by the wishes of the elderly people for whom their families should provide nursing care (Figure 6). It used to be true that many elderly people were cared for by daughters or daughters-in-law because they lived together in a family. But it is no longer realistic to ask for the help of a daughter or daughter-in-law because they live elsewhere in a different family.

This is partly due to the change in women's lifestyle from the old traditional one to the modern lifestyle. Before World War 2, Japanese women were expected to be married by arrangement of their parents, to be a good wife, to support their husbands, to be a good housekeeper, to raise children, to take care of their old parents-in-law, and to dedicate themselves to the family. But now the younger women seek jobs outside the house in society and are no longer expected to confine themselves to the house.

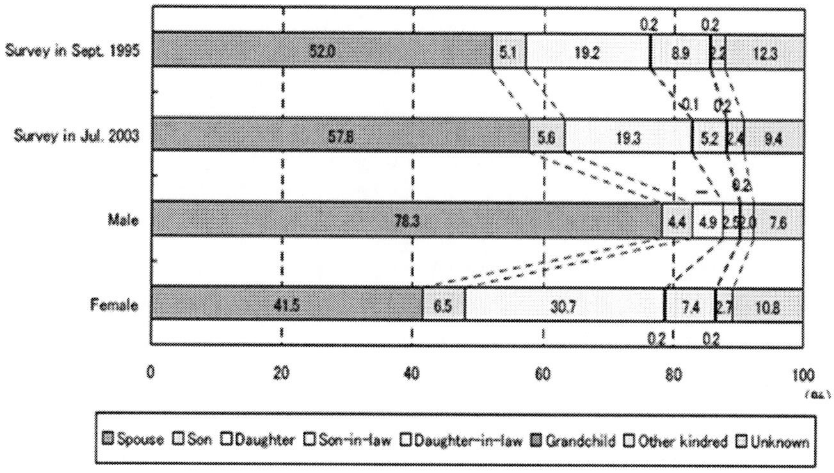

Japanese elderly is dependent to the spouse now, indicating decreasing role of daughter-in-law.

Figure 6. Who in the family will hopefully provide nursing care?

It is a drastic change for the Japanese elderly, especially the men who think they can rely on their wife and not on the daughter-in law.

It is good to observe the change in attitude as the elderly become more independent of children and grandchildren. But, in reality, the social system is not functioning well as far as supporting the life of the elderly is concerned. Survey data of primary caregivers to elderly people requiring long-term care is shown in Figure 7, clearly indicating that more than half (56%) of caregivers to the elderly are elderly themselves. In Japan's super-aged society, care of the elderly rests upon the elderly.

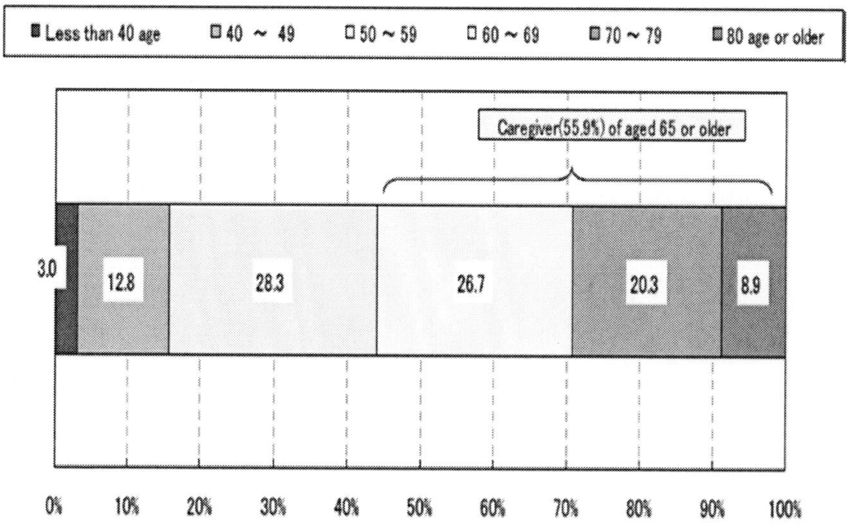

Figure 7. Constituent ratio by age group of primary caregivers of elderly people requiring long-term care.

CONCLUSION

In the Asia-Pacific region alone there were 13.7 million dementia patients in 2005, a figure which is expected to rise to 64.6 million by 2050, growing by a factor of 4.7 in 45 years. In addition to the high prevalence rate, severe disability in the patients' daily life, the burden on caring persons, and the long duration of the disease make dementia the heaviest burden on society.

In order to implement a social system in which the elderly people, including dementia patients, can live active lives, social determinants for the mental health of the elderly should be investigated in greater detail because the societal system should be designed and built for the elderly, giving full consideration to a society's cultural and traditional background.

I want to conclude this chapter by presenting a few proposals for designing the new social system.

First of all, we should change the wrong, backward-looking concept in which the elderly people used to be regarded as of little use to society. Considering the fact that a significant portion (15-30%) of society will be composed of elderly people in the near future, they should be a major component of society. The elderly should not be dependent on society; they should be the manpower supporting it. No society can survive without giving consideration to the elderly in its economy, its value code, and its government policy.

However, it is also true that the elderly are physically fragile, and it is not realistic to think of them as working all day long. It is advisable for the elderly to contemplate a balance between working and lifestyle. We need to implement a working environment in which the elderly can voluntarily share working opportunities. This is the only way in which the super-aged society can survive.

Jobs are not the only activity in which the elderly should participate. Even where those who do not need money are concerned it is still important to promote commitment to community activities to fulfill an active life. For this purpose, municipal service arrangements are highly recommended. Physical and mental isolation is the greatest evil for the elderly. Elderly people should be included in societal activity.

It is important to communicate to the people that we are responsible for leading a healthy life in our old age. To do so, we should plan our lives as elderly persons well in advance, no later than the age of fifty, giving full consideration to various social determinants.

In: Social Determinants and Mental Health
Editor: Sabine Bährer-Kohler
ISBN: 978-1-61324-353-4

Chapter 20

Lifespan Perspective – Loneliness in Older Persons: Correlates and Outcomes

Jiska Cohen-Mansfield
Department of Health Promotion, School of Public Health, Herczeg Center on Aging, Tel-Aviv, Israel
Department of Health Care Sciences and of Prevention and Community Health, George Washington University Medical Center and School of Public Health, US

Abstract

This chapter reviews the literature regarding loneliness in relation to the Model of Depression and Loneliness (MODEL) theoretical framework. The relationship between loneliness in old age and 1) demographic characteristics (age, marital status, gender, etc.), 2) personal characteristics (e.g., health, cognitive function, and psychological attributes), 3) environmental characteristics (e.g., social support, social network), 4) outcomes (morbidity, mental health, and mortality) is examined. Cross sectional findings, and longitudinal trends in and predictors of loneliness, are presented separately. Loneliness from a cross cultural perspective and implications for interventions are discussed.

Introduction

Loneliness is a sentiment experienced by a person defining his or her form or level of relationships as inadequate (Weiss, 1973), or an unpleasant subjective state of sensing a discrepancy between the desired amount of companionship or emotional support and that which is available in the person's environment (Blazer, 2002). Loneliness is a relatively common emotion experienced by older persons, and it is estimated that 40% of older persons are lonely at least sometimes - a rate that has apparently not changed much for several decades (Havens, Hall, Sylvestre, & Jivan, 2004; Routasalo, Savikko, Tilvis, Strandberg, & Pitkälä, 2006; Savikko, Routasalo, Tilvis, Strandberg, & Pitkälä, 2005; Weeks, 1994). Studies suggest that loneliness has both social and emotional dimensions (Russell, Cutrona, Rose, & Yurko, 1984). Creecy, Berg, and Wright (1985) and Larson (1990) described social loneliness as stemming from the absence of a meaningful friendship. Emotional loneliness has been described as the absence of an enduring intimate attachment to another (Russell, et al., 1984; Weiss, 1973). Other related terms refer to a more objective state than loneliness. Specifically, social isolation, which refers to having no or minimal contact with other people, or with specific types of others (Chappell & Badger, 1989; Wenger, Davies, Shahtahmasebi, & Scott, 1996), and social disconnectedness which involves a lack of contact with other people, as indicated by a small size of social network, or low frequency of social interactions (Cornwell & Waite, 2009). While loneliness has been contrasted with belonging, social isolation is opposite to social participation (Dykstra, 2009).

Theoretical Framework

In this chapter, we examine loneliness in relation to the Model of Depression and Loneliness (MODEL; Cohen-Mansfield & Parpura-Gill, 2007) theoretical framework, which describes environmental, health, and psychological reasons for loneliness in old age (see Figure 1). Specifically, *environmental factors* that contribute to loneliness include lack of opportunities to meet people, living arrangements, and diminished financial resources. *Health factors* consist of poor health and mobility difficulties. Lastly, *psychological factors* relate to insufficient social skills and low social self-efficacy. Studies of demographic, personal (health and psychological), and environmental contributors to loneliness in older persons are presented next.

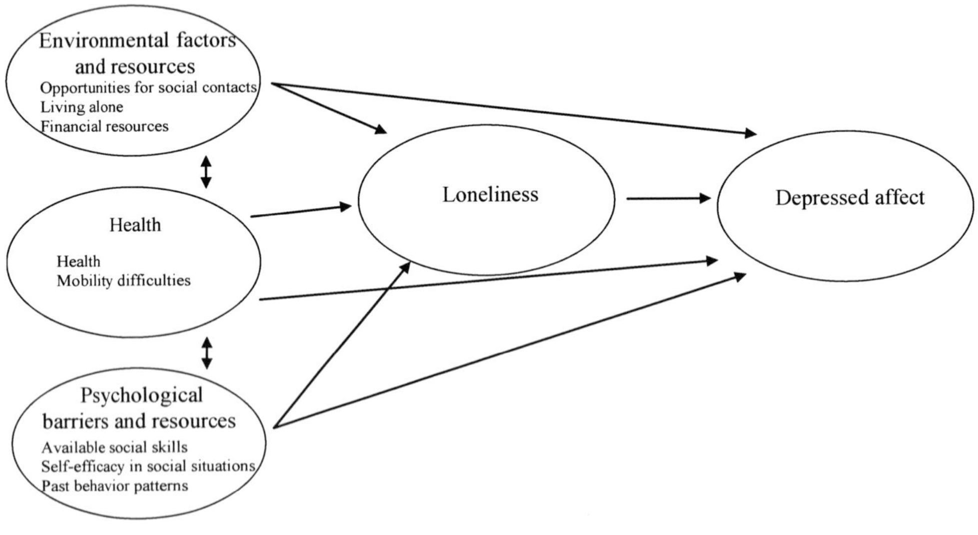

Figure 1. MODEL – Model of Depression and Loneliness © Cohen-Mansfield.

CROSS-SECTIONAL FINDINGS

Loneliness and Demographic Characteristics

Cross-sectional studies on demographic factors associated with loneliness in old age have yielded varied results. Regarding marital status, being unmarried was the most potent predictor of loneliness in a national sample of 75-94 year olds in Israel (Cohen-Mansfield et al.,2009), and marital status (widowhood\ nonmarried\ separated\ divorced\ widowed but not remarried) is commonly found to be related to loneliness (Dugan & Kivett, 1994; Havens, et al., 2004; Holmén, Ericsson, Andersson, & Winblad, 1992; Paul, Ayis, & Shah, 2006; Routasalo & Pitkala, 2003; Routasalo, et al., 2006; Steed, Boldy, Grenade, & Iredell, 2007; Stessman, et al., 1996; Theeke, 2010; Tijhuis, De Jong-Gierveld, Feskens, & Kromhout, 1999; Victor, Scambler, Bowling, & Bond, 2005; Wenger & Burholt, 2004). However, marital status was unrelated to loneliness in one study (Kim, 1999), while in other studies, marital status was related to loneliness through a mediating social network factor (Barron, Foxall, Von Dollen, Jones, & Shull, 1994; Dykstra & de Jong Gierveld, 2004).

Regarding age, associations between older age and loneliness have been found in several studies (Golden, et al., 2009; Savikko, et al., 2005; Victor, et al., 2005), though in one study these became insignificant after adjusting for age-related variables (Golden, et al., 2009) and a relationship with younger age was also reported (Theeke, 2010). Findings regarding gender are also inconclusive, as some associate loneliness with female gender (Beal, 2006; Golden, et al., 2009; Holmén, et al., 1992; Pinquart & Sörensen, 2001) and others with male gender (Andersson & Stevens, 1993; Chang & Yang, 1999; Mullins & Mushel, 1992). In another study, no gender differences were found (Tiikkainen, 2004).

Loneliness and Personal Characteristics: Health and Psychological

Regarding personal characteristics, a number of health factors have been found to relate to loneliness. These include poor subjective health (Cornwell & Waite, 2009; Havens, et al., 2004; Holmén, et al., 1992; Routasalo, et al., 2006; Savikko, et al., 2005; Steed, et al., 2007; Theeke, 2010; Tijhuis, et al., 1999; Victor, et al., 2005), a larger number of chronic illnesses (Theeke, 2010), impaired hearing (Dugan & Kivett, 1994; Victor, et al., 2005), functional disability (Jylhä, 2004; Kim, 1999; Korporaal, Broese van Groenou, & van Tilburg, 2008; Theeke, 2010), lack of mobility (Mellor & Edelmann, 1988), motor decline (Buchman, et al., 2010), poor self-reported functioning (Routasalo, et al., 2006; Savikko, et al., 2005), psychiatric morbidity (Bowling, Edelmann, Leaver, & Hoekel, 1989; Victor, et al., 2005), and depression (Luanaigh & Lawlor, 2008; Routasalo, et al., 2006; Stessman, et al., 1996; Tiikkainen, 2004). Traumatic events may also serve to increase loneliness. Specifically, older persons who had lost a partner experienced greater emotional loneliness shortly after the loss compared to their pre-loss scores (Van Baarsen, Smit, Snijders, & Knipscheer, 1999).

While some studies have found cognitive decline to be related to loneliness (Conroy, Golden, Jeffares, O'Neill, & McGee, 2010; Havens, et al., 2004; Holmén, et al., 1992), others have found no such relationship (Fees, Martin, & Poon, 1999; Stessman, et al., 1996; Tijhuis, et al., 1999). In yet another study, findings indicated that better cognition of centenarians was related to lower levels of loneliness in a Swedish sample, though not in an American sample (Martin, Hagberg, & Poon, 1997).

Several psychological characteristics have been linked with loneliness. Past behavior patterns (i.e., never having good friends) significantly correlated with loneliness (Cohen-Mansfield & Parpura-Gill, 2007). Self-efficacy inversely predicted loneliness among older persons, varying by gender. Specifically, less loneliness was predicted by stronger social, interpersonal, and emotional self-efficacy in women, and stronger financial, physical, and instrumental self efficacy in men (Fry & Debats, 2002). In line with that, self-efficacy in social situations was found to be the most important predictor of loneliness (Cohen-Mansfield & Parpura-Gill, 2007). Perceptions of social competence skills are inversely related to persons' experience of loneliness (DiTommaso, Brannen-McNulty, Ross, & Burgess, 2003; Wittenberg & Reis, 1986). Yet, it is unclear whether self-evaluations of one's skills and behavior reflect one's actual performance. Thus, in one study, lonely persons were reported to have less adequate skills of forming and maintaining relationships (Wittenberg & Reis, 1986). In contrast, in another study the social performance of lonely persons in experimentally assigned roles did not differ from that of non-lonely persons within each role, but a difference was found in the self-evaluation of one's performance, with lonely persons rating it more poorly than non-lonely persons (Vitkus & Horowitz, 1987).

Loneliness and Environmental Characteristics

Environmental factors with the potential to affect loneliness in older adults include the quality and quantity of social networks, appropriateness of the environment to an individual's cognitive and functional capabilities, accessibility, living arrangements, and the availability of resources (e.g., financial, entertainment, transportation). Cohen-Mansfield and Parpura-Gill (2007) found that the environmental barriers of financial resources and lack of opportunities for social contact were potent predictors of loneliness. The impact of financial resources was demonstrated in other studies as well, showing that low levels of income and educational attainment (Routasalo, et al., 2006; Savikko, et al., 2005; Victor, et al., 2005) and low socio-economic status (Pinquart & Sörensen, 2001) were associated with loneliness.

The presence of social support, social networks, and social participation, were associated with decreased loneliness (Jylhä, 2004; Wu, et al., 2010). Quality and frequency of social contact were also linked with loneliness. Less contact with close friends as well as lower levels of satisfaction with the quality of family and friend relations were associated with loneliness among older persons (Mullins & Dugan, 1990). This last finding is not surprising as loneliness intrinsically involves dissatisfaction with amount or quality of social contacts. Accordingly, it was also reported to be positively related to being poorly understood and to having unfulfilled expectations of one's social contacts (Routasalo, et al., 2006), and to lack of social fulfillment (Creecy, et al., 1985).

Most studies found loneliness to be negatively related to frequency of contact with others (e.g., Iecovich, et al., 2004) although one found no such relationship (Routasalo, et al., 2006). The relationship between loneliness and social support may be mediated by other factors. For example, findings of a meta-analysis (Pinquart & Sörensen, 2001) indicated that an inverse relationship between friendship and loneliness was significant for unmarried participants, but not for married participants. The authors suggest that friendship may be less crucial to married persons who have sufficient support from their spouse. Yet, inverse associations between loneliness and variables of social relationships were found, even among married adults (Shiovitz-Ezra & Ayalon, 2010). The impact of marital status may be indirect, as married persons are more likely to have children, who tend to belong to the social support network of their parents. Similarly, and in line with the MODEL (Cohen-Mansfield & Parpura-Gill, 2007), married persons were found healthier across health indicators, which enabled them to be more mobile and more socially engaged in activities (Cohen-Mansfield, Shmotkin, & Goldberg, 2009). Additional differences relating to loneliness and one's marital status have been reported. Specifically, while among the married, lonelier persons more commonly experienced a larger number of traumatic events, had more doctor's visits, and were less cognitively vital, among the unmarried, those with financial difficulties, poor health, and less support from their social network, showed higher levels of loneliness. Thus loneliness may have different etiologies in these subgroups (Cohen-Mansfield, et al., 2009).

Residential status, such as residing in a nursing facility, in a residential home, or moving into these residencies was associated with loneliness (Pinquart & Sörensen, 2001; Savikko, et al., 2005; Tijhuis, et al., 1999) ,as was living alone (Golden, et al., 2009; Havens, et al., 2004; Routasalo & Pitkala, 2003; Savikko, et al., 2005; Steed, et al., 2007) and living with fewer persons in the household (Theeke, 2010). Also, of those with living in sheltered housing more than half were reported to experience loneliness (Holmén, et al., 1992). In contrast, living in an adult child's household or near a child's home is protective of loneliness (Wenger & Burholt, 2004).

Loneliness is more common among rural older adults than among those living in cities (Dong & Simon, 2010; Savikko, et al., 2005). The decision to stop driving, usually out of necessity and due to a slowed response to driving cues, can also have significant implications for the loneliness and wellbeing of older adults (Johnson, 1998; Kihl, 1993). This may be particularly true for rural older adults, who often equate an automobile and driver's license with mobility and quality of life (Kihl, 1993).

LONGITUDINAL TRENDS AND PREDICTORS OF LONELINESS

Longitudinal findings on loneliness in old age show divergent results. Loneliness was found to significantly increase with age in several studies (Cohen-Mansfield, et al., 2009; Dykstra, van Tilburg, & Gierveld, 2005; Jylhä, 2004; Wenger & Burholt, 2004), though non-significant trends of increase were also reported (Tiikkainen, 2004; Tijhuis, et al., 1999), as well as a significant decrease (Holmén, et al., 1992). According to Demakakos et al. (Demakakos, Nunn, & Nazroo), loneliness progresses non-linearly across middle and old age, and peaks among persons over 80 years of age. In line with that, a recent review suggests that loneliness in older adults is most prevalent in those aged 80 and over and less common among middle-aged and young-old persons (Dykstra, 2009).

In contrast with the numerous aforementioned studies that examined the factors associated with loneliness in old age cross-sectionally, only a few dealt with its longitudinal predictors. These predictors include the absence of a spouse or partner (Dykstra, et al., 2005; Jylhä, 2004), lower financial status, poorer health, female gender (Cohen-Mansfield, et al., 2009), and decreased functional capacity (Dykstra, et al., 2005). Among older adults who experienced partner loss, greater levels of loneliness were predicted by a combination of psychological factors, i.e., being unable to anticipate the partner's death, and difficulties with establishing personal social contacts; health factors, i.e., worse physical condition, and social network factors, i.e., receiving less support from the social network prior to the loss (Van Baarsen, et al., 1999).

Outcomes

According to cross-sectional findings, loneliness is associated with hopelessness, depressed mood, lower levels of wellbeing (Golden, et al., 2009), poor quality of life (Paul et al., 2006), and is a potential risk factor for depression (Luanaigh & Lawlor, 2008). Furthermore, loneliness predicts poor quality of life (Chalise, Saito, & Kai, 2007), and psychological stress (Paul, et al., 2006). A review from 2008 concluded that loneliness is associated with various adverse physical health outcomes, such as higher blood pressure, poor sleep, immune stress responses, and cognitive deterioration over time in older adults (Luanaigh & Lawlor, 2008). In line with that, loneliness in older persons is linked with increased risk for late-life dementia (Wilson, et al., 2007). In a recent study, persons who were lonely in 2 waves of the study, two years apart, were reported to exercise less, use less alcohol, smoke more, score higher on depression, have more chronic illnesses and a larger average number of nursing home stays, compared with those who were not lonely on one of the waves, or both (Theeke, 2010).

Regarding the life-expectancy of lonely persons, loneliness was identified as a predictor of mortality (Penninx, et al., 1997; Shiovitz-Ezra & Ayalon, 2010), found to increase all-cause mortality risk (Seeman, 2000), and to have an indirect effect on mortality via associations with chronic disease, functional status, and self-rated health (Sugisawa, Liang, & Liu, 1994). Stek et al. (2005) found a circa twofold higher mortality risk for the oldest-old who suffered from feelings of both loneliness and depression. Finally, loneliness was an independent predictor of suicide among 65-74 year olds. Among persons aged 75 and above, loneliness was linked to suicide and marginally predicted suicide (Waern, Rubenowitz, & Wilhelmson, 2003).

Cross-Cultural Comparisons of Loneliness

Loneliness has been documented in many countries worldwide (Perlman, 2004; Stack, 1998; Sundström, Fransson, Malmberg, & Davey, 2009). Cross-cultural studies have shown that there are differences in the prevalence of reported loneliness in adults across cultures (see Routasalo & Pitkala, 2003). Cultural factors are related to and perhaps affect the very essence of the phenomenon (Perlman, 2004) as well as the acceptability of reporting it. Recent findings of a study comparing social network and wellbeing of older persons across two regional settings, one consisting of 5 Mediterranean countries and the other of 7 non-Mediterranean countries support this notion. The authors concluded that social network is a contextually bound phenomenon which may differ in its manifestation across different geographical regions (Litwin, 2010). Similarly, in a study of older persons aged 70-89 who live in the Netherlands, Tuscany, Italy, and Manitoba, Canada differences in the intensity of loneliness by location were found. Emotional loneliness was high for the Manitobans while social loneliness was high for the Tuscans. However, the determinants of loneliness were similar across the three countries. One exception was having a partner which served as a protector from loneliness to a greater extent in the Netherlands, compared to Italy and Canada (van Tilburg, Havens, & de Jong Gierveld, 2004).

CONCLUSION

The study of loneliness in older adults is imperative because the associated health risks may be especially severe for the older segment of the population (Luanaigh & Lawlor, 2008; Sorkin, Rook, & Lu, 2002; Tomaka, Thompson, & Palacios, 2006; Wilson, et al., 2007). Interventions which involve educational and social activity may be particularly helpful (Cattan, White, Bond, & Learmouth, 2005). Intervention programs targeting the quality of the older person's social network may yield additional benefits including improved cognitive function, decreased depression, and a better quality of life (Winningham & Pike, 2007). The finding of different predictors of loneliness in subgroups of the older populations, such as married and unmarried (Cohen-Mansfield, et al., 2009) supports the notion of tailoring different interventions for specific groups (Cattan, et al., 2005), targeting different issues such as grief over trauma or cognitive decline among the married vs. opportunities to access social events and contacts for the unmarried. Therefore, in line with the MODEL (Cohen-Mansfield & Parpura-Gill, 2007), it seems that a combination of psychological interventions, such as those addressing issues of social skills or self efficacy and social interventions increasing appropriate social opportunities as well as addressing environmental issues, such as access to available opportunities are needed. Future studies of correlates of and interventions for loneliness in older adults are needed in order to better understand how to mollify the impact of loneliness in old age.

REFERENCES

Andersson, L., & Stevens, N. (1993). Associations between early experiences with parents and well-being in old age. *Journal of Gerontology, 48*(3), P109-P116.

Blazer, D. G. (2002). Self-efficacy and depression in late life: A primary prevention proposal. *Aging and Mental Health, 6*(4), 315.

Bowling, A. P., Edelmann, R. J., Leaver, J., & Hoekel, T. (1989). Loneliness, mobility, well-being and social support in a sample of over 85 year olds. *Personality and Individual Differences, 10*(11), 1189-1192.

Buchman, A. S., Boyle, P. A., Wilson, R. S., James, B. D., Leurgans, S. E., Arnold, S. E., et al. (2010). Loneliness and the rate of motor decline in old age : The rush memory and aging project , a community-based cohort study. *Bmc Geriatrics, 10*(1), 77.

Cattan, M., White, M., Bond, J., & Learmouth, A. (2005). Preventing social isolation and loneliness among older people: A systematic review of health promotion interventions. *Ageing & Society, 25*(01), 41-67.

Chalise, H. N., Saito, T., & Kai, I. (2007). Correlates of loneliness among older newar adults in Nepal. *Nippon Koshu Eisei Zasshi, 54*(7), 427-433.

Chang, S. H., & Yang, M. S. (1999). The relationships between the elderly: Loneliness and its factors of personal attributes, perceived health status, and social support. *Kaohsiung Journal of Medical Sciences, 1999*(15), 337-347.

Chappell, N. L., & Badger, M. (1989). Social isolation and well-being. *Journal of Gerontology, 44*(5), S169-S176.

Cohen-Mansfield, J., & Parpura-Gill, A. (2007). Loneliness in older persons: A theoretical model and empirical findings. *International Psychogeriatrics, 19*, 279-294.

Cohen-Mansfield, J., Shmotkin, D., & Goldberg, S. (2009). Loneliness in old age: Longitudinal changes and their determinants in an Israeli sample. *International Psychogeriatrics, 21*(06), 1160-1170.

Cornwell, E. Y., & Waite, L. J. (2009). Social disconnectedness, perceived isolation, and health among older adults. *Journal of Health & Social Behavior, 50*(1), 31-48.

Creecy, R. F., Berg, W. E., & Wright, R. (1985). Loneliness among the elderly: A causal approach. *Journal of Gerontology, 40*(4), 487-493.

Demakakos, P., Nunn, S., & Nazroo, J. (2006). Loneliness, relative deprivation, and life satisfaction. In J. Banks, E. Breeze, C. Lessof & J. Nazroo (Eds.), *Retirement, health, and relationships of the older population in england: The 2004 English longitudinal study of aging*. London: Institute for Fiscal Studies.

DiTommaso, E., Brannen-McNulty, C., Ross, L., & Burgess, M. (2003). Attachment styles, social skills and loneliness in young adults. *Personality and Individual Differences, 35*(2), 303-312.

Dong, X., & Simon, M. A. (2010). Health and aging in a chinese population: Urban and rural disparities. *Geriatrics & Gerontology International, 10*(1), 85-93.

Dugan, E., & Kivett, V. R. (1994). The importance of emotional and social isolation to loneliness among very old rural adults. *The Gerontologist, 34*, 340-347.

Dykstra, P. (2009). Older adult loneliness: Myths and realities. *European Journal of Ageing, 6*(2), 91-100.

Dykstra, P. A., van Tilburg, T. G., & Gierveld, J. d. J. (2005). Changes in older adult loneliness. *Research on Aging, 27*(6), 725-747.

Fees, B. S., Martin, P., & Poon, L. W. (1999). A model of loneliness in older adults. *The Journals of Gerontology Series B: Psychological Sciences and Social Sciences, 54B*(4), P231-P239.

Fry, S. P., & Debats, D. L. (2002). Self-efficacy beliefs as predictors of loneliness and psychological distress in older adults. *The International Journal of Aging and Human Development, 55*(3), 233-269.

Golden, J., Conroy, R. M., Bruce, I., Denihan, A., Greene, E., Kirby, M., et al. (2009). Loneliness, social support networks, mood, and wellbeing in community-dwelling elderly. *International Journal of Geriatric Psychiatry, 24*(7), 694-700.

Havens, B., Hall, M., Sylvestre, G., & Jivan, T. (2004). Social isolation and loneliness: Differences between older rural and urban manitobans. *Canadian Journal on Aging, 23*, 129-140.

Holmén, K., Ericsson, K., Andersson, L., & Winblad, B. (1992). Loneliness among elderly people living in Stockholm: A population study. *Journal of Advanced Nursing, 17*(43-51).

Iecovich, E., Barasch, M., Mirsky, J., Kaufman, R., Avgar, A., & Kol-Fogelson, A. (2004). Social support networks and loneliness among elderly Jews in Russia and Ukraine. *Journal of Marriage and Family, 66*(2), 306-317.

Johnson, J. E. (1998). Older rural adults and the decision to stop driving: The influence of family and friends. [Article]. *Journal of Community Health Nursing, 15*, 205.

Jylhä, M. (2004). Old age and loneliness: Cross - sectional and longitudinal analyses in the Tampere longitudinal study on aging. *Canadian Journal on Aging La Revue Canadienne Du Vieillissement, 23*(2), 157-168.

Kihl, M. R. (1993). Need for transportation alternatives for the rural elderly. In C. N. Bull (Ed.), *Aging in rural America* (pp. 84-98). Newbury Park, CA: Sage.

Kim, O. (1999). Predictors of loneliness in elderly Korean immigrant women living in the United States of America. *Journal of Advanced Nursing, 29*, 1082-1088.

Korporaal, M., Broese van Groenou, M. I., & van Tilburg, T. G. (2008). Effects of own and spousal disability on loneliness among older adults. *Journal of Aging and Health, 20*(3), 306-325.

Larson, R. W. (1990). The solitary side of life: An examination of the time people spend alone from childhood to old age. *Developmental Review, 10*(2), 155-183.

Litwin, H. (2010). Social networks and well-being: A comparison of older people in Mediterranean and non-Mediterranean countries. *The Journals of Gerontology Series B: Psychological Sciences and Social Sciences, 65B*(5), 599-608.

Luanaigh, C. O., & Lawlor, B. A. (2008). Loneliness and the health of older people. *International Journal of Geriatric Psychiatry, 23*(12), 1213-1221.

Martin, P., Hagberg, B., & Poon, L. W. (1997). Predictors of loneliness in centenarians: A parallel study. *Journal of Cross-Cultural Gerontology, 12*(3), 203-224.

Mellor, K. S., & Edelmann, R. J. (1988). Mobility, social support, loneliness, and well-being amongst two groups of older adults. *Personality and Individual Differences, 9*(1), 1-5.

Mullins, L. C., & Dugan, E. (1990). The influence of depression and family and friendship relations on residents' loneliness in congregate housing. *The Gerontologist, 30*(3), 377-384.

Mullins, L. C., & Mushel, M. (1992). The existence and emotional closeness of relationships with children, friends, and spouses. *Research on Aging, 14*(4), 448-470.

Paul, C., Ayis, S., & Shah, E. (2006). Psychological distress, loneliness and disability in old age. *Psychology, Health and Medicine, 11*(2), 221-232.

Penninx, B., van Tillburg, T., Kriegsman, D., Deeg, D., Boeke, A., & van Eijk, J. (1997). Effects of social support and personal coping resources on mortality in older age: The longitudinal aging study in Amsterdam. *American Journal of Epidemiology, 146*(6), 510-519.

Perlman, D. (2004). European and Canadian studies of loneliness among seniors. *Canadian Journal on Aging La Revue Canadienne Du Vieillissement, 23*(2), 181-188.

Pinquart, M., & Sörensen, S. (2001). Influences on loneliness in older adults: A meta-analysis. *Basic and Applied Social Psychology, 23*, 245-266.

Routasalo, P., & Pitkala, K. H. (2003). Loneliness among older people. *Reviews in Clinical Gerontology, 13*(303-311).

Routasalo, P. E., Savikko, N., Tilvis, R. S., Strandberg, T. E., & Pitkälä, K. H. (2006). Social contacts and their relationship to loneliness among aged people - a population based study. *Gerontology, 52*(181-187).

Russell, D., Cutrona, C. E., Rose, J., & Yurko, K. (1984). Social and emotional loneliness: An examination of Weiss's typology of loneliness. *Journal of Personality and Social Psychology, 46*(6), 1313-1321.

Savikko, N., Routasalo, P., Tilvis, R. S., Strandberg, T. E., & Pitkälä, K. H. (2005). Predictors and subjective causes of loneliness in an aged population. *Archives of Gerontology and Geriatrics, 41*, 223-233.

Seeman, T. E. (2000). Health promoting effects of friends and family on health outcomes in older adults. *American Journal of Health Promotion, 14*, 362-370.

Shiovitz-Ezra, S., & Ayalon, L. (2010). Situational versus chronic loneliness as risk factors for all-cause mortality. *International Psychogeriatrics, 22*, 455-462.

Sorkin, D., Rook, K., & Lu, J. (2002). Loneliness, lack of emotional support, lack of companionship, and the likelihood of having a heart condition in an elderly sample. *Annals of Behavioral Medicine, 24*(4), 290-298.

Stack, S. (1998). Marriage, family and loneliness: A crossnational study. *Sociological Perspectives, 41*, 415-432.

Steed, L., Boldy, D., Grenade, L., & Iredell, H. (2007). The demographics of loneliness among older people in perth, western Australia. *Australian Journal on Aging, 26*, 81-86.

Stek, M. L., Vinkers, D. J., Gussekloo, J., Beekman, A. T. F., van der mast Roos, C., & Westendorp, R. J. G. (2005). Is depression in old age fatal only when people feel lonely? *American Journal of Psychiatry, 162*, 178-180.

Stessman, J., Ginsberg, G., Klein, M., Hammerman-Rozenberg, R., Friedman, R., & Cohen, A. (1996). Determinants of loneliness in Jerusalem's 70-year-old population. *Israel Journal of Medical Sciences, 32*, 639-648.

Sugisawa, H., Liang, J., & Liu, X. (1994). Social networks, social support, and mortality among older people in Japan. *Journal of Gerontology, 49*(1), S3-S13.

Sundström, G., Fransson, E., Malmberg, B., & Davey, A. (2009). Loneliness among older europeans. *European Journal of Ageing, 6*(4), 267-275.

Theeke, L. A. (2010). Sociodemographic and health-related risks for loneliness and outcome differences by loneliness status in a sample of US older adults. *Research in Gerontological Nursing, 3*(2), 113.

Tiikkainen, P., & Heikkinen, R. L. (2004). Associations between loneliness, depressive symptoms and perceived togetherness in older people. *Aging & Mental Health, 9*(526-534).

Tijhuis, M. A., De Jong-Gierveld, J., Feskens, E. J., & Kromhout, D. (1999). Changes in and factors related to loneliness in older men. The Zutphen elderly study. *Age and Ageing, 28*(5), 491-495.

Tomaka, J., Thompson, S., & Palacios, R. (2006). The relation of social isolation, loneliness, and social support to disease outcomes among the elderly. *Journal of Aging and Health, 18*(3), 359-384.

Van Baarsen, B., Smit, J. H., Snijders, T. A. B., & Knipscheer, K. P. M. (1999). Do personal conditions and circumstances surrounding partner loss explain loneliness in newly bereaved older adults? *Ageing & Society, 19*(04), 441-469.

van Tilburg, T., Havens, B., & de Jong Gierveld, J. (2004). Loneliness among older adults in the Netherlands, Italy, and Canada: A multifaceted comparison. *Canadian Journal on Aging La Revue Canadienne Du Vieillissement, 23*(2), 169-180.

Victor, C. R., Scambler, S. J., Bowling, A., & Bond, J. (2005). The prevalence of, and risk factors for, loneliness in later life: A survey of older people in Great Britain. *Ageing & Society, 25*(03), 357-375.

Vitkus, J., & Horowitz, L. M. (1987). Poor social performance of lonely people: Lacking a skill or adopting a role? *Journal of Personality and Social Psychology, 52*(6), 1266-1273.

Waern, M., Rubenowitz, E., & Wilhelmson, K. (2003). Predictors of suicide in the old elderly. *Gerontology, 49*, 328-334.

Weeks, D. J. (1994). Review of loneliness concepts, with particular reference to old age. *International Journal of Geriatric Psychiatry, 9*, 345-355.

Weiss, R. S. (1973). *Loneliness: The experience of emotional and social isolation.* Cambridge, MA: The MIT Press.

Wenger, G. C., & Burholt, V. (2004). Changes in levels of social isolation and loneliness among older people in a rural area: A twenty-year longitudinal study. *Canadian Journal on Aging, 23*(115-127).

Wenger, G. C., Davies, R., Shahtahmasebi, S., & Scott, A. (1996). Social isolation and loneliness in old age: Review and model refinement. *Ageing & Society, 16*(03), 333-358.

Wilson, R. S., Krueger, K. R., Arnold, S. E., Schneider, J. A., Kelly, J. F., Barnes, L. L., et al. (2007). Loneliness and risk of Alzheimer disease. *Arch Gen Psychiatry, 64*(2), 234-240.

Winningham, R. G., & Pike, N. L. (2007). A cognitive intervention to enhance institutionalized older adults' social support networks and decrease loneliness. *Aging & Mental Health, 11*(6), 716 - 721.

Wittenberg, M. T., & Reis, H. T. (1986). Loneliness, social skills, and social perception. *Personality and Social Psychology Bulletin, 12*(1), 121-130.

Wu, Z.-Q., Sun, L., Sun, Y.-H., Zhang, X.-J., Tao, F.-b., & Cui, G.-H. (2010). Correlation between loneliness and social relationship among empty nest elderly in Anhui rural area, china. *Aging & Mental Health, 14*(1), 108 -112.

In: Social Determinants and Mental Health
Editor: Sabine Bährer-Kohler
ISBN: 978-1-61324-353-4

Chapter 21

PREVENTION AND MENTAL HEALTH

Anand Ramakrishnan
Faculty of Old Age Psychiatry, Royal College of Psychiatrists, Nottinghamshire Healthcare NHS Trust, Kirkby-in-Ashfield, UK

ABSTRACT

Mental health and well being are fundamental to quality of life, enabling people to experience life as meaningful and to be creative (WHO 2005). Mental ill health is a major cause of disability and long term suffering to the affected individuals, their families and carers. Prevention strategies could be at primary, secondary or tertiary level. There are various community based interventions and also epidemiological and cohort based studies and randomised control trials. Health Promotion is essentially a constructive concept with a focus on process as much as outcome and an emphasis on appropriate methodologies drawn from a spectrum of social, behavioural and biomedical disciplines. (WHO 2004) There is evidence that mental disorders increase the risk of physical illness and vice versa. Preventive interventions work by focusing on reducing risk factors and enhancing protective factors associated with mental ill-health. However, many preventive and health promotion interventions address groups of people across the communities of all ages.

Older people have to deal with physical disabilities associated with age, co-morbidities and neurodegenerative conditions and psychosocial issues such as vulnerability and stigma of mental illness.

Chronic conditions such as diabetes, elevated blood cholesterol level in midlife and depression have been associated with increased risk of Alzheimer's disease. Similarly current smoking, never having been married, low education and lack of social support are all reported to be risk factors for Alzheimer's disease. Preventive measures can be aimed at these factors and their influence on preventing or delaying cognitive decline.

There are non-modifiable factors such as age, gender and genetic disposition, which are not currently amenable to preventive programmes although they may become feasible in the future. Current preventive strategies involve modifiable factors like physical exercise to reduce cardiovascular risks in developing dementia, depression and anxiety, controlling life style issues like smoking, alcohol use, dietary fat and nutrition, regular physical and mental exercise and managing obesity. Preventing head injury, early use of acetyl cholinesterase inhibitors and minimal or no use of antipsychotics have been implicated in delaying onset or slowing the progression of dementias like Alzheimer's disease.

Regular interventions to enhance a relatively stress free life by improvement of psychosocial factors, living conditions, healthcare and psycho-education may be helpful measures to prevent depression, reduce suicide rate and improve their quality of life. Combating stigma, discrimination and ageism, promoting intergenerational activities, good housing and the promotion of life style choices that foster independence are other interventions that are aimed at improving mental health of older people.

INTRODUCTION

About 450 million people suffer from mental disorders (WHO 2001). One in every 4 persons may be affected by some kind of mental disorder at some stage in their life. Health promotion involves people of all ages, classes, cultural diversities and happens in urban and rural settings. Prevention and promotion of mental health is inextricably linked to human rights and ethical issues, stigma and taboo associated with mental illnesses. Effective prevention can do a lot to alter perceptions and hence change the way mental disorders are looked upon by society.

The concept of risk and protective factors is important in dealing with these issues. Risk factors deal with increased probability, severity and duration of mental illness and protective factors relate to conditions that improve or prevent mental ill health such as self-esteem, emotional resilience, positive thinking, problem-solving and social skills, and management of stress. Both risk and protective factors can be individual, family-related, social, economic and environmental in nature (WHO 2004).

Mental ill health can be much more devastating in old age posing a double jeopardy. Apart from the psychosocial burden, mental illness can also be disabling for the sufferers, it can take a tremendous toll on the emotional and socio-economic wellbeing of family members and other carers. It is essential that attention is paid to the prevention and promotion in mental health at the level of policy formulation, legislation, decision making, resource allocation and overall health care system (WHO 2002). The national co-morbidity survey identified that later onset illness is mostly of co-morbid conditions, with estimated lifetime risk of any disorder at age 75 years (50.8%) only slightly higher than observed lifetime prevalence (46.4%) (Kessler et al 2005). Hence prevention of co-morbidity would substantially reduce prevalence of lifetime psychiatric disorders.

The WHO launched activities relating to the International Year of Older Persons in 1999 and the theme "Active Ageing" was selected for 1999 World Health Day. It is important to promote an energetic, healthy older generation to benefit from their rich social and emotional resilience and experience, to reduce cost due to multiple co-morbidity and prevent chronic mental illnesses like depression and dementia. Active healthy ageing is ensured through strategies and policies that help age friendly housing, access to healthy lifestyles, activities, promotion of social integration and the enhancement of spiritual and cultural satisfaction.

Traditionally prevention is considered at three levels:

1. Primary Prevention - treating or controlling the causative agent helps to prevent the occurrence of diseases. This is not very successful in mental health disorders as exact

causative mechanisms are not generally known. Most of the community based preventive measures are examples of primary prevention.

2. Secondary Prevention – here the emphasis is on early diagnosis and treatment so that the illness is treated early thereby preventing significant morbidity. Early diagnosis of schizophrenia and depressive disorders and effective treatment strategy are examples of secondary prevention. Secondary prevention is also about reducing risks of recurrence or relapse – eg using mood stabilisers in affective disorders
3. Tertiary Prevention - the negative impact of the illness is contained by treating complications and also by implementing rehabilitation so as to reduce disability and dependence.

Old age is a situation when people should be able to enjoy life without the worry of employment and bringing up of children. But old age brings psychosocial distress in the loss of status, changing roles and the likelihood of physical illness. This can lead to increased physical and emotional and sometimes financial stress to the carers. Mental health promotion should be quite helpful in old age improve quality of life and reduce disability. (ProMenPol Project Final 2009)

Community Based Interventions

Early regular screening of risk factors and mental disorders like depression and dementia, providing psycho-education methods among chronically ill elderly and their care givers, promoting activities and improving independence all are examples of community based interventions.

- Active exercise interventions: many cross-sectional studies and controlled trials have suggested that exercise such as aerobic exercise and Tai-chi provide physical and psychological benefits in older people (Li et al, 2001). The benefits include increased life satisfaction, improved happiness, positive mood states and a feeling of mental wellbeing. This also reduced psychological distress and depressive symptoms and lowered blood pressure and stress. The mobility and stability of walking also improved due to regular aerobic exercise. Research has demonstrated that physical exercise can stimulate release of neurotransmitters and neuronal growth factors in the brain. Social benefits associated with the exercise may also play an important part in explaining the health benefits associated with regular physical exercise (Harvey et al, 2010).
- Mental health First Aid is a model developed by Betty Kitchener and Tony Jorm in Australia. It is designed to teach members of the public how to support someone in a mental health crisis situation or who is developing a mental disorder and how they could improve mental health literacy, encourage appropriate and early help seeking and reduce stigma. Mental health first aid is taught in a 12 hour course that is usually run over four 3 hours sessions. This programme is now widely used in western countries and reviews have reported positive benefits (Kitchener & Jorm, 2008).

- "Moving forward: Bradford's older peoples mental health programme" is an initiative in England, providing community support in the areas of secondary and tertiary prevention of mental illness in older people. The community network comprises extending mental health support in the community and voluntary sector, with mental health cafes for those with dementia, anxiety and depression and virtual mental health cafés using Information Technology (DH Care networks, UK 2008).

Prevention of Depression

Depression is the most prevalent psychiatric disorder affecting around 340 million people worldwide (WHO 2004). It is common in the older people, perhaps due to their psychosocial-cultural situation; it imposes a heavy burden on sufferers as well as carers. Effective community programmes to prevent depression in the population have comprised of multiple actions including selective and indicated interventions. Controlled studies have shown a significant but small effect of 11% reduction in depressive symptomatology after interventions (WHO 2004) identifying and strengthening protective factors that prevent depression. These include counselling for the elderly and psychoeducation. Selective intervention leads to significant improvement in depressive symptoms after receiving adequate help and social support. Interventions may target a large group or population through the use of sufficient self help materials, such as information leaflets distributed by mass media and the internet. Education helps people at risk of depression by producing positive thinking, challenging negative thinking styles and improving problem solving skills. The evidence is weak for debriefing and bereavement counselling at times of natural calamities such as severe drought and floods situations, volcanic eruptions and tsunami are helpful to prevent depression and suicide.

The Royal Colleague of Psychiatrists, UK responding to the European Commission's white paper on mental health in 2006, put forward three proposals to improve mental health in Europe:

[1] Promoting mental health in the whole population
[2] Targeting vulnerable groups and preventing mental illness in such as those with a past history of mental illness (including alcohol and drug abuse), psychological trauma (including abuse at any age, combat and terrorism), learning/intellectual disability (including specific and pervasive developmental disorders), long term physical illnesses and disabilities, migrants, prisoners (pre and post conviction) and those at risk from discrimination or exploitation
[3] Each programme should encompass policy areas and include mental health promotion and prevention, impart knowledge and information, provide support carers. It should also include research, training, education and consider issues such as ethics and human rights.

Suicide in Older People

Suicide is a major risk in older people. A study in England (Howard et al, 2000) concluded that older men are at a higher risk of suicide than woman. About 70% of older persons in their sample who committed suicide were male, 50% had seen their GP in the month before death for physical complaints, and 15% were under psychiatric care at the time of death. They were also at risk of possible drug overdoses due to large number of medications taken for various co-morbid conditions. There are social factors including social isolation, being divorced, widowed or single and also physical disabilities (O'Connell et al 2004). The UK government set out a suicide prevention programme in 2004 with following goals.

1. To reduce risk in key high risk groups.
2. To promote mental well-being in the wider population.
3. To reduce the availability and lethality of suicide methods.
4. To improve reporting of suicidal behaviour in the media.
5. To promote research on suicide and suicide prevention.

Prevention of Dementia

Any type of dementia is a significant cause of mortality worldwide and results in severe psychosocial burden to the individuals, families and carers. A possible pandemic of dementia is predicted with 100% increase in incidences between 2001 and 2020 and 300% increase in China, India and other South Asian and Western Pacific countries. (Ferri et al 2005).

The Alzheimer's International report in 2010 estimated the world wide cost of dementia as US $ 604 billion, of which 70% is spent in Western Europe and America. In its report of 2009 it predicted prevalence of dementia worldwide in 2010 as 35.6 million, increasing to 65.7 millions by 2030 and 115.4 million in 2050. About two thirds of these people live in developing countries. The total cost of dementia care is enormous, not only for the dementia sufferers but also for their families/carers and society as a whole. It is difficult to calculate the indirect costs, like unpaid care by family and carers.

Global Costs of Dementia: Alzheimer's disease is the fifth leading cause of death for people over 65 years in the United States. It is difficult to estimate the burden it imposes on people with dementia and their families/carers. Reitz (2010) published a summary risk score for the prediction of Alzheimer's disease in older people, based on their vascular risk profile. He found that their summary score was able to predict the risk of late onset Alzheimer's disease. As the cost and burden of dementia increases every year it is sensible to develop measures to prevent onset of dementia or at least delay its occurrence. Delaying the onset of dementia by five years would half its prevalence (Jorm et al 1987). The commonest type of dementia is Alzheimer's disease; vascular dementia comes next in prevalence. The aetiology of various types of dementias are multifactorial and it has been difficult to develop an effective prevention strategy.

Possible preventive strategies for dementia require consideration of:

- Knowledge about risk factors for dementia and its subtypes
- The extent to which such risk factors are modifiable
- Evidence that modification of these risk factors does indeed result in subsequent reduction in the incidence of dementia (NICE, 2007).

Impairment in multiple domains of cognition may be observed several years before the clinical diagnosis of AD or other types of dementia. The shift from normal ageing to preclinical dementia is not clear, the neuropsychological changes of early dementia are not much different from the normal ageing process. Global cognitive deterioration occurs early, affecting episodic memory, executive functioning, verbal ability, visuospatial skills, attention and perceptual speed. (Backman et al 2004). The term Mild Cognitive Impairment (MCI) describes a condition where individuals' subjective symptoms and memory loss are apparent and measurable cognitive deficits are present but not severe enough to cause disruption to every day life. At a group level, worsening of episodic memory is a reliable predictor of conversion from MCI to AD.

The best known risk factors for dementia like hypertension and hypercholesterolemia mostly develop in middle age i.e. 15-20 years earlier than developing dementia, suggesting that neuropathological change happen a number of years before clinical symptoms appear. Perhaps prevention strategies should be aimed at middle aged people without cognitive impairment. It would be economically impractical as only a small percentage of them develop dementia later on (Purandare et al, 2005) but these are risk factors also for ischemic heart disease and stroke.

The prevention strategies to prevent or delay the onset of dementia especially AD are described in the broad categories as given below.

I. Non-modifiable risk factors

These are risk factors that are pre-determined and cannot be influenced much that includes age (most predictable factor), sex (AD is more in women), intelligence (AD occurs early in people with Learning Disability) and genetic make up (Chromosomes 1,14, 21 and 6 have been implicated) (Naj et al, 2010. Farrer et al, 1997).

II. Potentially Modifiable Risk Factors

There have been conflicting reports about these risk factors on its ability to prevent or delay onset of AD or other types of dementias. Notable risk factors are smoking (for vascular dementia and AD (Ott et al, 1998) and alcohol (moderate use of alcohol has been found useful in prevention of dementia (Letenneur, 2004). There is no convincing evidence for diabetes (Evans, Sastre, 2003) but some epidemiological studies suggested diabetes as a risk factor for vascular dementia and AD in individuals who lack the ApoE4 allele (Ahtiluoto et al, 2010). High blood pressure is a risk factor in stroke but there is no evidence for blood pressure lowering drugs in prevention of dementia (McGuinness 2009).

Other factors are obesity (obesity in middle age is associated with increased risk of dementia (Gustafson et al, 2003; Kivipelto et al, 2005), high cholesterol levels (there is no good evidence that statins help in preventing AD or dementia (McGuinness 2009), hormone replacement therapy (little evidence that oestrogen therapy enhanced overall cognitive functioning (Lethaby et al 2008) although some evidence exists for increased cognitive decline with hormone replacement therapy), anti inflammatory drugs (some epidemiological studies have shown long-term use of non -steroidal anti inflammatory drugs, to be associated with a two-to-four fold reduced risk of AD (Purandare 2005), but another study using celecoxib, rofecoxib and naproxen were found to increase the incidence (Meinert C et al, 2009). Anti oxidants in red wine and green tea may help to delay onset of AD (Savaskan et al, 2003) (Kuriyama 2006) but there is no consistent evidence for vitamin E (Boothby & Doering, 2005).

Folic acid was associated with improvement in the response of people with AD to cholinesterase inhibitors (Malouf 2008) and an Oxford study (Smith et al, 2010) showed that those who took folic acid, vitamin B6 and B12 (lowers homocysteine level in blood which is a risk factor for brain atrophy, cognitive impairment and dementia) had their brains shrink by 0.76 percent a year on average, while those on placebo had an atrophy rate of 1.08 percent. Ginkgo Biloba has not been found to be effective in reducing incidence of dementia (DeKosky 2008). Exercise- A recent review showed that 20 of 24 population-based studies showed a link between physical activity and reduced risk for dementia or cognitive decline (Tan, 2010). A low fat diet rich in Omega 3 polyunsaturated fatty acids and fish (Mediterranean diet) also was found to be effective in delaying onset of AD. Cognitive Training- Findings in relation to cognitive training to prevent or delay AD are mixed. Some studies have shown to delay cognitive decline by improving the cognitive reserve (Mowszowski 2010).

Elan AD vaccine clinical trial was suspended due to the toxicity of the vaccine when 5 percent patients developed 'cerebral inflammation' although current trials with a new vaccine developed against a non human protein is encouraging (Glabe et al 2010).

A consensus report by National Institute of Health, America (2010) has stated that there is currently no evidence exists to support the association of any modifiable factor with reduced risk of AD.

CONCLUSION

Mental health is affected by a variety of psychological, socio-cultural, biological and environmental processes. It is the principal cause of emotional, social and financial burden for all ages, especially older people due to their relative frailty, disability and co-morbidity. The mental health promotion is spurred and fostered by a growing understanding that health and social problems may be exacerbated by social and economic problems and individuals' life styles. (WHO 1992) Promotion of mental health and prevention of ill health may be assisted by improving the awareness of social, psychological and emotional issues of the whole population, especially health care and government organizations and other policy makers. Cultural, economic and commercial constraints play a prominent role in prevention and promotion; this may result in poor investment in prevention. Public health authorities and health professionals will need to take a leadership role here, even if they cannot find the necessary financial resources within the health sector to implement programmes. Collaboration between mental health, public health and other sectors is complex but necessary for making prevention programmes a reality (WHO 2004). National mental health policies should not be solely concerned with mental disorders, but should also recognize and address the broader issues which promote mental health. This should include mainstreaming mental health promotion into policies and programmes in government and business sectors including education, labour, justice, transport, environment, housing, and welfare, as well as the health sector (WHO, 2010)

Key Recommendations

- Mental health needs to be recognised as a community responsibility, not just an individual concern, as the evidence suggests that the social and economic costs of poor mental health are high and will continue to grow without community and government action.
- Cost effective measures that are evidence based, locally available, involving family members and other carers should form an integral part of daily practice. These interventions should help to reduce stigma and eradicate discrimination in access to health and social care for the elderly. Many more social and community based interventions to enhance social support and quality of life are necessary in the ever changing world of social, familial and financial insecurity.
- Safe, age friendly initiatives are necessary that prevent falls, foster social integration and maximise peoples' potential to achieve satisfaction and happiness in a stress free environment.
- Older people should be able to get help with physical care from primary health care as co-morbidity is common in older people which may have a negative impact on their mental health. This includes regular review of health and medication, help with mobility, activity and physical exercise and immunisations.
- Social care should be treated as a priority. Older people should have access to a choice of independent and supported living including smart house technology, day care facilities, help at home to maintain nutrition, clean environment and personal care; facilities for avoiding loneliness, recreation and opportunities for psychological stimulation and cultural enhancement.
- Create an environment that promotes healthy life choices, generate a living environment that are sensitive to the socio-economic, cultural and ethnic needs of older people; supports families, friendships and other forms of close personal relations between older people themselves and across generations, combat ageism and other discrimination and stigma of mental ill health.
- More future research is needed to prevent disabling depression and dementia, psychotic disorders and suicide in older people.
- International action is necessary for generating and disseminating further evidence, for assisting low and middle-income countries in implementing effective programmes (and not implementing those that are ineffective), and for fostering international collaboration

(Adapted from "Promoting mental health, a summary report by WHO 2005, Conclusion report of the Conference on mental health and well being, Europe 2010").

REFERENCES

Ahtiluoto,S; Polivikoski, M; Solomon, A et al. (2010). Diabetes, Alzheimer disease, and vascular dementia, a population-based neuropathologic study. Neurology, 75, 1195-1202

Appleby, L.,et al. (2004). *National Suicide Prevention Strategy for England,* Department of Health, UK.

Backman, L; Jones, S; Berger, A.K., *et al.* (2004). Multiple cognitive deficits during the transition to Alzheimer's disease. *Journal of Internal Medicine, 256,* 195–204.

Boothby, LA; Doering, PL. (2005). Vitamin C and Vitamin E for Alzheimer's disease. *The Annals of Pharmacotherapy,* 39, 2073–2080.

Conclusions from the conference.(2010). *"Mental health and Well-being in Older People-making it happen"* June 2010, Madrid, European Communities.

Daviglus,ML; Bell, CC; Berrettini,W et al. (2010). National Institutes of Health State-of-the-Science Conference Statement: Preventing Alzheimer's Disease and Cognitive Decline. *NIH Consens State Sci Statements.* 2010 Apr 26–28; 27(4):1–27.

DeKosky, ST; Williamson, JD; Fitzpatrick, AL; et al. (2008). Ginkgo Biloba for Prevention of Dementia: A Randomized Controlled Trial, *JAMA.* 300(19), 2253-2262

Evans, JG; Sastre, AA; (2003). Effect of the treatment of Type II diabetes mellitus on the development of cognitive impairment and dementia. *Cochrane Database of Systematic Reviews,* Issue 1. Art. No.: CD003804. DOI: 10.1002/14651858.CD003804

Farrer, LA; Cupples, LA; Haines, JL; et al. (1997). Effects of age, sex, and ethnicity on the association between apolipoprotein E genotype and Alzheimer disease. A meta-analysis. APOE and Alzheimer Disease Meta Analysis Consortium. *JAMA,* 278,1349-56.

Glabe, CG; Rasool, S; Coria, HM; et al. (2010). Non human amyloid oligomer epitope reduces Alzheimer's-like neuropathology in 3xTg-AD transgenic mice (725.6 abstract, presented at *Neuroscience 2010* conference)

Gustafson, D; Rothenberg, E; Blennow, K; *et al.* (2003). An 18-year follow-up of overweight and risk of Alzheimer disease. *Archives of Internal Medicine, 163,* 1524–1528.

Harvey, SB; Hotoph, M. (2010). *The British Journal of Psychiatry* 197: 357-364

Health Situation and Trends Assessment, Health Situation in the South-East Asia Region, 1998-2000, *Trends in Health Status* (WHO, 1999).

Hogervorst, E; Yaffe, K; Richards, M; *et al.* (2002). Hormone replacement therapy for cognitive function in postmenopausal women. *Cochrane Database of Systematic Reviews, 2,* CD003122.

Howard, C. (2000). Suicide in the elderly, *Adv. Psychiatr. Treat,* 6, 102-108

http://www.dhcarenetworks.org.uk/Prevention/type/Resource/?cid=4114 (Moving Forward, Bradford) accessed on 14/11/2010

http://www.rcpsych.ac.uk/press/collegeresponses/collegeeuresponsemay06.aspx accessed on 14/11/2010

http://www.searo.who.int/en/Section1243/Section1382/Section1386/Section1898_9436.htm accessed on 19/11/2010

Jorm, AF; Betty, A; Kitchener, BA; Kanowski, LG. *et al.* (2007). Mental health first aid training for members of the public. *International Journal of Clinical and Health Psychology,* 7(1), 141-151

Jorm, AF; Jolley, D. (1998). The incidence of dementia: a meta-analysis. *Neurology, 51*, 728–733.

Jorm, AF; Korten, AE; Henderson, AS. (1987). The prevalence of dementia: a quantitative integration of the literature. *Acta Psychiatrica Scandinavica, 76*, 465–479.

Kessler, RC; Berglund, P; Demle, O; et al.(2005). Lifetime Prevalence and Age-of-Onset Distributions of DSM-IV Disorders in the National Comorbidity Survey Replications, *Arch Gen Psychiatry*, 62, 593-602

Kitchener, BA; Jorm, AF. (2006). Mental health first aid training: review of evaluation studies, *Aust N Z J Psychiatry.* 40(1), 6-8.

Kivipelto, M; Ngandu, T; Fratiglioni, L.; et al. (2005). Obesity and vascular risk factors at midlife and the risk of dementia and Alzheimer disease. *Archives of Neurology, 62*, 1556–1560.

Kuriyama, S; Hozawa, A. et al.(2006). Green tea consumption and cognitive function: a cross-sectional study from the Tsurugaya Project. *The American Journal of Clinical Nutrition,* 83, 355-61.

Lethaby, A; Hogervorst, E; Richards, M; Yesufu, A; Yaffe, K. (2008). Hormone replacement therapy for cognitive function in postmenopausal women. *Cochrane Database of Systematic Reviews*, Issue 1. Art. No. CD003122.

Letenneur, L. (2004). Risk of dementia and alcohol and wine consumption: a review of recent results. *Biological Research*, 37, 189–193.

Li, F; Harmer, P; McAuley, E; Fisher, KJ. et al. (2001). Tai chi, self-efficacy, and physical function in the elderly. *Prevention Science, 2*(4), 229-239.

Malouf, R; Evans, GJ. (2008). Folic acid with or without vitamin B12 for the prevention and treatment of healthy elderly and demented people. *Cochrane Database of Systematic Reviews*, Issue 4. Art. No. CD004514.

McGuinness, B; Craig, D; Bullock, R; Passmore, P. (2009). Statins for the prevention of dementia. *Cochrane Database of Systematic Reviews*. Issue 2,Art. No. CD003160.

McGuinness, B; Todd, S; Passmore, P; Bullock, R. (2009). Blood pressure lowering in patients without prior cerebrovascular disease for prevention of cognitive impairment and dementia. *Cochrane Database of Systematic Reviews*, Issue 4. Art. No.: CD004034.

Meinert. C L; McCaffrey, L D; Breitner. C S J. (2009). Alzheimer's Disease Anti-inflammatory Prevention Trial (ADAPT). *Alzheimers Dement* , 5(2), 93–104.

Mental Health Action for Europe. (2005). *WHO European ministerial conference on Mental Health:* January, 2005.

Mowszowski, L; Batchelar, J; Naismith, L. (2010). Early prevention for cognitive decline: can cognitive training be used as a selective prevention technique? *International Psychogeriatrics*, 2010, 22:4, 537-548.

Naj, AC; Beecham, GW; Martin, ER. et al. (2010). Dementia Revealed: Novel Chromosome 6 Locus for Late-Onset Alzheimer Disease Provides Genetic Evidence for Folate-Pathway Abnormalities. *PLoS Genetics*, 6 (9): e1001130 DOI: *10.1371/journal.pgen.1001130.*

NICE–SCIE *Guideline on supporting people with dementia and their carers in health and social care National Clinical Practice Guideline Number 42, National Collaborating Centre for Mental Health. 2007.* Published by the British Psychological Society and Gaskell, the Royal College of Psychiatrists.

Position of Mental Health Europe on Mental health and well being of older people, Mental health Europe – Sante Mentale Europe, June 2010. *http://www.mhe-sme.org* accessed on 1/12/2010.

Prevention and Promotion in Mental Health. (2002). *WHO Meeting on Evidence for Prevention and Promotion in Mental Health: Conceptual and Measurement Issues* World Health Organization.

ProMenPol Project Final, 2009. A Manual for Promoting Mental Health and Wellbeing: Older Peoples Residences. *http://www.mentalhealthpromotion.net/resources/toolit-manuals/manual-for-older-people-setting.pdf*, accessed on 1/12/2010.

Purandare,N; Ballard, C; Burns, A.(2005), *Adv. Psychiatr. Treat.* 2005 11: 176-183.

O'Connell, H; Chin, A; Cunningham, C; et al. (2004). Recent developments: Suicide in older people *BMJ,* 329:895.

Ott, A; Slooter, A J C; Hofman, A: et al (1998) Smoking and the risk of dementia and Alzheimer's disease in a population-based cohort study: the Rotterdam study. *Lancet*, 351, 1840–1843.

Reitz, C; Tang, M.X; Schupf, N; Manly, J J; et al. (2010). A Summary Risk Score for the Prediction of Alzheimer Disease in Elderly Persons. *Arch Neurol,* 67(7), 835-841.

Savaskan, E; Olivieri, G; Meier, F; et al (2003) Red wine ingredient resveratrol protects from beta-amyloid neurotoxicity. *Gerontology*, 49, 380–383.

Shapiro, A; Taylor, M. (2002). Effects of a community based early intervention program on the subjective well-being, institutionalization, and mortality of low-income elders. *Gerontologist*, 42(3), 334-341.

Smith AD; Smith SM; de Jager CA; et al. (2010) Homocysteine-Lowering by B Vitamins Slows the Rate of Accelerated Brain Atrophy in Mild Cognitive Impairment: A Randomized Controlled Trial. *PLoS ONE* 5(9): e12244. doi:10.1371/journal.pone.0012244.

Stevens, N; Tilburg ,VT. (2000). Stimulating friendship in later life: A strategy for reducing loneliness among older women. *Educational Gerontology,* 26(1), 15-35.

Tan, Z. (2010) . *Presented the results from Framingham study results at the Alzheimer's Association International Conference on Alzheimer's Disease*, July 2010.

Wimo, A; Prince, M. (2010). *Alzheimer's Disease International World Alzheimer Report* 2010, The Global Economic Impact of Dementia : Alzheimer's Disease International (ADI), 21 September 2010.

World Health Report 2001. *Quoted in Prevention and Promotion in Mental Health*, WHO 2002.

WHO (2001). *Evaluation in Health Promotion. Principles and Perspectives. Rootman I, Goodstadt M, Hyndman B. et al. (eds). WHO Regional Publications, European Series, No. 92, pp. 533.*

WHO (2004). Prevention of mental disorders, effective interventions and policy options. *http://www.who.int/mental_health/evidence/en/prevention_of_mental_disorders_sr.pdf.*

WHO (2004). *Prevention of mental disorders : effective interventions and policy options : summary report / a report of the World Health Organization Dept. of Mental Health and Substance Abuse ; in collaboration with the Prevention* Research Centre of the Universities of Nijmegen and Maastricht .

WHO (2010). *Media centre, Fact sheet* 220.

In: Social Determinants and Mental Health
Editor: Sabine Bährer-Kohler
ISBN: 978-1-61324-353-4

Chapter 22

SELF-MANAGEMENT AND MENTAL HEALTH

Henrike Wolf
University of Zurich, Department of Old Age Psychiatry and Psychiatry Research, Zurich, Switzerland

INTRODUCTION

While self-management is a well-established and evidence-based approach to a number of long-term medical conditions, it is still relatively new in the context of mental health. Self-management in the context of mental health involves 1) coping and managing the stressors of daily life in healthy people, 2) preventing and managing milder psychiatric conditions 3) self-management programs targeting on people with psychiatric diagnoses, including conditions that are regarded as relatively severe.

Currently, the WHO and the European Commission are co-funding a project aimed at supporting Member States to improve strategies and actions to empower people with mental health problems and their carers. The project started in April 2008 and runs to March 2011 [1].

HISTORY AND CONCEPT OF SELF-MANAGEMENT

Self-management has become a broad generic term in the Anglo-American literature for such interventions that aim to train health service users and enable them to actively solve problems and improve their self-regulation and –efficacy. If this systematic learning and change process is successful, individuals (re-)gain their ability to manage their lives without external professional support services. This view is closely related to approaches of social learning theory, self-control and –regulation, and cognitive behavioral therapy.

Self-management has now become an approved terminus in the international scientific community, and the term has entered the THESAURUS OF PSYCHOLOGICAL INDEX TERMS [2].

The term self-management originated in the chronic disease and medical rehabilitation literature. One of the first uses of the term appeared in 1976 in a book written by Thomas Creer on the rehabilitation of chronically ill children. According to Creer and Christian, the term "self-management" was coined to encourage patients to become active participants in their treatment. [3]

Today, an increasing number of self-management programs are becoming available for chronic medical conditions, such as arthritis, diabetes, heart disease, COPD, inflammatory bowel disease, HIV and many others.

For example, the Stanford Patient Education Research Centre has developed and evaluated a range of Self-management based interventions for a number of chronic health conditions. Their programs are aimed at chronic somatic rather than psychiatric conditions. Such programs have rapidly gained world-wide perception and have been adopted, in many countries, e.g. in Spain, Australia, and the United Kingdom [4,5].

An example of a Stanford Self-Management Program is "The Chronic Disease Self-Management Program", a non-condition-specific program aiming at people with different chronic health problems. It is given as a workshop of two and a half hours duration, once a week, for six weeks, in community settings such as senior centers, churches, libraries and hospitals. Workshops are facilitated by two trained leaders, one or both of whom are non-health professionals with a chronic diseases themselves.

Subjects covered include: 1) techniques to deal with problems such as frustration, fatigue, pain and isolation, 2) appropriate exercise for maintaining and improving strength, flexibility, and endurance, 3) appropriate use of medications, 4) communicating effectively with family, friends, and health professionals, 5) nutrition, and, 6) how to evaluate new treatments.

According to the online advertisement of the program, „it is the process in which the program is taught that makes it effective" and a highly participative atmosphere is intended, „where mutual support and success build the participants' confidence in their ability to manage their health and maintain active and fulfilling lives" (http://patienteducation.stanford.edu/programs/, 2011).

Generally, self-management in such programs involves the person with the chronic disease "engaging in activities that protect and promote health, monitoring and managing the symptoms and signs of illness, managing the impact of illness on functioning, emotions and interpersonal relationships and adhering to treatment regimes"(Center for the Advancement of Health, 1996)[6].

According to Lorig [5] self-management is also about enabling participants to make informed choices, to adapt new perspectives and generic skills that can be applied to new problems as they arise, to practise new health behaviors, and to maintain or regain emotional stability. In chronic medical conditions, this process involves management <u>tasks</u> –medical management, role management, and emotional management as well as essential management <u>skills</u> - problem solving, decision making, resource utilization, the formation of a patient–provider partnership, action planning, and self-tailoring [5].

Expected Benefits of Self-Management

According to the WHO global report on preventing chronic disease, self-management is now a necessary part of any treatment which tries to improve the coping ability of patients and their caregivers [7].

In a number of well-designed and prospectively studied interventions, for example those of the Stanford Self-Management Program, the self-management intervention improved health-promoting behaviors, such as length of physical or mental relaxation exercise per week. Participants reported a significantly improved communication with the physicians. In studies of painful conditions (for example arthritis or back pain), there was significant pain or even disability reduction, and in addition less reported fatigue, health stress or worry about health status [5].

Fewer studies focused on the outcome of self-management intervention with regards to cost effectiveness. Evidence is accumulating from a number of randomized controlled studies that self-management is cost effective and may even reduce health care costs [5,8,9].

In light of the world-wide dramatic increase in chronic conditions [10], such studies greatly trigger the growing public-health interest in self-management as it currently takes place in many countries.

Scientific Evidence

There is a growing interest in non-pharmacological interventions in chronic conditions and despite natural disadvantages to study such interventions under controlled and blinded conditions, the methodological quality of the published studies has improved greatly in the last decade.

A current search in the Cochrane database reveals an impressive study quantity in the field of self-management. The search term self-management in title currently identifies 18 active systematic metaanalyses evaluating self-management approaches in various somatic conditions, five of which have been completed.

Some of the completed systematic reviews report overall significance of self-management interventions in highly relevant aspects of disease-management.

For example, a total of 18 randomized trials were identified that compared self-monitoring and self-management of oral anticoagulation with standard monitoring. The combined results of these trials showed a halving of thromboembolic events and all-cause mortality with self-monitoring and self-management [11].

A systematic review on group-based training for self-management strategies in people with type 2 diabetes showed improved diabetes control as measured by blood markers as well as improved knowledge of diabetes. Self-management interventions also led to a reduced need for diabetes medication. Self-empowerment, quality of life, self-management skills and treatment satisfaction improved after self-management interventions [12].

On the other hand, the scientific studies and existing meta-analyses reveal considerable conceptual and methodological heterogeneity in studies published under the label of self-management.

For example, the Cochrane review on lay-led self-management education programs in chronic conditions [13] included seventeen trials that involved 7442 participants. The combined analyses of these studies suggest only small and short-term effects of lay-led self-management improvements in participants' self-efficacy, self-rated health, cognitive symptom management, and frequency of aerobic exercise". The authors concluded that there was currently "no evidence to suggest that such programs improve psychological health, symptoms or health-related quality of life, or that they significantly alter healthcare use". Because few such studies were designed to measure longer-term outcomes, it was suggested by the authors that future research should focus on long-term effects.

Lorig [5] commented that in examining self-management evidence one must distinguish between programs that meet the criteria outlined previously and those that are called self-management but do not meet the criteria. Small or absent effects in meta-analyses might be due to heterogeneous criteria for self-management. For example, goal setting may be one of the key components that need to be used in order to make self-management successful [5].

Thus, when evaluating self-management evidence, it is important to scrutinize the intervention and evaluation methods that were used in each particular study.

On the other hand, it may be necessary and useful to integrate related concepts and interventions into the field of self-management, as for example wellness and recovery [14], empowerment [15], or psychoeducation.

SELF-MANAGEMENT IN THE CONTEXT OF MENTAL HEALTH

Health and Mental Health Definitions

The World Health Organization defines health as "a state of complete physical, mental and social well-being, and not merely the absence of disease or infirmity" [16]. This definition implies that perfect "health" is an unattainable ideal. On the other hand the WHO definition provides the basis for health promotion outside and independent of disease (health is never perfect, it is changeable and hence can be influenced by intervention even independent of formal disease severity).

This point of view is also reflected in the concept of mental health. Freud's simple and accurate definition of health as the capacity "to work and to love" is widely accepted by mental-health specialists and it is clearly reflected in the WHO definition of "mental health".

Thus, self-management in the context of mental health covers a broad spectrum of possible strategies that range from improving coping with and managing the stressors of daily living, via preventing and managing milder psychiatric conditions, such as burn-out or mild depression, up to preventing of or intervening in severe psychiatric conditions.

Needs and Expected Benefits of Self-Management in Mental Health

The promotion of mental health and the prevention of mental illness form part of national policy in many countries. Self-management in this context is an obvious focus of current initiatives by the WHO and national health programmes in many countries.

For example, self-management has been propagated in the context of empowerment initiatives in mental health [15,17]. Empowerment has been defined as the level of choice, influence and control that people can exercise over events in their lives [17]. Empowerment is seen as a multidimensional social process through which individuals and groups gain better understanding and control over their lives. As a consequence, they are enabled to change their social and political environment to improve their health-related life circumstances. Self-management is one of the key developments that allow empowerment to happen [15].

The WHO has recognized empowerment as a core element of health promotion and disease prevention in various international instruments such as the Ottawa Charter on Health Promotion [18] and the Bangkok Charter for Health Promotion in a Globalized World [7].

Beyond formal efficacy in terms of health or economic effects, self-management initiatives may also help challenge existing perceptions and reduce stigmatization by enhancing the reputation of people with a psychiatric diagnosis as being capable citizens [19].

Another strong impulse for self-management initiatives in the context of mental health originates in current trends for deinstitutionalization in many countries. Most European countries have policies on developing community-based services and reducing the use of large psychiatric hospitals (WHO, 2008).

Reduced reliance on institutional care can only be achieved by replicating it in community settings, and self-management interventions could support this process by easing the transition of institutional care to community. A randomized study suggested that self-management can successfully support the process of deinstitutionalization [20]. Thus, it has been suggested to include self-management in deinstitutionalization related policy if more such evidence arises [15]. Similar studies appear to be under way [21].

The Scientific Situation

There are fewer published studies in the field of self-management and chronic mental health conditions as compared to chronic somatic disorders. Since the interest in self-management interventions in the mental health field has developed only recently, there is currently no meta-analytical evidence for self-management with regard to mental health. From promising work in progress, there is a small but growing evidence for the usefulness of self-management in the context of mental health conditions.

Primary Prevention Programs

The use of self-management in healthy people to prevent stress-related disorders, burnout and the mental and physical consequences is self-evident. It is well known that mental health problems and stress cause a significant portion of healthcare costs, and also complicate the management of other chronic conditions. Self-management should become a part of primary prevention programs, which should ideally start early in life [22].

While the need and value of early interventional preventive trials based on self-management have been clearly described [22], published studies using self-management intervention with the focus on primary prevention of mental disorders appear to be scarce.

The P4Well (Pervasive Personal and PsychoPhysiological management of WELLness concept for working-age citizens) study program is one of the few published studies following a preventive approach. The study was designed to support the stress and recovery management in working-age citizens. It aims at improving health management strategies by combining psychological methods with personal health technologies, such as modern mobile phone applications and different measurement devices, and using these strategies on a daily basis. The study is ongoing and first published results provide a preliminary assessment of the role and importance of experts, technologies, and peer-support in the concept [23].

Self-Management in the Context of (Severe) Psychiatric Diseases

Because the self-functions are affected by psychiatric conditions, it may at a first glance appear counterintuitive to use self-management approaches in such conditions. In fact, self-management programs have only recently shifted their focus from chronic somatic conditions to mental conditions and have now began to involve people with psychiatric diagnoses.

Interestingly, first support for the usefulness and feasibility of self-management support strategies appears to derive from the body of self-management publication in the field of chronic somatic conditions.

For example, self-management interventions were successful in individuals with chronic somatic conditions and co-morbid depression. In the study by Jerant et al. [24], depressive symptoms moderated the effect of chronic illness self-management training on self-efficacy. Individuals with more depressive symptoms seemed to be more likely to express self-efficacy gains from self-management training than individuals with lower depressive symptom severity. In another study, psycho-educational treatment appeared to be beneficial in diabetic patients with mild to moderate depressive symptoms [25]. Similar observations were made in patients with schizophrenia in a study that primarily assessed the adherence to medications in type 2 diabetes [26]. While among veterans with diabetes, overall hypoglycemic medication adherence was low, individuals with co-morbid schizophrenia were more likely to be adherent to these medications.

There are a number **of** studies indicating that self-management interventions in chronic somatic conditions may also reduce or prevent depressive symptoms in many somatic conditions. In a randomized controlled trial assessing self-management in elderly subjects with macular degeneration, the self-management program prevented depression during a 6-month follow-up in poorly sighted elderly patients [27].

Another study reported that a nurse-led minimal psychological intervention improved disease-specific quality of life in depressed patients with COPD [28].

Feasibility of Self-Management Interventions in the Treatment of Psychiatric Conditions

There is an increasing, though yet limited number of studies describing and evaluating self-management strategies in persons with various psychiatric diseases.

Principally, it seems to be possible to improve medical self-management in persons with serious mental illness. The HARP study focused on persons with severe mental illness

(Schizophrenia, mono- and bipolar depression, PTSD) and comorbid chronic medical illness [29]. In this peer-led intervention program, medical self-management was feasible and showed promise for improving a range of health outcomes among mental health consumers with chronic medical co-morbidities. However, self-management interventions specifically designed and focused on mental health outcomes are still rare.

Some examples of studies of self-management interventions in patients with psychiatric diagnoses are described in the following section.

Mood Disorders (Depression and Mania)

Because of their high prevalence and the associated burden for health care systems, there is naturally a strong public health focus on improving interventions in mood disorders [30].

Health service patterns in Canada were noted to support the use of self-management for depression in primary care [31].

While nonpharmacological interventions exist many of which use self-management components, they have not been published and evaluated under the label of self-management. Examples are the Psychoeducation for mono – and bipolar disorder as developed in Spain by the Bipolar Disorders Programme of the Institut d'Investigacions Biomèdiques August Pi I Sunver (IDIBAPS[32], or the course by MDF (The BiPolar Organization in the UK) that has been running self-management training for people with bipolar disorder since 1998 [15].

More recently, randomized trials using self-management interventions in affective disorders have been designed to show not only the effectiveness but also the cost-effectiveness [33]. The study by Lamers et al. [33] is ongoing and will use psychological outcome measures. The primary outcome measure is depression using the Beck Depression Inventory. Secondary outcome measures include quality of life, daily functioning, self-efficacy, autonomy, and participation. In the economic evaluation, cost-effectiveness and cost-utility ratios will be calculated. Furthermore, a process evaluation will be carried out.

Some robustly designed studies have been performed in the field of comorbidity of chronic pain and depression [34-36]. Optimized antidepressant therapy followed by a pain self- management program resulted in substantial improvement in depression as well as moderate reductions in pain severity and disability [37,38].

While such studies greatly support the use of self-management in affective disorders, more research appears to necessary to evaluate and understand the mechanisms through which self-management is specifically effective in affective disorders.

From some recent publications in the field, it is indicated that peer support may be useful in some conditions, such as post-partum depression [39]. Other studies support the use of written and computer-based self-help treatments for depression [40,41].

Schizophrenia

A recently published study suggests that self-management education may be useful to influence directly the psychopathology in schizophrenia. A 10-session Behavioral Management of Persistent Auditory Hallucinations Course was developed based on the University of California—San Fransisco's (UCSF) Symptom Management Model, an existing model of self-control of psychotic symptoms, and an extensive literature review of strategies to manage auditory hallucinations. The 10-session course was tested and found to reduce negative characteristics of auditory hallucinations, anxiety, and depression as well as intensity of auditory hallucinations and commands to harm [42].

At the background of the slow transition to a community-based mental health system in Japan, there is currently a special interest in programs to support this process. Anzai et al. at the Matsuzawa Psychiatric Hospital in Tokyo have adapted an empirically validated skills training program to prepare patients with schizophrenia for life in the community after discharge from the hospital. The Community Re-entry Module consists of sessions on medication and how to self-administer it, warning signs of relapse and how to develop and implement an emergency plan to deal with relapse, how to find and secure housing and continuing psychiatric care in the community, and how to reduce stress and promote coping after discharge.

The participants were 32 inpatients meeting ICD-10 and DSM-IV criteria for schizophrenia who were transferred to rehabilitation wards at Matsuzawa Psychiatric Hospital in Tokyo because of persistent and refractory symptoms of psychosis and poor insight into their illness. For the patients who received skills training, the improved scores on a scale, which measured patients' functioning in naturalistic situations on the wards, and the longer community tenure suggest that patients were able to generalize the skills learned in the module to everyday life, both in the hospital and in the community.

Other Psychiatric Disorders

Litz et al. [43] published a randomized, controlled proof-of-concept trial of an internet-based, therapist-assisted self-management treatment for posttraumatic stress disorder.

The self-management cognitive behavior therapy was designed to teach patients strategies to help them cope and manage their reactions to situations that triggered recall of traumatic experiences (and negative affect and arousal). The intervention taught, promoted, and prompted stress and negative affect management strategies that were applied to a personalized hierarchy of trauma triggers (stressful contexts). The goal was to reduce PTSD symptom burden and to promote greater self-efficacy and confidence in coping capacities. One-third of those who completed self-management cognitive behavior therapy achieved high-end state functioning at 6 months [43].

Limits of Self-Management in the Context of Severe Mental Disorders

Some studies dealt specifically with limits of using self-management interventions in severe mental health conditions. Understanding such limits is essential to design appropriate interventions in the mental health field. Corrigan et al. showed that learning medication self-management skills in schizophrenia was significantly associated with recall memory and visual vigilance, but not with conceptual flexibility. Skill learning was not influenced by psychotic symptoms [44].

In another study, the efficacy of self-management appeared to be hampered by psychological symptoms, such as depression [36,45]. However, in the study by Bell and colleagues, individual self-management skills were evaluated without applying a specific intervention [45].

Self-Management in Dementia and Mild Cognitive Impairment

Alzheimer's disease (AD) is one of the most common chronic diseases in the older segment of the population. It should thus naturally be a focus of self-management interventions. However, there is an astonishing lack of self-management programs or intervention studies involving people with AD or dementia [46]. At first glance, the symptoms of AD may be incompatible with the demands of self-management. However, AD is more and more recognized as a chronic and gradual disease that involves less severe stages, when disease-management decisions can still be made. Due to the revolutionary development of diagnostic tools in the dementia field, the diagnosis of AD is now possible at an earlier time point and before severe cognitive symptoms of dementia have developed [47,48].

At the early stage of the illness, people with AD are capable of engaging in key components of self-management, such as acquiring knowledge of their condition, agreeing on a treatment plan, sharing in medical decision-making, and adopt life styles and daily routines that reduce the impact of the illness on their emotional, social and physical life [49]. Because many disease-management decisions need to be made in AD at a later stage, when the affected individual can no longer participate in the decision-making, self-management in AD is even more pro-active than in other chronic conditions [50]. This fact stresses the importance of advance directives, but it also means that a relative or proxy should preferably be involved in the disease-management from an early stage. From a first study of persons with MCI and their caregivers, it was concluded that persons with MCI and their partners are able to minimize the threat of AD by perceiving that the progression of symptoms can be controlled and possibly prevented with health promotion activities [51]. More such studies are needed, and it is foreseeable that such results can help to trigger the development of concrete intervention programs for people affected with MCI and early dementia disorders.

Conclusion and Future Perspectives

Self-management is relatively new in the field of mental health. Evidence is currently accumulating that self-management is a feasible and effective strategy in mental health conditions, both in the context of primary and secondary prevention as well as in empowering people with chronic and severe mental illness.

In the future, the focus of self-management initiatives and trials in the mental health field should be centered even more on preventive interventions, both in adolescence and more advanced age.

REFERENCES

[1] WHO, Regional Office Europe. User empowerment in mental health - a statement by the WHO Regional Office for Europe *www.euro.who.int/en/what-we-do/health-topics. 2010*

[2] APA. *Thesaurus of Psychological Index* Terms®, Eleventh Edition,. Eleventh Edition ed; 2007

[3] Creer TL, Christian WP. *Chronically ill and handicapped children, their management and rehabilitation*: Research Press Co.; 1976

[4] 4. Lorig KR, Sobel DS, Ritter PL, Laurent D, Hobbs M. Effect of a self-management program on patients with chronic disease. *Eff Clin Pract*; 2001:256-262

[5] Lorig KR, Holman H. Self-management education: history, definition, outcomes, and mechanisms. *Ann Behav Med;* 2003:1-7

[6] Center. An indexed bibliography on self-management for people with chronic disease, Center for the Advancement of Health. In: *Center for the Advancement of Health and Center for Health Studies Group Health Cooperative of Puget Sound* 1996

[7] WHO. *Preventing chronic disease, a vital investment: WHO global report.* . Geneva: WHO; 2005

[8] Kennedy AP, Nelson E, Reeves D, et al. A randomised controlled trial to assess the effectiveness and cost of a patient orientated self management approach to chronic inflammatory bowel disease. *Gut*; 2004:1639-1645

[9] Bourbeau J, Collet J-P, Schwartzman K, et al. Economic benefits of self-management education in COPD. *Chest*; 2006:1704-1711

[10] Parker MG, Thorslund M. Health trends in the elderly population: getting better and getting worse. In, *Gerontologist*; 2007:150-158

[11] Garcia-Alamino JM, Ward AM, Alonso-Coello P, et al. Self-monitoring and self-management of oral anticoagulation. *Cochrane Database Syst Rev*; 2010:CD003839

[12] Deakin T, McShane CE, Cade JE, Williams RDRR. Group based training for self-management strategies in people with type 2 diabetes mellitus. *Cochrane Database Syst Rev*; 2005:CD003417

[13] Foster G, Taylor SJC, Eldridge SE, Ramsay J, Griffiths CJ. Self-management education programmes by lay leaders for people with chronic conditions. *Cochrane Database Syst Rev*; 2007:CD005108

[14] Sterling EW, von Esenwein SA, Tucker S, Fricks L, Druss BG. Integrating wellness, recovery, and self-management for mental health consumers. *Community Ment Health J*; 2010:130-138

[15] Crepaz-Keay D. User Empowerment in Mental Health: a statement by the WHO Regional Office for Europe *(http://www.euro.who.int/__data/assets/pdf_file/0020/113834/E93430.pdf.* 2010

[16] WHO. *Preamble to the Constitution of the World Health Organization as adopted by the International Health Conference.* New York, 19-22 June, 1946; signed on 22 July 1946 by the representatives of 61 States (Official Records of the World Health Organization, no. 2, p. 100) and entered into force on 7 April 1948. 1946

[17] WHO. World Health Organization & European Commission. User Empowerment in Mental Health: a statement by the WHO Regional Office for Europe *(http://www.euro.who.int/__data/assets/pdf_file/0020/113834/E93430.pdf)*. 2010

[18] WHO. World Health Organization. Ottawa Charter for Health Promotion. *(http://www.who.int/hpr/NPH/.../ottawa_charter_hp.pdf*. 1986

[19] Thornicroft G. *Actions Speak Louder... Tackling Discrimination against people with mental illness*. London, Mental Health Foundation; 2006

[20] Naoki K, Nobuo A, Emi I. *[Randomized controlled trial on effectiveness of the community re-entry program to inpatients with schizophrenia spectrum disorder, centering around acquisition of illness self-management knowledge]*. Seishin Shinkeigaku Zasshi; 2003:1514-1531

[21] Stevens S, Sin J. Implementing a self-management model of relapse prevention for psychosis into routine clinical practice. *J Psychiatr Ment Health Nurs*; 2005:495-501

[22] Viner RM, Barker M. Young people's health: the need for action. *BMJ* (Clinical research ed) 2005;330:901-903

[23] Happonen AP, Kaipainen K, Väätänen A, et al. A concept to empower self-management of psychophysiological wellbeing: preliminary user study experiences. *Conf Proc IEEE Eng Med Biol Soc*; 2009:312-315

[24] Jerant A, Kravitz R, Moore-Hill M, Franks P. Depressive symptoms moderated the effect of chronic illness self-management training on self-efficacy. *Med Care;* 2008:523-531

[25] Pibernik-Okanovic M, Begic D, Ajdukovic D, Andrijasevic N, Metelko Z. Psychoeducation versus treatment as usual in diabetic patients with subthreshold depression: preliminary results of a randomized controlled trial. *Trials*; 2009:78

[26] Kreyenbuhl J, Dixon LB, McCarthy JF, et al. Does Adherence to Medications for Type 2 Diabetes Differ Between Individuals With Vs Without Schizophrenia? *Schizophrenia Bulletin*;36:428-435

[27] Brody B, Roch-Levecq A, Kaplan R, Moutier C, Brown S. Age-related macular degeneration: Self-management and reduction of depressive symptoms in a randomized, controlled study. *Journal of the American Geriatrics Society*; 2006:1557-1562

[28] Lamers F, Jonkers CCM, Bosma H, et al. Improving quality of life in depressed COPD patients: effectiveness of a minimal psychological intervention. *COPD*; 2010:315-322

[29] Druss BG, Zhao L, Esenwein SAv, et al. The Health and Recovery Peer (HARP) Program: A peer-led intervention to improve medical self-management for persons with serious mental illness. *Schizophr Res;* 2010:264-270

[30] Murray G, Suto M, Hole R, et al. Self-management strategies used by 'high functioning' individuals with bipolar disorder: from research to clinical practice. *Clin Psychol Psychother*; 2010

[31] Bilsker D, Goldner EM, Jones W. Health service patterns indicate potential benefit of supported self-management for depression in primary care. In, *Can J Psychiatry;* 2007:86-95

[32] Colom F, Vieta E. A perspective on the use of psychoeducation, cognitive-behavioral therapy and interpersonal therapy for bipolar patients. *Bipolar Disord;* 2004:480-486

[33] Lamers F, Jonkers CCM, Bosma H, Diederiks JPM, van Eijk JTM. Effectiveness and cost-effectiveness of a minimal psychological intervention to reduce non-severe

depression in chronically ill elderly patients: the design of a randomised controlled trial [ISRCTN92331982]. *BMC Public Health*; 2006:161

[34] Kroenke K, Bair MJ, Damush TM, et al. Optimized Antidepressant Therapy and Pain Self-management in Primary Care Patients With Depression and Musculoskeletal Pain A Randomized Controlled Trial. *Jama-Journal of the American Medical Association* 2009;301:2099-2110

[35] Kerns RD. Antidepressants combined with self-management of pain improves outcomes in people with comorbid pain and depression. *Evid Based Ment Health*; 2010:13

[36] Bair MJ, Matthias MS, Nyland KA, et al. Barriers and facilitators to chronic pain self-management: a qualitative study of primary care patients with comorbid musculoskeletal pain and depression. *Pain Med;* 2009:1280-1290

[37] Kroenke K, Bair MJ, Damush TM, et al. Optimized antidepressant therapy and pain self-management in primary care patients with depression and musculoskeletal pain: a randomized controlled trial. *JAMA*; 2009:2099-2110

[38] Kroenke K, Bair M, Damush T, et al. Stepped Care for Affective Disorders and Musculoskeletal Pain (SCAMP) study design and practical implications of an intervention for comorbid pain and depression. *General Hospital Psychiatry;* 2007:506-517

[39] Dennis C-L. Training health visitors to identify and treat depressive symptoms with psychological approaches reduces postnatal depression. *Evid Based Ment Health;* 2009:83

[40] Williams C, Whitfield G. Written and computer-based self-help treatments for depression. *British Medical Bulletin* 2001;57:133-144

[41] Cuijpers P. Bibliotherapy in unipolar depression: a meta-analysis. *J Behav Ther Exp Psychiatry;* 1997:139-147

[42] Buccheri RK, Trygstad LN, Buffum MD, Lyttle K, Dowling G. Comprehensive evidence-based program teaching self-management of auditory hallucinations on inpatient psychiatric units. *Issues Ment Health Nurs*; 2010:223-231

[43] Litz BT, Engel CC, Bryant RA, Papa A. A randomized, controlled proof-of-concept trial of an Internet-based, therapist-assisted self-management treatment for posttraumatic stress disorder. *Am J Psychiatry*; 2007:1676-1683

[44] Corrigan PC, Wallace CJ, Schade ML, Green MF. Learning Medication Self-Management Skills in Schizophrenia: Relationships with Cognitive Deficits and Psychiatric Symptoms. *Behavior Therapy*; 1994:5-15

[45] Bell RA, Andrews JS, Arcury TA, et al. Depressive symptoms and diabetes self-management among rural older adults. *Am J Health Behav;* 2010:36-44

[46] Bährer-Kohler S, Krebs-Roubicek E. Management and Self-Management Programs for Chronic Disease - Tools, Tranformation and Promotion. Bährer-Kohler S ed, Self-Management of Chronic Disease - *Alzheimer's disease.* Heidelberg: Springer; 2009

[47] Dubois B, Feldman HH, Jacova C, et al. Research criteria for the diagnosis of Alzheimer's disease: revising the NINCDS-ADRDA criteria. *Lancet Neurology* 2007;6:734-746

[48] Gertz HJ, Kurz A. *[Diagnosis without therapy : Early diagnosis of Alzheimer's disease in the stage of mild cognitive impairment.].* Der Nervenarzt

[49] Markwick M, Reece M, Battersby MW. The development and implementation of a generic assessment tool in chronic disease self-management. In: *Health Outcomes 2002: Current Challenges and Future Frontiers*. Canberra; 2002

[50] Kurz A. Self-management of patients with Alzheimer's disease. In: Bährer-Kohler S ed, Self-management of chronic disease: *Alzheimer's disease.* Heidelberg: Springer; 2009

[51] McIlvane JM, Popa MA, Robinson B, Houseweart K, Haley WE. Perceptions of Illness, coping, and well-being in persons with mild cognitive impairment and their care partners. A*lzheimer disease and associated disorders* 2008;22:284-292

CONCLUSION

The interaction between social determinants and mental health as well as the complex nature of the latter has been known for a long time.

There are comprehensive scientific findings and assessments regarding social determinants in the context of mental health which have been described again and again by the WHO.

In the mental health context, biological and social markers belong together. It is understandable that critical questions should be asked about why the influence of this insight should be as restricted as it is today.

Qualified studies on social determinants and mental health should be promoted more extensively. The subject should be given more sustained and forward-looking consideration in teaching, training and professional development.

The subject has many facets and, as stated in the introduction to this book, it is *perhaps the most complex and challenging of all* in the field of health (Tsouros, 2003). It affects and/or concerns all of us to a greater or lesser extent. There is a codified right to health for every one of us (United Nations, 1948). One field in which this right is implemented is decision-making, where consultants and public bodies are involved. This calls for knowledge, skills, and often funds, plus the commitment of every one of us. We must be the change that we want to see in the world, as Mahatma Gandhi once said. I think there is much that remains to be done in the field of mental health for all, especially in the context of social determinants.

REFERENCES

Tsouros, A.D. (2003). Foreword. In Marmot, M. Wilkinson, R. (Editors) (2003). *Social Determinants of Health, The solid facts, second edition,* p.5.

United Nations (1948). *Universal Declaration of Human Rights*. New York: United Nations.

INDEX

A

B

C

D

E

F

G

H

I

J

K

L

M

N

O

P

Q

R

S

T

U

V

W

Y